# CARE AESTHETICS AND DEMENTIA STUDIES

AF739699

Building on several pioneering projects and aspects of lived experience, *Care Aesthetics and Dementia Studies: New Directions for Person-Centred Practices* presents a new vision for dementia studies where care aesthetics is situated as the language for the doing of person-centred care and the processes of everyday evaluation.

Presented over four interconnected Parts, this book shares a collection of studies and conceptual thinking that spotlights the sensory, embodied, and relational aspects of person-centred practices and focuses on both the macro- and micro-processes of care, elevating such interactions into a seen and visible craft. It contains contributions from a range of interdisciplinary authors, including those with backgrounds in philosophy, psychiatry, theatre and performance studies, neuroscience, improvisation studies, sociology, gerontology, design, health and social care, and the Royal Horticultural Society. People living with dementia and family carers are also represented within the chapter authorship.

This book should be of interest to a range of readers, from those living with dementia to practitioners in any setting of dementia care, and to students and trainees who are interested in knowing more about the evolving field of aesthetic practices in dementia studies.

**John Keady** is Professor of Mental Health Nursing and Older People at The University of Manchester, a post he holds jointly with Greater Manchester Mental Health NHS Foundation Trust, UK.

**Jackie Kindell** is Clinical Senior Lecturer in Speech and Language Therapy at The University of Manchester, UK.

**James Thompson** is Professor of Applied Theatre at The University of Manchester and Co-Director of the Care Lab, UK.

## Routledge Studies in Care Aesthetics

Series Editor: James Thompson

*Routledge Studies in Care Aesthetics* brings together cutting-edge research in care and its interactions with disciplines across humanities and arts. Building on the existing work of applied theatre and socially engaged arts, this series provides text-books, research and practitioner texts in the growing field of care aesthetics.

Volumes currently available in the series are:

**Care Aesthetics**
For Artful Care and Careful Art
*James Thompson*

**Care Aesthetics and the Arts**
*Kate Maguire-Rosier, Réka Polonyi, and James Thompson*

**Care Aesthetics and Dementia Studies**
New Directions for Person-Centred Practices
*John Keady, Jackie Kindell, and James Thompson*

For more information about this series, please visit: https://www.routledge.com/Routledge-Studies-in-Care-Aesthetics/book-series/RSSiCA

# CARE AESTHETICS AND DEMENTIA STUDIES

## New Directions for Person-Centred Practices

*Edited by*
*John Keady, Jackie Kindell, and James Thompson*

Routledge
Taylor & Francis Group
LONDON AND NEW YORK

Designed cover image: "Music in Mind Vinyl Record Cover" © 2024 A Studio Called Jane

First published 2027
by Routledge
4 Park Square, Milton Park, Abingdon, Oxon OX14 4RN

and by Routledge
605 Third Avenue, New York, NY 10158

*Routledge is an imprint of the Taylor & Francis Group, an informa business*

© 2027 selection and editorial matter, John Keady, Jackie Kindell, and James Thompson; individual chapters, the contributors

The right of John Keady, Jackie Kindell, and James Thompson to be identified as the authors of the editorial material, and of the authors for their individual chapters, has been asserted in accordance with sections 77 and 78 of the Copyright, Designs and Patents Act 1988.

The Open Access version of this book, available at www.taylorfrancis.com, has been made available under a Creative Commons Attribution (CC BY) 4.0 International license.

Any third party material in this book is not included in the OA Creative Commons license, unless indicated otherwise in a credit line to the material. Please direct any permissions enquiries to the original rightsholder.

For Product Safety Concerns and Information please contact our EU representative GPSR@taylorandfrancis.com. Taylor & Francis Verlag GmbH, Kaufingerstraße 24, 80331 München, Germany.

*Trademark notice*: Product or corporate names may be trademarks or registered trademarks, and are used only for identification and explanation without intent to infringe.

*British Library Cataloguing-in-Publication Data*
A catalogue record for this book is available from the British Library

ISBN: 9781041033509 (hbk)
ISBN: 9781041033493 (pbk)
ISBN: 9781003623441 (ebk)

DOI: 10.4324/9781003623441

Typeset in Times New Roman
by codeMantra

***John:*** *To Mike Nolan who put the theory, belief, supervision, and time behind the ambition and to all those I have worked with and been alongside over the years.*

***Jackie:*** *To all the people living with dementia, family members, and staff I have worked with.*

***James:*** *To my parents-in-law, Stan and Judy Witton, with love.*

# CONTENTS

*List of box* *xiii*
*List of figures* *xv*
*List of images* *xvii*
*List of tables* *xix*
*Notes on contributors* *xxi*
*Foreword* *xxv*
*Emeritus Professor Mike Nolan*
*Acknowledgements* *xxix*
*Abbreviations used in the book* *xxxi*

Introduction 1
*James Thompson, Jackie Kindell and John Keady*

**PART 1**
**A critical and personal appreciation of care aesthetics and living with dementia** **19**

1 Thinking behind an aesthetic approach to dementia 21
*Julian C. Hughes*

2 Sketching with my mum: visual autoethnographic reflections on 'care-ful' art and 'art-ful' care 43
*Christina Buse*

PART 2
Care aesthetics and creative practices 67

3 Creating aesthetic objects with people living with dementia 69
*Henry McPherson, Rebecka Fleetwood-Smith, Robyn Dowlen, Cathy Riley, Jane Bowyer and John Keady*

4 Care aesthetics and the experience of living with semantic dementia over time 100
*Jackie Kindell, Caroline Swarbrick, Sion Williams and John Keady*

5 Doing care aesthetics: dress, grooming, and appearance-related practices in dementia care settings 118
*Sarah Campbell and Rebecka Fleetwood-Smith*

6 Exchanging moments: what happens if we integrate language describing the 'care work' of artists with that of healthcare support workers? 144
*Kate Maguire-Rosier and Réka Polonyi*

7 Creative moments and dementia: fostering relational, aesthetic approaches in care home settings 160
*Rebecka Fleetwood-Smith and Robyn Dowlen*

8 Integrating aesthetics, neuroaesthetics, and Polyvagal Theory to develop a novel conceptual framework for person-centred dementia care 180
*Sarah Fox*

PART 3
Care aesthetics, outside spaces, and everyday design 203

9 Gardening as an aesthetic practice for people living with dementia 205
*Rita Newton, Daniel Atherton, Ozichi Brewster, Emmanuel Tsekleves and John Keady*

10 Care aesthetics or the aestheticisation of care? Reminiscence rooms and the tensions of dementia-friendly design 235
*Daryl Martin, Christina Buse and Sarah Nettleton*

11 Care-full neighbourhoods: exploring the aesthetic dimension of neighbourhoods for people living with dementia 256
*Andrew Clark*

PART 4
**New beginnings in care aesthetics** **275**

12 Concluding thoughts and next steps 277
*John Keady, Jackie Kindell and James Thompson*

*Afterword: Caring for my husband Frank who lived and died with advanced semantic dementia* *287*
*Sue Ennis*
*Index* *289*

# BOX

8.1 Glossary of Key Terms 197

# FIGURES


2.1 North Wales seaside resort, summer 2017 47
2.2 Storm clouds gathering, North Wales bird reserve, summer 2017 48
2.3 Forget-me-nots in the garden, 19 May 2021 48
2.4 'The roses are my favourite', 1 July 2021 50
2.5 Leaf printing with mum (sort of!), 19 September 2021 52
2.6 Sketching on my own nearby my parents' home, 26 January 2022 55
2.7 Sketching on the bench while my mum and dad are walking, 26 September 2022 58
3.1 Examples of 'playful' object handling session boxes 74
3.2 Example knitted textile sample 80
3.3 Example knitted pocket sample 81
3.4 Developing designs. Left, bookmark concept. Right, keyhole cut out for outer sleeve 86
3.5 Completed design. Top (outer cover). Bottom (sleeve insert) 89
3.6 The Open Doors Research Groups' co-created vinyl record sleeve cover, posed with vinyl record 90
4.1 Doug's A4 sheet – Making Connections 111
8.1 Mapping aesthetic moments 196

# IMAGES


| | | |
|---|---|---|
| 9.1 | A view of the Community Wellbeing Garden at RHS Garden Bridgewater | 213 |
| 9.2 | Advertising postcard for the ESRC FOSS event at RHS Garden Bridgewater | 216 |
| 9.3 | The position of the oak poster boards and exhibition posters adjacent to the Community Wellbeing Garden | 217 |
| 9.4 | The 'blackboard and chalk' advertising for the ESRC FOSS exhibition at RHS Garden Bridgewater | 218 |
| 9.5 | Exhibition introductory poster | 219 |
| 9.6 | Spring poster | 221 |
| 9.7 | Summer poster | 222 |
| 9.8 | Autumn poster | 223 |
| 9.9 | Winter poster | 224 |
| 9.10 | Rita and Ozichi seated in the Community Wellbeing Garden | 226 |

# TABLES

9.1 Participating household demographics and property type 211
9.2 The number of Rita's visits to each household 212

# CONTRIBUTORS

**Daniel Atherton** is Interpretation Manager North at Royal Horticultural Society Garden Bridgewater, Salford, Greater Manchester.

**Jane Bowyer** is a Designer and Director of 'A Studio Called Jane', a Manchester-based creative practice; her work spans branding, campaigns, and public art projects rooted in co-design and collaboration.

**Ozichi Brewster** is Therapeutic Gardener at Royal Horticultural Society Garden Bridgewater, Salford, Greater Manchester.

**Christina Buse** is Lecturer in Sociology at the University of York, with research interests in the areas of embodiment, ageing, dementia, and sensory methodologies.

**Sarah Campbell** is Senior Lecturer in Health and Social Care at Manchester Metropolitan University and her research in ageing, dementia, and care uses participatory and creative methods.

**Andrew Clark** is Professor at the Institute for Lifecourse Development, University of Greenwich.

**Robyn Dowlen** is Research Fellow based in the Research Centre for Arts and Wellbeing at Edge Hill University and specialises in creative involvement and engagement practices with people living with dementia.

**Sue Ennis** cared for her husband Frank who practised as an academic and was later diagnosed with semantic dementia; she lives in the Northeast of England.

**Rebecka Fleetwood-Smith** is a creative researcher and textile artist predominantly working in health and social care settings and is Senior Research Associate on the UKRI-funded project 'Sensing Spaces of Healthcare: Rethinking the NHS Hospital' at the University of Bristol.

**Sarah Fox** holds a PhD in Cognitive Neuroscience and has built an interdisciplinary career spanning neuroscience, public involvement, dementia policy, and aesthetic research.

**Julian C. Hughes** is Honorary Professor at the University of Bristol, where he was previously Professor of Old Age Psychiatry. He was formerly an NHS consultant and Honorary Professor of Philosophy of Ageing at Newcastle University.

**John Keady** is Professor of Mental Health Nursing and Older People at The University of Manchester, a post he holds jointly with Greater Manchester Mental Health NHS Foundation Trust.

**Jackie Kindell** is Clinical Senior Lecturer in Speech and Language Therapy at The University of Manchester.

**Kate Maguire-Rosier** is Assistant Professor of Disability Studies and the Arts at Maastricht University.

**Daryl Martin** is Lecturer in Sociology at Maynooth University, with interests in the intersections of architecture, embodiment, and healthcare.

**Henry McPherson** is a musician and researcher and is currently a Bicentenary Fellow in music at The University of Manchester where his work focuses on improvisation and 'in the moment' creativity.

**Sarah Nettleton** is Emeritus Professor of Sociology at the University of York, with research interests relating to medical knowledge and practice, sociology of the body and embodiment, and healthcare architecture.

**Rita Newton** is a final year ESRC CASE PhD student at The University of Manchester where she is completing longitudinal ethnographic research on gardening at home and the lived experience of dementia.

**Open Doors Research Group,** run by Greater Manchester Mental Health NHS Foundation Trust's Memory and Dementia service, leads on a range of initiatives to support people living with dementia and their carers across Greater Manchester.

**Réka Polonyi** is Research Fellow at the Drama Department, The University of Manchester.

**Cathy Riley** is Manager of the Open Doors and Reach Beyond Services, a self-advocacy group of people living with dementia and their carers based in the city of Salford and funded by Greater Manchester Mental Health NHS Foundation Trust.

**Caroline Swarbrick** is Senior Lecturer in Ageing at Lancaster University and has researched and published widely in the field of dementia studies.

**James Thompson** is Professor of Applied Theatre at The University of Manchester and Co-Director of the Care Lab and is the editor of the Routledge 'Studies in Care Aesthetics' series.

**Emmanuel Tsekleves** is Professor of Global Health Design Innovation and Director of Future Cities Research Institute at Lancaster University, and academic career mentor from PhD to Professorial level.

**Sion Williams** is Reader in Health Research at Bangor University and has a long-standing interest in participatory work with older people.

# FOREWORD

*Emeritus Professor Mike Nolan*

'When I use a word', Humpty Dumpty said in a rather scornful tone, 'it means just what I choose it to mean – neither more nor less' (Carroll, 1872, p. 186).

If we all adopted Humpty Dumpty's degree of latitude, then effective communication would be impossible for it relies on a shared understanding of what words mean. Of course, language evolves over time and words fall out of common usage and new ones are added. If we are unsure as to their meaning, then we can always consult a dictionary. The meaning of some words however seems so intuitively obvious that we do not question them.

Care, a notion central to this important new book, is one such word. But as Reich (1995), in his seminal review of the history of the notion of care argues, although care is 'the glue' that binds society together, a unified meaning remains elusive. The authors of this volume therefore face a formidable task in seeking to provide a better understanding of the role of care in making 'life feel pleasant, meaningful, or emotionally rich' (Andrew Clark, Chapter 11) for people living with dementia. But their ambition does not end here. Rather, they seek to create a 'new beginning' for dementia care by opening up an 'interdisciplinary and multi-directional dialogue' that unites the notions of care and aesthetics.

'Aesthetics' is not a word in such everyday usage as 'care' but is, perhaps, commonly associated in most peoples' minds with notions of 'Art' and 'Beauty'. As the editors share in the Introduction, this book aims to provide a broader definition in which care aesthetics is concerned primarily with the 'sensory engagement between people and between people and their worlds'; and in this context, people mainly refers to people living with dementia and their carers. This volume, as the editor's note, is the first time that such an undertaking has been attempted. High ambition indeed!

In addressing this challenging task, the editors bring together a diverse range of contributors that extends well beyond the 'usual suspects' and draws on insights from such varied disciplines as horticulture, dance, music, art, and theatre. This is a major strength of this book. Another is that, whilst of necessity, the authors draw on the theoretical and conceptual literature, multiple descriptions of real-life examples of care aesthetics in practice are presented throughout the various chapters. It is these that bring the authors' arguments to life, dealing, as they sometimes do, with the seemingly mundane but nonetheless 'small scale *but* significant' (editors, introduction; original emphasis) 'moments' in which care aesthetics are made manifest.

Although this book is rich in detail and presents several cogent and valuable insights, for this reader two jumped out as being of central import. The first is the observation made several times, and by a number of different contributors, is the need 'to recognise the reciprocal nature of human interdependence at the heart of care aesthetic concepts' (Andrew Clark, Chapter 11). For as the editor's note in their introductory chapter, care is 'always in relation with others'. This raises the possibly vexed, but intriguing question, of whether the continued reliance on the discourse of person-centred adequately captures such reciprocity?

The second is the emphasis placed at numerous points on the importance of 'moments' of care. As both Henry McPherson and his colleagues in Chapter 3 and Andrew Clark in Chapter 11 state, it is often the small things experienced 'in the moment' that enrich the lives of people living with dementia. In their concluding chapter, the editors identify 'moments' as a key concept underpinning their vision of care aesthetics. As Rebecka Fleetwood-Smith and Robyn Dowlen contend in Chapter 7, such 'moments' usually occur in everyday interactions and are often improvised and unpredictable rather than planned. They argue that a key challenge for the future is to shift the emphasis from measuring programme outputs to recognising the importance of the 'micro-interactions' of care. They pose the searching question 'who do we need to convince' that such 'moments' are of value? Anyone who reads this book will need little convincing.

As noted earlier, this is an ambitious volume intended to herald a 'new beginning' for discourse around care for people living with dementia. At the heart of this new beginning is the need to provide a broader understanding of the nature of care aesthetics. This, it is suggested, will allow us to 'turn a new page' that opens up 'new opportunities and connections' so as to enable us to embark upon a 'continuous journey of inter-disciplinary learning and discovery' (editors, concluding chapter). This book has considerable potential to initiate such a 'moment'. However, whilst the 'moments' discussed within this volume are primarily fleeting and temporally limited, a moment also has other meanings. One such relates to matters of 'moment', that is, import, hence the term 'momentous'. The publication of Tom Kitwood's (1997) seminal work was indeed momentous in the history of dementia care. The editors hope that this volume will create 'ripples' that reveal new opportunities and connections across time, thereby potentially creating another such 'moment'. I would be very surprised if it did not.

## Personal postscript

Relatively early in my academic career I had the privilege of establishing the first post-graduate qualification in Gerontology in Wales for practitioners in health and social care working with older people and their carers. One of the students on the inaugural programme at Bangor University was a young community psychiatric nurse working with people living with dementia and their carers in rural North Wales. It was clear from the outset that he was a person passionate about his field and driven to promote better care and support. Needless to say he excelled on the course and went on to become my first PhD student. Since then, I have heard it said that he has created a few 'ripples' of his own! His name: John Keady.

Mike Nolan, Emeritus Professor of Gerontological Nursing, University of Sheffield.

1 March 2026

## References


Carroll. L. (1872). *Through the Looking Glass and What Alice Saw There*. Oxford: Macmillan.

Kitwood, T. (1997). *Dementia Reconsidered: The Person Comes First*. Buckingham: Open University Press.

Reich, W.T. (1995). History of the notion of care. In W.T. Reich (ed.) *Encyclopedia of Bioethics. 5 Volumes*. New York: Simon & Schuster Macmillan, pp. 319–313. Available: https://care.georgetown.edu/Classic%20Article.html; accessed 1 March 2026.

# ACKNOWLEDGEMENTS

We would like to thank the following people and personnel without whom none of the text would have been possible:

- All the contributors to this book for your friendship, inspiration, and skills and for meeting all the submission deadlines in such a busy work, practice, and everyday life environment. This book is built on your shoulders.
- Tassia Watson, Josie Brown, and Heather Doquiatan, Editorial Assistants at Routledge, for all their help in getting this book together and for the behind-the-scenes encouragement and liaison since the time this book was first commissioned in December 2024. Thanks also to Stacey Walker, publisher of 'Theatre & Performance Studies' at Routledge, and to Steph Hines, editor of the 'Theatre & Performance Studies' list at Routledge, for their support of this book and ourselves in our editorial role.
- Matthew Fox, Divisional Support Assistant at the Division of Nursing, Midwifery and Social Work, The University of Manchester, for his invaluable and skilled help in assembling this book.
- The three reviewers of the original book proposal for helping to shape the flow, context, and content of this book, and for their overall support for the ambition of the text.
- Jane Bowyer, Designer and Director of 'A Studio Called Jane Ltd' [https://studiocalledjane.co.uk/; accessed 1 March 2026], for her permission to use the co-produced vinyl record sleeve design with the Open Doors Research Group as the front cover image for this book. Further information about the steps leading to the co-production of this image can be found in Chapter 3 of this book. As Cathy Riley, the facilitator of the Open Doors Research Group shared about its development, the co-produced vinyl record sleeve design 'beautifully captures

the spirit of collaboration, creativity, and care that underpins everything we have done together'. We are especially honoured to be able to take forward that legacy in partnership with Jane.

- The Arts and Humanities Research Council of the United Kingdom for their funding of the 'Care Aesthetics: Research Exploration' project, colloquially known as the CARE project, that brought the editors of this book together and allowed us time to develop some of the ideas and networks shared in this book. Grant number: AH/W003104/1.
- Our respective families.

Finally, please note that whilst every possible effort has been made (in good faith) to seek permissions where these were required in this book, have any been overlooked the fault would be rectified at the earliest possible opportunity.

John Keady, Jackie Kindell and James Thompson, 1 March 2026

# ABBREVIATIONS USED IN THIS BOOK

| | |
|---|---|
| ANS | Autonomic Nervous System |
| ARC-GM | Applied Research Collaboration-Greater Manchester |
| AI | Artificial Intelligence |
| CARE | Care Aesthetics: Research Exploration [project] |
| CD | Compact Disc |
| CLG | Collaborative Learning Group |
| DMN | Default Mode Network |
| ESRC | Economic and Social Research Council |
| ESRC CASE | Economic and Social Research Council Collaborative Studentship Competition |
| EU | European Union |
| FOSS | Festival of Social Sciences |
| HCSW | Healthcare Support Worker |
| HRA | Health Research Authority |
| NIHR | National Institute for Health and Care Research |
| NHS | National Health Service |
| PPIE | Patient and Public Involvement and Engagement |
| PWD | People Living with Dementia |
| RHS | Royal Horticultural Society |
| SSCR | School for Social Care Research |
| UK | United Kingdom |
| UKRI | UK Research and Innovation |

# INTRODUCTION

*James Thompson, Jackie Kindell and John Keady*

Welcome to *Care Aesthetics and Dementia Studies: New Directions for Person-Centred Practices* – this book is the third in the 'Routledge Studies in Care Aesthetics' series following James Thompson's (2023) *Care Aesthetics: For Artful Care and Careful Art* and then the edited book *Care Aesthetics and the Arts* (Maguire et al., 2025). We are grateful for the generous contributions of all the authors featured in this book, for their willingness to explore different aspects of dementia studies through the lens of care aesthetics, and for the way they have challenged the boundaries and possibilities for the idea so dynamically. The editors of this text come from very different practice and academic backgrounds – Applied Theatre (James), Speech and Language Therapy (Jackie), and Mental Health Nursing (John) – and we are all based at The University of Manchester in the UK, although John has a joint university – National Health Service (NHS) appointment with the Greater Manchester Mental Health NHS Foundation Trust. We have been brought together through a common interest in the importance of an aesthetic approach to health and social care through the experience of collaborating on a research project (more below) and through the commitment to maintaining a close connection to practice within academic contexts. Our different disciplinary perspectives have helped to shape the selection of the authors in this book and have ensured that each editor has enjoyed seeing care aesthetics being tested in very different ways and in diverse contexts. We hope that this interdisciplinary starting point has created a dialogue between dementia studies, person-centred care, and care aesthetics that is multi-directional. Indeed, our ambition is for the theoretical and practical vision of person-centred care to be pushing how care aesthetics might be understood and used in everyday contexts and, simultaneously, for how a focus on the aesthetics of care might extend and, at times, trouble, what we understand by person-centredness.

DOI: 10.4324/9781003623441-1
This chapter has been made available under a (CC BY) 4.0 license.

Whilst care aesthetics as a concept draws on a broad range of disciplinary research areas – including feminist care ethics, everyday aesthetics, socially engaged arts, and health and social care research – this is its first detailed application and development in the field of dementia studies. Each editor here collaborated on the UK's Arts and Humanities Research Council-funded 'Care Aesthetics: Research Exploration' (CARE) project at The University of Manchester (2022–2025) which examined how care aesthetics could be used to examine caring practice in different older people care contexts. This project is discussed in more detail in Chapter 6 by Kate Maguire-Rosier and Réka Polonyi and will shortly be mentioned in further detail. However, whilst this was the first funded research project on care aesthetics specifically, it is important to acknowledge that an aesthetic orientation within dementia studies is prefigured by a number of writers and scholars, some of whom appear in this book. For example, Honorary Professor of Psychiatry, Julian C. Hughes (2014), has written about 'the aesthetic approach to people living with dementia' and Christina Buse and Julia Twigg (2018) referred to an 'aesthetic of care' (p. 341) in their analysis of dressing older people in the context of dementia care. Julian and Christina's separate opening chapters in this book develop this existing work on the importance of noticing the aesthetic aspects of dementia care practice including, in Christina's case, in the context of an autoethnography about her mother's lived experience of dementia. Similarly, there has been a long tradition of using creative and ethnographic practices to explore work related to people living with dementia, particularly connected to different art forms, notably music (see, for example, Dowlen et al., 2022) and through analysis of sensory practices, such as grooming, gardening, or everyday care (Ward et al., 2016a, 2016b; Buse et al., 2023). Again, some of the authors responsible for this pioneering work are featured in the pages that follow. Moreover, recent scholarship on the neighbourhoods of people living with dementia (Keady, 2024), and an appreciation of valuing quality experiences 'in the moment' (Keady et al., 2022), have become important topics in dementia research and which have considerable overlap with the ideas that are inherent in care aesthetics (Thompson, 2023). Consequently, these themes open opportunities for an aesthetic analysis and are taken up by Andrew Clark in Chapter 11 and other authors across this edition.

Building on these examples of existing scholarship, and as shown in the 'Contributors' section at the start of this book, the editors have sought to bring together a range of stakeholders to showcase a diverse collection of perspectives. The aim has been to combine theoretical, empirical, and practice-orientated works, with different styles to bridge both the traditionally academic and then more personal or intimate registers. We have invited colleagues whose work explicitly or implicitly connects to care aesthetics – some extending an orientation that was already present in their work, and others bringing a care aesthetical orientation for the first time. Through the sensory, embodied, and relational language of aesthetics, the overall intention has been to develop a direction for dementia studies that will have applied as well as theoretical relevance. We hope, of course, that this is the start of a growing interest in aesthetic approaches to care for, and with, people living with dementia, rather than the final word.

Before introducing the chapters specifically, the Introduction offers an overview of care aesthetics itself and then raises some of the key concerns or questions that are emerging in a care aesthetical approach to dementia studies, including its connection to person-centred care. The Introduction ends with an overview of the structure of this book and the chapters that follow, and the writing style used in this book.

## Care aesthetics: framework, approach, concept, or a thing that is done?

As is referenced in several of the chapters in this book, there have been a range of articles that have used care aesthetics either fully or partly as a means of understanding aspects of dementia care. These have involved both the editors of this edition and several of the authors of the chapters (see, for example, Campbell et al., 2024; Dowlen et al., 2024; Fox et al., 2025; Jones et al., 2025). Care aesthetics in these different examples has been used to re-examine data from previous studies, to look again at the practice of certain staff and family members, or to re-evaluate aspects of care practice that are often missed in other studies. Always, in these examples, there is a shift between using care aesthetics as a somewhat fixed framework for exploring care's sensory and affective elements, to a more loosely conceived approach that points to the different qualities of care in certain circumstances. The former might be called a capital CA 'Care Aesthetics' approach, and the latter, perhaps, an orientation in research searching for a more elusive quality. Writers across this book use 'care aesthetics' in both these ways – and then in others. The editors of course welcome these variations and in no way seek to close down the differences in how an attention to the intricate relations between care and aesthetics in dementia studies plays out. For some, it is a clear framework of analysis, for others, a more general orientation for an analysis of case studies, and then for others, it is a very loose, somewhat tentative concept used alongside other complementary modes of enquiry. Finally, in addition to these variations in use of care aesthetics as an 'approach', there are those that position it more as a description of a practice – for them, care aesthetics is something that is done. This is particularly perceptively argued in Chapter 5 of this book entitled 'Doing care aesthetics: dress, grooming, and appearance-related practices in dementia care settings' which is authored by Sarah Campbell and Rebecka Fleetwood-Smith.

Before illustrating these different ways of using care aesthetics, we will outline briefly some of the definitions being used for its two component words. Clearly, the aim here is not to repeat previous work – and long philosophical traditions – but to give some pointers to how the editors, and authors of the chapters, are using these terms. First *care* is used to refer to a practice that is completed informally (in families, between friends, and in communities) and formally (in health and social care settings, in homes, and in medical contexts) that seeks to support a person or persons to live positive, socially meaningful lives. This might be linked to health and wellness, but it is also connected to more general social concerns and connection to others. In this framework, cleaning a wound is care and so is preparing a meal for your friend. This might be highly technical, professional care or everyday practices of care between people that requires 'doing something' but with no particular training or qualification. Care is, of course, given and received, and individuals over a life course will often shift between both roles. Then, in addition, it is an activity not only between individuals, but also between groups and within wider social contexts that provide and receive care at institutional or social levels. Care is also a word used in everyday speech and therefore contains many different and, at times, contradictory implications. It is important to note that it is used both descriptively and evaluatively, and sometimes the clarity of which usage is in operation is not obvious. Descriptions of care contain no assumption that it is referring to a positive or negative. When we say 'care home', there is no immediate sense whether that home is of high or low quality. However, when it is used evaluatively – 'I care for my mother' – there is a sense of something positive, perhaps nurturing. The key point here is that evaluatively care is used as a critical tool to examine the inequalities and poor execution of care as well as when it is done with high quality or distributed more fairly.

In stating that care is a thing done, it should be emphasised that it is always in relation to others. Care is reciprocal and contains within it multiple, intersecting tensions between power and control alongside collaboration and solidarity. And, of course, as mentioned above, different people at different times in their lives, for multiple reasons, shift between requiring and being required to care. It is universal – we all will have been cared for (whether well or poorly) to grow from childhood – but the experience of it is highly particular and differentiated according to multiple contextual, geographic, and temporal factors. The reality of universality with particularity means that care's organisation and execution is fraught with dynamics of inequality and discrimination alongside examples of practices that are extraordinarily life-affirming. And these examples can be found within the structural systems of care as well as the micro acts of interpersonal caring practice.

The short overview above of course owes much to different care theorists' accounts. Whilst many in this book draw from writers across health, social care, sociologies of care, and other disciplines, this willingness to examine both care practice and the social contexts that enable or impede it draws heavily on the history of feminist care ethics. This is a community of scholars, practitioners, and activists who have brought care into the centre of political, social, and health debates. Starting with the pioneering work of Nell Noddings (2013) and Carol Gilligan (2009) in education and psychology respectively, more recent work has examined the ethics of care within politics and democracy (Robinson, 2011; Tronto, 2013), disability (Held, 2006), the posthuman (Puig de la Bellacasa, 2017), and, of course, in health (Mol, 2008) and the care of older people (Mol et al., 2010). The attention to care as a bodily practice is seen in the work of Maurice Hamington (2004) and Annmarie Mol (2008), demonstrating that questions of responsibility, relatedness, and vulnerability can be examined within the specifics of interhuman practice. However, care theorists also examine care as an ethical enquiry that has a system-wide potential for rethinking human and more-than-human relations. Drawing this into the context of dementia care as developed by the authors here, care becomes a practice with complex ethical implications for the lives of those living with dementia and their carers and, simultaneously, a critical term that makes demands on what systems and structures properly permit those communities to be looked after with the dignity they deserve.

To complement this brief overview, we now turn to *aesthetics* and how it is being used within the phrase 'care aesthetics' and, more broadly, in how it features in the work of the different authors in this book. If we take care as a complex word due to the frequency it is used across everyday speech as well as in academic discourses, we can see that aesthetics is similarly problematic as a concept that shifts between informal usage and more technical or philosophical contexts. By way of an example, when doing an internet search on 'care aesthetics', one is as likely to get directions to the local high street beautician as one is to an analysis of the sensory practices of a carer in a dementia care context. Aesthetics can refer to the everyday sense of beautification, making something 'aesthetic' and, therefore, when used within healthcare and specifically dementia care, it is important to recognise this lay sense of the term is often present. The aim here is to offer an overview of some of the assumed definitions attached to the word and to respond in two different ways. First, the link to beauty salons and similar aesthetic care enterprises adopts what we would argue is a narrow version of aesthetics, only using it within a visual register – aesthetics becomes restricted to a judgement of what something looks like. Aesthetics in 'care aesthetics' is interested in visual qualities but extends this single sensory concern with sight to include all the senses within its terms of reference. So, rather than the colloquial usage which concerns making something look more appealing, care aesthetics is focused on the contribution of all the senses to human (and non-human) well-being. That means that the use of touch, smell, hearing, and movement are all part of the aesthetics of care. Second, care aesthetics seeks to have a more circumspect relation to beauty. Whilst the beauty of care might be an objective (including a claim, which is itself subject to debate, that the more beautiful, the better the care), we expand the remit of aesthetics to include an attention to a full range of sensory qualities of a care experience, including those which are unpleasant or ugly. Again, this comes with the testable claim that ugly care is connected, if not synonymous, with poor care. As with the word 'care', as described above, aesthetics works as both an evaluative and descriptive term.

This account has started from a lay understanding of aesthetics. This is of course relevant within dementia care settings, as we are working where there are existing uses of the term and often nervousness about what it seeks to designate. This is noted in the work of Sarah Fox and colleagues (2025) where the term 'meaningful moment of connection' was preferred by people living with dementia to 'everyday aesthetics' (p. 3) due to these varied associations with the word and its inherent complexity; and see also Chapter 8 in this book. It is, however, also important to acknowledge the broader history of aesthetics and note where the more inclusive version adopted here originates. There is, in fact, a long history where aesthetics refers to the experience of all the senses in response to an engagement with the world – whether other people, the immediate material context, or the wider environment. The first usage of the word aesthetics comes from the 18th century with the German writer and philosopher Alexander Baumgarten who coined the word in 1735 to refer to sensory knowing as a counterpoint to reason or logical knowledge (for a good overview, see: Miller et al., 2022, p. 3). This drew on the Greek word *aesthesis* referring to sensory perception or experience. Aesthetics, in this early formulation, does not start from an appreciation of the appearance of an object, but a sensory experience that includes the whole body.

Whilst a long history of aesthetic theory has predominantly focused on how human society has responded to the arts, and to a lesser degree to nature or the environment, the ambition of care aesthetics is to draw on this original, more expansive definition, but take it in a somewhat different direction. Aesthetics, of course, might connect to the arts, and to a visual register, but for care aesthetics, it aims to go beyond this to examine the sensory engagement between people and between people and their worlds. The pragmatist philosopher Richard Shusterman (2000) refers to this as a version of aesthetics that is concerned with 'enriched experience' (p. 114), something that is embedded in our daily lives, rather than a reified activity connected to artists and the arts only. This more expansive version of aesthetics has been taken up in the important field of 'everyday aesthetics' that again seeks to widen aesthetics from a study of beauty or art to a close examination of the sensory practices of everyday life. Cleaning your house, doing the laundry, and cooking your meals – and caring for each other – become practices that are examined for their aesthetic qualities. These concerns have been explored in detail in the work of Yuriko Saito (2008, 2017), Richard Shusterman (2000, 2012) and Ben Highmore (2011), amongst others. Whilst there are debates in this field over whether aesthetics refers to a heightened everyday moment or a way of capturing the totality of routine or mundane experiences, the importance for care aesthetics is that this field takes ordinary interhuman experience as significant for exploration or analysis. Its ambition is, therefore, to take aesthetics out of the exclusive terrain of art appreciation and help to situate it within the ordinary lives of communities – and, of course, how they give and receive care.

Whilst everyday aesthetics is a vital point of reference for care aesthetics, one slight difference of emphasis (besides the particular focus on care itself) is on the importance of examining relations between people, and not only between people and their material worlds. Ultimately, of course, an experience relies on body-to-body, and bodies to material (whether that is personal clothes, hospital beds, or the walls of a building), relations. The emphasis in care aesthetics on the interhuman is largely the result of human-to-human relations rarely being taken seriously in aesthetic theories. A notable exception to this is in the field of relational aesthetics (Bourriaud, 2002) where the making of relations between people is considered for the sensory experience it elicits. Care aesthetics (as an approach) is seeking to explore how an aesthetic experience, therefore, does not only reside within the body of a person but also is an experience in relation to another. The carer and the cared for are both the creators of that experience. Traditional aesthetics has focused predominantly on human's experience of objects or non-human others (sounds, pictures, and so forth), whereas care aesthetics' emphasis is to include interhuman experiences as a site of significance.

Of course, these accounts of both care and aesthetics are summaries which necessarily give little space for the many complexities and controversies in both areas. By bringing care and aesthetics together, the aim is to suggest that the relational practices of caring – from the small scale to the societal – can be understood for their complex combination of sensory, embodied practices. The histories and controversies surrounding both words do not disappear as they are brought together in this way. Not only are there obvious points of connection between the two words – a focus on relations, an attention to bodily practices, an interest in sensory experience – but also there are unresolved tensions. For example, 'What is the role of beauty in care?'; 'How does an ethic of care connect to an aesthetic?' and so forth. These questions are not to be resolved here, but the hope is that through the chapters, some of these will be addressed. Whilst we, as the editors, have a sense of *what we mean by the term*, we are also keeping its definition open to extend what it might reveal in different practices, and where it needs to be questioned or challenged.

To illustrate some of the benefits and then also some tensions in this openness, the next part of the Introduction will offer three examples of care practice from different contexts. The purpose is both to draw out some of the themes that arise when care aesthetics is brought into dialogue with dementia care and then to look at what claims it makes as a mode of analysis. It is important to note that whilst more theoretical work on care aesthetics has appeared in four different monographs – Donovan (2016), Mihai (2022), Saito (2022), and Thompson (2023) – as James Thompson (2023) is an editor of this book and oversees the 'Care Aesthetics Series' for Routledge, it is his work that will be drawn upon particularly in this text. That said, each of these four authors has developed complementary accounts of what it means to argue for an aesthetic dimension to care, and their work has influenced different perspectives and directions for this emerging field. The three examples here go backwards to the moment when James first encountered what he understood as an example of an aesthetic of care in his witnessing of the physiotherapy sessions for a colleague. Then, we move onto an example from contemporary literature where a chiropodist is caring for the feet of an elderly client. Finally, we include examples taken from the work of a Dutch arts organisation called 'The Genetic Choir' and their work with people living with dementia, and data linked to the CARE research project mentioned earlier. These are deliberately eclectic but hopefully a sense of the ambitions, and some of the parameters of a care aesthetic approach, can be demonstrated through them.

### *Physiotherapy*

When James' Congolese colleague was injured in 2011, he came to live with him and his family, and they became involved both in supporting his recuperation from an operation and subsequent physiotherapy. James gives a detailed account of this experience in his book *Care Aesthetics: For Artful Care and Careful Art* (Thompson, 2023) and the purpose here is not to repeat its general argument that there was an aesthetic element in the care that was given. The aim here is just to focus on what this early argument suggests as some central tenets of the overall approach. First, perhaps an obvious, but somewhat less acknowledged aspect of this example is that it was a healthcare relationship that inspired a curiosity about what it might mean to claim that care has an aesthetic. Whilst James is a researcher and practitioner from the arts, care aesthetics does not come from, nor wholly belong to, the arts community. In commenting on the bodily practices of the physiotherapist and the close embodied responses of his friend, James was bringing an attention of an arts researcher – someone who was trained to draw attention to the way a body moves in space, much like Chapter 6 in this book from Kate Maguire-Rosier and Réka Polonyi – but the starting point of this version of care aesthetics is not found in what might be traditionally called an 'arts in heath' project. A key principle for care aesthetics, therefore, is that it starts from care and is not necessarily concerned with an arts practice. Of course, arts and artists might be involved in a practice that has a certain aesthetics of care, but the ambition of the idea is that it is located first and foremost in the experience and expertise of people caring (in multiple settings) and the responses of those for whom they care.

The second orientation suggested by this first example is that there were highly skilled sensory practices that combined to create a relationship between a health professional and a patient. The care aesthetic 'lens' noticed the sophisticated interplay of the different sensory practices – so, the subtle variations and different qualities of touch, the shifts in eye contact, the alignment of breath, and the movement between the two bodies. Watching them repeatedly, James noticed the minute adaptations to different needs of his friend, the subtle changes in pressure of a touch, or shift in posture. This was not formulaic care but precisely executed responsive care that changed and always seemed to flow between the two people present. Attending to these embodied qualities was therefore an attention to the quality of the care – and again an important claim, the greater the fluency or even elegance of the movements between them, the better the care appeared to be. Of course, 'appeared' is an important disclaimer here, but it goes without saying that the quality of the relationship and the gradual improvement in the movement of James' colleague's hand and arm suggest the extraordinary skill of the physiotherapist had positive results. So, these first two claims combined to argue for a certain type of noticing and then valuing elements of a care practice that were both embedded in a care practitioner's technical skills, her virtuosic execution of them, and then in the sensitive and collaborative responses from the person being cared for. An artist's sensibility to the practices of bodies and the affective experiences they allow might have been part of this orientation, but it is in no means a claim that artists and arts researchers are key to this particular focus.

The final point to take from this first example is related to care aesthetics' critical use. James was implicitly using care and aesthetics in an evaluative sense in this example, drawing attention to the extraordinary, embodied practices of the physiotherapist. It was, in his words, an example of beautiful care. This might be explained by the fact that having seen a colleague badly injured, a search for a positive human practice was an important counterpoint to the violence of the original event that caused the injury. This tendency for care aesthetics to point to the exceptional – and particularly the exceptionally positive – is not, however, a given. An analysis of aesthetics of care can focus on the ugly, painful, and poorly executed as much as what might be experienced as positive. Many accounts of care aesthetics in the pages that follow do still document the subtle, mostly enriching practices of care, but there is also ambivalence. Care can of course be beautiful and ugly simultaneously; it can have moments of warmth with terrible pain. As care aesthetics develops, these nuanced accounts of the complexity of the sensations of care are a vital part of its analytic work.

### *Marzahn, Mon Amour*

*Marzahn, Mon Amour* is a novel by the German writer Katja Oskamp (2022) which narrates the experience of a writer turned chiropodist in the Marzahn area of east Berlin. She writes in astounding detail of older people's feet where 'everything feels so delicate, so easily broken' (Oskamp, 2022, p. 56). The argument here is that her book is an impressive account of care aesthetics. The reason for choosing it is to make two points about a care aesthetic focus. The first relates to the significance of the attention to the smallest details of care and the second concerns the hidden, perhaps less than glamorous parts, of care practice. Care aesthetics is arguing that just because in some examples of analysis the attention is on a micro act of care, this should not be taken as an indication of the scale of its importance. We would argue that this attention to the small scale *but* significant is a positive feature of many of the chapters in this book. Oskamp (2022) writes in astonishing detail about the intimacies of foot care, but the result is always a commentary on the importance of building relationships and seeking sustenance for broken lives. Here is, by way of example, her narrator's account of her care work with her client called Frau Noll:

> I take her […] left foot and steadily stroke from the base joints of her toes along her instep towards her ankle joints. Everything feels so delicate, so easily

> broken. I draw on what I've learned over the course of many massages: contact over a wide surface area gives more pleasure than a targeted touch. One hand must always remain on the foot to avoid the sensation of abandonment. A moderate tempo shows I'm not in a hurry. Suddenly [...] Frau Noll cries out [...] 'Beautiful.' And again: 'Beautiful.' And once more: 'Beeeaaauuutiful!'
>
> *(Oskamp, 2022, p. 56)*

Earlier in this chapter, Oskamp's (2022) narrator explained that it was 'physical contact and voice' that were 'the best things to use when approaching someone whose field of vision' (p. 54) is greatly reduced. This is an expert who knows about touch, tone of voice, and the moderation of tempo to create a particular experience for her client. These are exactly the modulations of sensation with which care aesthetics is concerned. There is clearly an aesthetic in her care of Frau Noll, but the delicateness of the woman's feet, the sense that they can be easily broken, and the demand that a person such as her should not be abandoned also illustrate that this practice is a vital act of support in a world where too many people are left isolated. Pointing to the significance of expertly organised touch, simultaneously demonstrates how a more careful society starts from the embodied practices of expert carers. A focus on care aesthetics – here, a minute account of the massage of the delicate feet of an older person – is not separate from wider social issues of loneliness but an intimate part of their repair.

The second point to emphasise here is that Oskamp's account of chiropody – including scraping dead skin, cutting fungus from nails, and easing the pain of bunions – is rarely the topic of literature and far from an attention to the beautiful that might be assumed to be the focus of aesthetics. Care work deals with complex, difficult, and at times messy bodies, and that practice is too often not documented or given value. It might be unglamorous, but that in no way means that it is done without skill, expertise, and extraordinary attention to the dignity of another person. The experience for Frau Noll is *beautiful*, the activity is richly and elegantly described by the author, and we therefore note a certain poetry in the complexity of the work. This does not deny the range of complex sensations always involved in any care practice but illustrates the frequent ambivalent emotions that surround intimate care acts. Messy bodies can still be handled beautifully. *Marzahn, Mon Amour* offers a vision of the aesthetics of a chiropodist's care and the relations she created with a diverse community of elders. It is a novel that acknowledges the extraordinary craft of a healthcare professional, an aesthetics in the micro details of foot care, and the dignity of the older people who deserve not to be abandoned.

### *The Genetic Choir (Amsterdam) and the CARE project*

There is a moment in the short film 'Beyond Words' (https://kimbrand.nl/beyond-words-english/; accessed 1 March 2026), about The Genetic Choir's work in dementia settings, when their artistic director, Thomas Johannsen, sits next to a woman in a care home and seemingly does very little. He sings or hums quietly, looking at her and she both looks back and seemingly ignores him. He is shoulder to shoulder with her but does not appear to need a response or force one. In the empirical work of the CARE project in Manchester, there was a moment from the observation data where a healthcare support worker (HCSW) sat for some time with a patient living with dementia on a settee holding their hand whilst apparently doing little else. This moment continued for some minutes and was noted by the researcher for the sense of calm and intimate attention that was being practised. As a research team, we became interested in this because the observer felt it was important, but it did not fit into standard designations of significance. The HCSW was spending time with a patient and using bodily proximity and the touch of her hand to acknowledge the presence of the person. They were not distracted by a temporal rhythm that was demanding the completion of particular care tasks but practising a form of care that recognised the importance of being with this person, in the here and now. Both this care worker and Johannsen were prepared just to be with another person. The exemplar nature of these moments was thus found in their attention to the here and now, the sensory quality created between two people, and the acceptance of the quietness of the patient, not as a signal automatically of some form of loss.

These examples are chosen to illustrate three themes within care aesthetics. First is that they illustrate that close attention to the bodily practice of care, noticing the subtleties of touch, body position, or movement, is a mode of analysis just as appropriate to examine the actions of a care worker, or a family carer, as it is an artist. In fact, in seeking to notice the micro sensory aspects of a care practice, we see how different communities demonstrate a range of strengths and weaknesses in their work. However, there is no suggestion that artists can automatically practice an exemplary aesthetic of care in their 'arts in health' initiatives, and similarly, there is no guarantee that carers have a highly attuned bodily practice. The second point to draw out from this example is the relation between what might be called 'task-based' and 'non-task-based' care and closely connected to this, 'technical' and 'non-technical' care. Sometimes, the sensory and embodied practices that we are focused on here are referred to as the soft skills of a care professional. A key suggestion of care aesthetics is that the value hierarchy between soft and hard should be challenged. There are multiple skills that make up a care practice, with different demands and different forms of complexity. At times, a division between technical task and non-technical/non-task is a relevant division to notice, but this is not always the case. For example, fitting a cannula in a patient's arm or the back of their hand might be viewed as a 'technical/task', whilst sitting with the patient by their bed to reassure them about the procedure to come could be viewed as 'non-technical/non-task'. In the earlier examples above, it is easy to see how sitting with the two older individuals could be viewed as a 'non-technical/non-task' care moment.

Care aesthetics seeks to complicate these divisions. In all tasks in a care setting, from highly complex to more straightforward and everyday, there are a range of bodily skills and sensory ways of practice that impact on how it happens and how it is experienced. Fitting a cannula still involves a quality of attention, an understanding of touch and a delicate set of movements that are at one and the same time technically and sensorily complex. Changing a person's continence pad or washing a patient are both care tasks, but filled with emotional, embodied, and sensory relations that must be attended to for the task to run smoothly. So, care aesthetics is not arguing that the technical and task-based activities need to be mindful of an additional layer of the 'aesthetic' skill but pointing out that the 'aesthetic/technical' are intimately interwoven in everyday caring practices. And then, of course, the same can be said of those moments that are apparently 'non-task'. The argument of a care aesthetic approach is that the attention to the body and life of another requires a high degree of sensory awareness. Sitting with someone, apparently doing nothing, is a highly skilled moment of meeting someone's needs for company, calm, and an acknowledgement of their personhood. Doing nothing is never doing nothing.

The final point to make regarding these two examples – which we would argue demonstrate immense skill by both professionals – is that they recognise the importance of presence when working with people living with dementia. This term comes from the work of Andries Baart and Gus Timmerman (2024) which argues that the starting point for care work is establishing a relationship of presence with another. Rather than starting from an intervention mindset – how must I try to change the other? – they argue that being present for someone recognises them as a person who deserves acknowledgement and attention. The urge to do, to act, or to intervene, is so strong in the health and social care sectors that their insistence on a starting point of being present and creating a relationship, challenges many of the hierarchies that place 'task-based/technical' against the apparently 'non-technical/non-task-based' work. Being present for someone, as a starting point for a care relationship, suspends the distinctions and prejudices inherent in these divisions and argues instead that an embodied awareness of the value of the other person is a starting point. Being present with someone is not the *soft extra*, or doing nothing, but we would argue the starting point for person-centred care.

This brings us neatly to the subtitle of this collection: *New Directions for Person-Centred Practices*. This is, of course, a reference to the pioneering work of the social psychologist Tom Kitwood who, in his seminal text *Dementia Reconsidered: The Person Comes First* (Kitwood, 1997), argued for a movement away from a purely medical or disease-focused model, to one that recognised the personhood of the individual living with dementia. His interest was in care work that sought to maintain a person's sense of self, that acknowledged their life story, and that recognised the importance of warmth and love in caring relationships. Kitwood (1997) also identified the five core psychological needs of people living with dementia as attachment, comfort, identity, inclusion, and occupation and the need to foster positive person work in everyday interactions with people living with dementia. This overall ethos has clearly inspired the research and practice of many of the writers in this collection. In giving the example of Johannsen from The Genetic Choir and the HCSW, we are illustrating that person-centredness in dementia care does not necessarily start from something recognised as an activity, or intervention. It also requires this willingness to slow down and be present with another. One emphasis we are interested in this edition is how and why this is done. How does a carer make time, understand their body and another's body, and discover a way of recognising the person in front of them? Person-centredness, therefore, for this book is an ethos but, crucially, it is also a set of *practices* that needs to understand the complexity and crafted nature of all moments of attentive care.

We are suggesting these are new directions, not as a way of challenging the orientation of person-centredness in Kitwood's body of work, but to point to multiple, different contexts where the difficulty of creating a person-centred relationship plays out. Whether in neighbourhoods, in gardens, in domestic spaces, in hospital wards, or in music groups, creating a relationship of care demands a highly skilled set of practices – a set of aesthetic practices – that need to be valued and acknowledged as an integrated part of care work. Sitting for a moment, washing, dancing with a resident to reassure them, singing together, shaving, or helping to feed are all examples where a claim to person-centredness needs to be tested with a close examination of the sensory, embodied (aesthetic), and relational practices that are used. This is present in the research on person-centredness, but we believe care aesthetics brings a precise language for its exploration. Kitwood (1997) had his own term 'timalation' to refer to the sensory practices involved in positive person work, and whilst not developed fully in his early work, the attention implied by this word to the management and coordination of a sensory relationship for the person living with dementia, overlaps with the emphasis of care aesthetics. Kelly and colleagues (2023) discuss 'timalation' in relation to an analysis of music therapy with people living with dementia, particularly outlining how it refers to the multiple senses to be explored in arts work. The emphasis in care aesthetics is that all activities in a care context require an attention to the different sensory modalities that shape a person's well-being. Learning to sit, wait, and connect requires an acute sensitivity to the highly differentiated needs of another, as does understanding how to wake someone, bathe them, or complete multiple other daily activities. Detailed exploration of the aesthetics of a care experience, between people living with dementia and their carers, whether family members or professional staff, gives us the descriptive, analytic language for the complex practical work of relationship building – of doing person-centred care.

## The chapters

This now brings us to the chapters. As we said at the top of the Introduction, we are grateful to the different authors for their willingness to write for this book and their interest in examining how care aesthetics works across multiple different areas of their research and practice. The benefits, we feel, of collecting these perspectives in book form, are that we have more freedom to accept contributions made in different registers and formats. So, here you will find traditional research articles alongside reflective analyses and then accounts of personal experience.

This book is broken down into four parts. Part 1, 'A critical and personal appreciation of care aesthetics and living with dementia', brings together the psychiatrist and philosopher Julian C. Hughes and sociologist Christina Buse, two people, as mentioned earlier, who have already brought an aesthetic language into their research and practice work in the field of dementia studies. Julian reassesses his earlier work on an aesthetic approach to dementia (Hughes, 2014), a piece of analysis that both prefigured care aesthetics and also established a number of its terms of reference. Here, he explores some of its assumptions and theoretical origins. This piece sits alongside the moving account from Christina that documents her experience of caring for her mother in North Wales. Her own art practice of sketching becomes a practice that connects to her caring relationship with her mother, both as a form of self-care and one that maintains her mother's care for her. These opening chapters, we feel, set the tone of this book – one that is intimate, reflective, and theoretically probing but simultaneously caring in the way the chapters are presented.

In Part 2, 'Care aesthetics and creative practices', this book switches to a series of chapters exploring different 'creative' practices. This starts with Henry McPherson and colleagues' analysis of two case studies of object creation with people living with dementia. The first is activities based on textile work and the tactile relationships that are realised in giving people the opportunities to touch, feel, and manipulate different textures. The second case study is a music group where the Open Doors Research Group (a self-advocacy group of people living with dementia) collectively co-created and co-designed an album cover sleeve that celebrated their different musical tastes and memories. We are delighted that the final album cover is featured as the cover of this book and see also the Acknowledgements at the start of this text. The next chapter is led by Jackie Kindell, who is a co-editor of this book, and draws on her background in semantic dementia as a speech and language therapist. This chapter explores how a focus on aesthetic moments can reveal new understanding about the potential for maintaining relationships alongside difficulties in communication. Next, Sarah Campbell and Rebecka Fleetwood-Smith focus on the 'doing' of care aesthetics using participatory and social research methods to illustrate their creative method of working. Kate Maguire-Rosier and Réka Polonyi then draw on their backgrounds as arts researchers and trained artists (in dance and clowning, respectively) to illustrate how their knowledge of bodily practices helped them to document the skills of HCSWs working with people living with dementia admitted to NHS mental health wards for older people. Their trained 'aesthetic sensibility' allowed them to notice in minute detail how bodies worked in the spaces of dementia care. The penultimate chapter in Part 2 is written by Rebecka Fleetwood-Smith and Robyn Dowlen and explores different forms of everyday aesthetic engagement. Rather than the more formal context of an arts group, Rebecka and Robyn examine dress, grooming, and then everyday moments, to explore the importance of sensory practices in enabling quality life experiences – and a sense of creative citizenship – for people living with dementia and their families. The final chapter in Part 2 of this book is by Sarah Fox and combines three fields – neuroaesthetics, everyday aesthetics, and Polyvagal Theory – to argue for a new approach to examining the everyday lives of people living with dementia and their families. The ambition of this chapter is to outline an interdisciplinary proposal for improving people's well-being through enhancing their opportunities for meaningful aesthetic moments.

Part 3 of this book, 'Care aesthetics, outdoor spaces, and everyday design', changes context and rather than dealing with particular practices, takes dementia studies into different social environments. The first chapter explores gardening, and how living in, and continuing to take pleasure from interaction with a garden, can provide immense support and feelings of well-being. Rita Newton and colleagues, including co-authors from the Royal Horticultural Society, give a beautiful account of the importance of gardens and gardening and a detailed commentary on the way people living with dementia care for their natural spaces and are, in turn, cared for by them. Daryl Martin and his colleagues' chapter is similarly about relations with a materiality, in this case, the role of reminiscence rooms in dementia contexts and the problems associated with 'dementia-friendly' design. This chapter is an account of the challenges in design and architectures of care, and again how spaces shape the opportunity for or possibility of living well within them. The final chapter in Part 3 takes people living with dementia out into their neighbourhoods to argue for the need to go beyond the concept of 'dementia-friendly' design to a more expansive idea of 'neighbourhood aesthetics'. Recontextualising and drawing upon his previous research collaborations, Andrew Clark's chapter explores how people make their neighbourhoods through the relations that are possible within them. These relationships in turn help to connect people living with dementia to others in their communities and to the spaces they inhabit, both in the present and through lived time.

The final part of this book, Part 4, is called 'New beginnings in care aesthetics' and includes one concluding chapter and an Afterword. The concluding chapter is written by the editors and offers a brief summary of the key themes that emerged across all the different chapters and how they present opportunities for future research and practice. We outline some new possibilities for the dialogue between dementia studies and care aesthetics and suggestions as to what types of questions we should, or could, be asking. The final piece in the book is an Afterword and a personal account from Sue Ennis describing the experience of her care for her husband Frank and drawing on the language of care aesthetics for its presentation. We are indebted to Sue for her willingness to write so powerfully and movingly about this experience – one where the complex realities of intimate care are laid bare. The aesthetic lens here shows the multisensory experiences of care include the smells, textures, emotions, the sights, and the sounds. This chapter alone demonstrates that care aesthetics is not seeking to gloss care as 'the beautiful', but to show determinedly the sensory complexity of any intimate care relationship. The honesty and warmth with which this account is written about something so personal is a fitting way to end this book, and we want to thank Sue for her permission to publish it.

### *Writing style and presentation*

Each of the main chapters in this book (except Chapter 12) includes, at the end, 'Three Key Further Reading References' and a brief description of each shared reference as a way of quickly focusing down on the key debates and issues in its substantive area. In the writing style and across all the chapters, authors have been encouraged to use people/person living with dementia unless referring to 'the person with dementia living at home' or suchlike, when 'living' will be removed from the descriptive terminology, or when people/person with dementia is cited from source material. We will use dementia studies as terminology that should be read to include dementia care when it is not specifically spelled out as such. Authors will also use carers as a descriptive term during this book to refer to both 'formal' and 'informal' caregiving relationships. In-text references for each chapter in this book are presented at the end of each chapter.

One final point to make about all the chapters is to acknowledge how many joint and repeated authors there are. As you will notice, some names appear more than once. Whilst this of course demonstrates the collaborative nature of much dementia studies and health and social care research, it is also an indication of the strong interest in this field from a closely associated group of researchers, practitioners, and writers, including people living with dementia and family carers. We hope these overlapping interests and authorial perspectives enrich the overall book and show it to be the result of a group of stakeholders who have a common commitment to person-centred care in the field of dementia. Indeed, all authors who have taken part in this book believe that commitment is enhanced by an attention to the aesthetics of care, and how this can lead to more fulfilled lives of all those affected by the experience of living with dementia.

## References

Baart, A. and Timmerman, G. (2024). *Relational Caring and Presence Theory in Health Care and Social Work: A Care-Ethical Perspective*. Bristol: Bristol University Press.

Bourriaud, N. (2002). *Relational Aesthetics*. Trans. Pleasance, S. and Woods, F. with Copeland, M. Dijon: Les Presses du Réel.

Buse, C. and Twigg, J. (2018). Dressing disrupted: Negotiating care through the materiality of dress in the context of dementia. *Sociology of Health & Illness*, 40 (2): 340–352. https://doi.org/10.1111/1467-9566.12575

Buse, C., Balmer, A., Keady, J., Nettleton, S. and Swift, S. (2023). 'Ways of being' in the domestic garden for people living with dementia: Doing, sensing and playing. *Ageing & Society. First View* 1–25. https://doi.org/10.1017/S0144686X22001489

Campbell, S., Dowlen, R., Keady, J. and Thompson, J. (2024). Care aesthetics and 'being in the moment' through improvised music-making and male grooming in dementia care.

*International Journal of Education & the Arts*, 25 (si1.13). Available: https://journals.psu.edu/ijea/article/view/63522; accessed 1 March 2026.

Donovan, J. (2016). *The Aesthetics of Care: On the Literary Treatment of Animals*. London: Bloomsbury.

Dowlen, R., McPherson, D.H.J., Swarbrick, C., Hoskin, L., Thompson, J. and Keady, J. (2024). Creating and reliving the moment: Using musical improvisation and care aesthetics as a lens of connection and self-expression for younger people living with dementia. *International Journal of Environmental Research and Public Health*, 21 (8): 972. Available: https://doi.org/10.3390/ijerph21080972; accessed 1 March 2026.

Dowlen, R., Keady, J., Milligan, C., Swarbrick, C., Ponsillo, N., Geddes, L. and Riley, B. (2022). In the moment with music: An exploration of the embodied and sensory experiences of people living with dementia during improvised music-making. *Ageing & Society*, 42 (11): 2642–2664. https://doi.org/10.1017/S0144686X21000210

Fox, S., Thompson, J. and Keady, J. (2025). Meaningful moments of connection: How people affected by dementia and their carers living at home understand, interpret and experience everyday aesthetics. *International Journal of Geriatric Psychiatry*, 40 (8): e70136. Available: https://doi.org/10.1002/gps.70136; accessed 1 March 2026.

Gilligan, C. (2009). *In a Different Voice: Psychological Theory and Women's Development*. Cambridge: Harvard University Press.

Hamington, M. (2004). *Embodied Care: Jane Addams, Maurice Merleau-Ponty, and Feminist Ethics*. Chicago: University of Illinois Press.

Held, V. (2006). *The Ethics of Care: Personal, Political, and Global*. Oxford: Oxford University Press.

Highmore, B. (2011). *Ordinary Lives: Studies in the Everyday*. London: Routledge.

Hughes, J.C. (2014). The aesthetic approach to people with dementia. *International Psychogeriatrics*, 26 (9): 1407–1413. https://doi.org/10.1017/S1041610214001100.

Jones, L., Cullum, N., Watson, R., Thompson, J. and Keady, J. (2025). 'Only my family can help': The lived experience and care aesthetics of being resident on an NHS psychiatric/mental health inpatient dementia assessment ward – a single case study. *Ageing & Society*, 45 (6): 1143–1164. https://doi:10.1017/S0144686X24000096

Keady, J. (ed.) (2024). *Reconsidering Neighbourhoods and Living with Dementia: Spaces, Places, and People*. Maidenhead: Open University Press/McGraw-Hill.

Keady, J.D., Campbell, S., Clark, A., Dowlen, R., Elvish, R., Jones, L., Kindell, J., Swarbrick, C. and Williams, S. (2022). Re-thinking and re-positioning 'being in the moment' within a continuum of moments: Introducing a new conceptual framework for dementia studies. *Ageing & Society*, 42 (3): 681–702. https://doi.org/10.1017/S0144686X20001014

Kelly, L., Ahessy, B., Richardson, I., Moss, H. (2023). Aligning kitwood's model of person-centered dementia care with music therapy practice. *Music Therapy Perspectives*, 41 (2): 198–206. https://doi.org/10.1093/mtp/miad015

Kitwood, T. (1997). *Dementia Reconsidered: The Person Comes First*. Buckingham: Open University Press.

Maguire-Rosier, K., Polonyi, R. and Thompson, J. (eds.) (2025). *Care Aesthetics and the Arts*. London: Routledge.

Mihai, M. (2022). *Political Memory and the Aesthetic of Care: The Art of Complicity and Resistance*. Stanford: Stanford University Press.

Miller, B.J., Glaser, J. and Burke, J. (2022). Palliative aesthetics. In W. Breitbart and H. Chochinov (eds.) *Handbook of Psychiatry in Palliative Medicine: Psychosocial Care of the Terminally Ill*. Third edition. Oxford: Oxford Academic, Chapter 23: https://doi.org/10.1093/med/9780197583838.003.0023

Mol, A. (2008). *The Logic of Care: Health and the Problem of Patient Choice*. London: Routledge.

Mol, A. Moser, I. and Pols, J. (eds.) (2010). *Care in Practice: On Tinkering in Clinics, Homes and Farms*. Bielefeld: Transcript.

Noddings, N. (2013). *Caring: A Relational Approach to Ethics and Moral Education*. Berkeley: University of California Press.

Oskamp, K. (2022). *Marzahn, Mon Amour*. Trans. J. Heinrich. Bath: Peirene Press.

Puig de la Bellacasa, M. (2017). *Matters of Care: Speculative Ethics in More than Human Worlds*. Minnesota: University of Minnesota Press.

Robinson, F. (2011). *The Ethics of Care: A Feminist Approach to Human Security*. Philadelphia: Temple University Press.

Saito, Y. (2008). *Everyday Aesthetics*. Oxford: Oxford University Press.

Saito, Y. (2017). *Aesthetics of the Familiar: Everyday Life and World-Making*. Oxford: Oxford University Press.

Saito, Y. (2022). *Aesthetics of Care: Practice in Everyday Life*. London: Bloomsbury.

Shusterman, R. (2000). *Performing Live: Aesthetic Alternatives for the Ends of Art*. New York: Cornell University Press.

Shusterman, R. (2012). *Thinking through the Body*. Cambridge: Cambridge University Press.

Thompson, J. (2023). *Care Aesthetics: For Artful Care and Careful Art*. London: Routledge.

Tronto, J. (2013). *Caring Democracy: Markets, Equality, and Justice*. New York: New York University Press.

Ward, R., Campbell, S. and Keady, J. (2016a). Assembling the salon: Learning from alternative forms of body work in dementia care. *Sociology of Health & Illness*, 38 (8): 1287–1302. https://doi.org/10.1111/1467-9566.12461

Ward, R., Campbell, S. and Keady, J. (2016b). 'Gonna make yer gorgeous': Everyday transformation, resistance and belonging in the care-based hair salon. *Dementia: The International Journal of Social Research and Practice*, 15 (3): 395–413. https://doi.org/10.1177/1471301216638969

# PART 1

# A critical and personal appreciation of care aesthetics and living with dementia

# PART I

# 1

# THINKING BEHIND AN AESTHETIC APPROACH TO DEMENTIA

*Julian C. Hughes*

## Introduction

This chapter looks at the underlying philosophical basis to the notion of aesthetics in relation to people living with a diagnosis of dementia. My interest more broadly is in the relevance of aesthetics to human beings. But an important part of my thesis is that dementia shows or reveals the aesthetic nature of humanity or of persons. It is not solely people living with dementia who make this manifest – we all do – but dementia acts as a focus. And I am interested in how this aesthetic nature is fleshed out in practice.

I am going to suggest it is fleshed out in nine ways:

1 It means we are sentient as well as cognitive beings.
2 It means we are embodied.
3 It means we are interrelated and interdependent.
4 It means that, as humans, we are situated persons.
5 It also means that we are active agents in the world with which we engage.
6 It means that we engage in particular ways, in ways that cannot but be caring.
7 But it is more than simply caring or concern: it is solicitude.
8 And because of its deep connections with how we are as persons, our aesthetic nature cannot be conceived without the context of ethics.
9 Finally, it is also connected with notions of friendship and love.

These nine ways are almost an argument, although they form a very loose sort of argument. In what follows, I hope – at least I wish to suggest – that the nine ways outline aspects of our humanity which should seem obvious. If I am stating the obvious, I shall be pleased.

DOI: 10.4324/9781003623441-3
This chapter has been made available under a (CC BY) 4.0 license.

## Sentient beings

In a very moving account of her husband's dementia, Barbara Pointon (2007) talked about how, as his dementia worsened, she felt she saw more of the essence of Malcolm. 'Does it matter what we call it', she asked, '– spirit, soul, inner self, essence, identity – so long as we have experienced it?' (p. 119). In the absence of Malcolm's dementia, she would never have had this experience. She found 'the real Malcolm' in the 'revelation of his essential self because of the loving care he receives and the trust that this engenders' (p. 119).

I suspect that not every family carer of someone living with dementia would say that they had experienced such a positive encounter with the person for whom they cared. But many do describe a sense of growth or a deepening of their relationships. It is worth noting that the revelation of Malcolm's essential self occurs in the context of care, where this is a mutual experience (by the bye, Malcolm was an extremely talented musician: a man of great aesthetic sensitivity). The second point worth noting is that the essential Malcolm emerges at a stage when cognitive abilities were most impaired. So, this encounter was based more on the senses and the emotions than on any intellectual or cognitive engagement, which is the point I wish to emphasise. For, aesthetics is – as well as anything else it might be – about the senses and our sentient being.

As James Thompson and his colleagues also indicated in the Introduction to this book, it was Alexander Gottlieb Baumgarten (1714–1762) who is credited with the emergence of aesthetics in modern times. Of course, interest in theoretical considerations to do with art has been around at least since the Greeks. But Musalek and Scheibenbogen (2025) suggest that thinkers such as Parmenides of Elea, Plato, and Aristotle, as well as more modern philosophers, have undervalued 'emotional-aesthetic knowledge' in favour of 'cognitive-rational knowledge'. Baumgarten (1970) stated: 'The end of aesthetics is the perfection of sense cognition as such. This, however, is beauty' (§14). By 'sense cognition', he meant knowledge derived from the senses. Whilst he accepted a rationalist account of knowledge – that we gain knowledge through the use of reason – he felt that this needed to be complemented by the knowledge we accrue from the senses. Gregor (1983) suggested that Baumgarten's claim is a modest one: '…given the nature of man, his perfection requires the development of his potentialities for both perception and discursive reasoning' (p. 364). Baumgarten's use of the word 'aesthetics', after all, reflects its Greek etymology, suggesting 'things perceptible by the senses'. It is a basic tenet of empirical philosophy that knowledge starts with sensory experiences. But even a rationalist, who holds that knowledge is in some way innate, will admit that our senses are important in terms of informing, shaping, or confirming what we know. To the average person on the Clapham omnibus, it will not be egregious to be told that we shall do better as human beings if we take note of the things we see, touch, smell, hear, or taste.

Aesthetics is not solely about art and not solely about beauty. At a basic level, it is about how we perceive (or sense) the world:

> I may value a rose bush because it is hardy, prolific, disease-resistant and the like, but if I value the rose aesthetically the most obvious relevant grounds will be the way it looks, …, and the way it smells; the same grounds may be a basis for aesthetic dislike.
>
> *(Urmson, 2004, pp. 24–25)*

Now, there is every reason to believe that a person living with even advanced dementia still engages with the world sensorily.

It is for this reason that there has been a burgeoning of interest in how people living with dementia might be helped by, or benefit from, arts interventions. This literature is now so vast that it would be a Herculean task to review it systematically. But there are a good number of previous reviews (and reviews of the reviews, such as Manji and Fallavollita (2022)) ranging from scoping to systematic, and covering a range of different art forms (e.g., Vink et al., 2004; Beard, 2012; Guzmán-García et al., 2013; Hughes, 2014; Livingston et al., 2014; Zeilig et al., 2014; Young et al., 2016; Karkou and Meekums, 2017; Livingston et al., 2017; Deshmukh et al., 2018; Dowlen et al., 2018; van der Steen et al. 2018; Dorris et al., 2021; Hughes, 2025). The arts include, amongst other things (with convenient examples of relevant studies), the visual arts (Newman et al., 2019; Boutoleau-Bretonnière et al., 2024), public art (Kelson et al., 2017), music (Sonntag, 2016; Dowlen et al., 2024), dance (Coaten and Newman-Bluestein, 2013; Guzmán et al., 2017), literature (Rollason et al., 2024) including poetry (Killick, 2017), as well as photography (Dooley et al., 2021), sculpture (Chauhan, 2020), theatre (Gray, 2019; Dalby et al., 2024), design (Walker, 2022), and jewellery (Wallace et al., 2013). If we broaden our understanding to include all aesthetic practices, that is those that rely on sentient experience, we can also include, *inter alia*, play (Li, 2022), the use of clowns (Kontos et al., 2016), pets (Li et al., 2023), museums (Hendriks et al., 2021), and even walking (Kohler et al., 2021) and gardening (Murroni et al., 2021; Newton et al., 2021– and see Chapter 9 in this book by Rita Newton and her colleagues for an applied example of everyday gardening practices and living with dementia).

Although reviews show some positive results (for example, in the use of music), despite the large number of studies and the many reviews, there is a recurring problem. Almost all the studies can be criticised on methodological grounds (i.e., the samples are too small, the studies are not controlled and not replicated). There are two responses to this. First, as was wisely said by Beard (2012), 'strictly allopathic methodologies will continue to fall short of adequately evaluating what are deeply idiosyncratic psychosocial issues' (p. 633). Responses to the arts will always be 'deeply idiosyncratic' and 'psychosocial'. Innovative ways to evaluate these interventions are necessary. In Guzmán-García et al. (2016), for example, which was a study of a dance intervention in care homes, each resident was used as his or her own control. In other words, the measures to be used for each person were particular to that person. In one, it might have been that she was depressed; in another, it might have been that he was agitated. Having assessed the person multiple times before the intervention, as well as during it, further multiple assessments of the particular behaviour or mood were taken after the dancing intervention. Improvement was demonstrated for nine out of ten participants.

Qualitative studies are obviously useful for art interventions, but they must be undertaken rigorously (Shoesmith et al., 2021). They are often disparaged on the grounds that it is quantitative data that will win the day with those who control research funding. But we know that 'arts on prescription' is becoming more fashionable and politically acceptable, including for people living with dementia, albeit subject to the general difficulty of underfunding (O'Connor et al., 2025).

The second response to the accusation that the methodology of arts studies is generally poor is more radical. It is to say that we do not really need randomised controlled studies, or any formal empirical research (although studies may be helpful in securing funding), to tell us that the arts have beneficial effects for people living with dementia. We can simply see it. We can see people enjoying the visit to the art gallery or museum. We can see them tapping their feet to the music. We can watch them participating in the dance. Nevertheless, we must recall that our responses to art are always 'deeply idiosyncratic'. Pet therapy will do nothing for one person but will be a tonic to another. Some of us like Ludwig Beethoven, but not Elvis Presley; some might like both. So, the use of the arts must be undertaken with caution and only after careful conversations with the person and with those who know him or her well. But the bottom line is that we are sentient beings, so an aesthetic approach will always be relevant, especially when intellectual (cognitive) functions are compromised.

Henry, a man with marked dementia who hardly spoke, responded with enthusiasm to music on an iPod ('Alive Inside: A Story of Music and Memory'; available: https://www.youtube.com/watch?v=8HLEr-zP3fc; accessed 1 March 2026). When asked what music did for him, Henry replied: 'It gives me the feeling of love. … You've got beautiful music here … I feel a band of love, of dreams'. Our aesthetic sense makes up our being as human beings, not as a frippery, but as an essential.

## Embodied beings

If aesthetics implies perception by the senses, then the fact of our embodiment is clearly crucial. Our bodies are the means by which we see, hear, smell, touch, and taste the world. But they are not simply mechanisms. Philosophers have recognised this for some while. Charles Taylor (1995), for instance, wrote: 'Our understanding is itself embodied … My sense of myself, of the footing I am on with others, is in large part also embodied' (pp. 170–171).

It is worth contemplating this for a moment, partly because it undermines the far too commonly held dualistic misconception that we are bodies and minds, two separate sorts of stuff, as René Descartes (1596–1650) proclaimed. The whole issue of the mind and body (or brain) is discussed with great clarity by Eric Matthews (2005). If mind and body were separate, it would be ridiculous to suggest that a mental function, such as understanding, is a bodily one. But it is not ridiculous at all, as is shown by the commonly used example of cycling a bike. I know how to go round a corner on a bike, even though I would be totally unable to explain this in terms of its physics. I might be able to teach my grandchildren how to do this by telling them what it feels like and the movements they must make (you need to lean into the turn a bit and keep your speed up), but not by giving them a purely cognitive account (whatever that would be!).

Instead, we need to recognise that human beings form a unitary whole: we are minded bodies or embodied minds. We understand some things in a bodily manner, and we sometimes show our understanding by bodily means. As the late Alasdair MacIntyre (1929–2025) once wrote: 'The primary expressions … of mind are bodily expressions and human minds exist only as the minds of this or that particular body' (MacIntyre, 2006, p. 89). In the second edition of *Dependent Rational Animals* (MacIntyre, 2009), he said: '… it is true of us that we do not merely have, but are our bodies' (p. 6). This sort of philosophical expression undoubtedly reflects the profound impact of Maurice Merleau-Ponty (1908–1961) who wrote in *Phenomenology of Perception* (Merleau-Ponty, 1962) that: 'The body is our general medium for having a world' (p. 169).

The second part of the quotation above from Taylor, which my sense of myself is also embodied, is relevant to people living with dementia. Phinney and Chesla (2003) picked this up when they sought to explore how dementia is 'experienced as a phenomenon of the lived body' (p. 285). In a now seminal paper describing ethnographic research in a care home for people living with dementia, Kontos (2004) wrote: 'During interactions, words assume a gestural significance to the extent that their conceptual meaning is formed by inference from the gestural meaning' (p. 840). The phrase 'gestural significance' is striking and clearly suggests how meaning between people is embodied, as is shown specifically in the interactions of people living with dementia. Subsequently, Kontos (2005) has pushed the notion of 'embodied selfhood' where: 'Personhood persists as an embodied dimension of human existence and, as such, must be embraced in dementia care' (p. 567). Continuing the theme of embodiment, Kontos et al. (2021) examined how dance can 'enhance social inclusion by supporting embodied self-expression, creativity, and social engagement of persons living with dementia and their families' (p. 714). They highlighted two themes: playfulness and sociability, both of which make use of, and depend on, our bodily engagements.

If our embodied natures suggest metaphysical realities and an enhanced status for aesthetics, they also suggest the many ways in which our engagements are also physical in a more mundane sense. Julia Twigg, whose work in the dementia field has always been innovative and illuminating, has summed this up by her talk of 'bodywork', which she describes as 'ambivalent':

> At times it verges on areas of taboo in connection with sexuality or human waste. It is potentially demeaning work, and when undertaken by high status individuals it is typically accompanied by distancing techniques.
>
> *(Twigg, 2000, p. 391)*

Building on this sort of account, James Thompson (2023) has outlined his account of 'care aesthetics' as emphasising that bodies act and respond to each other, 'in particular cultural, social, economic, and political contexts' (p. 62). Our aesthetic nature as human beings is fleshed out in bodily ways, as is shown by the interactions with and of people living with dementia, but this also suggests how interrelated and interdependent we are.

## Interrelated and interdependent beings

We are not simply sentient and embodied beings; we also relate to and depend on others. In answering the question, 'What is a human body?', MacIntyre (2006) put it this way: 'Human bodies ... are partially constituted by their social relationships, just because their movements can only be intelligently characterized and represented in terms of social interaction' (p. 95). The point to notice is that our social relationships are said *to constitute* what the human body is; in other words, there is something essential about our sociality. It is this: only in the context of our social embeddedness do the movements of human bodies make sense or meaning. I shall return to this in the next section, whereas for now, I shall focus on just two aspects of our essentially social nature.

The first is our interrelatedness. Our aesthetic nature is shown by the ways in which we relate. We look after each other in ways that can be intellectual but are mostly embodied and rely on the senses. Through the senses, we pick up that someone needs help; and then the help we give (for good or ill) is mostly through our bodies, by our movements which make sense in the context of human society.

Furthermore, the possibility and the importance of our relationships are maintained even into advanced dementia. In his conversations with Dr. B, the psychologist Steven Sabat (2001) asked whether people can still have good relationships even when one of them has dementia. Sabat's own relationship with Dr. B, who has Alzheimer's disease, demonstrates the importance of relationships and the way in which such relationships can be mutually satisfying (Sabat frequently thanks Dr. B for comments he makes or the help he gives with the research project). In response to Sabat's question, Dr. B says: 'Definitely ... why not?'; and when Sabat clarifies with him that it is his wife and children who give him happiness, Dr. B replies: 'Oh ya! So the world to me still lives' (Sabat, 2001, p. 282). Sabat comments that the family were still 'the cornerstone of meaning' (Sabat, 2001, p. 282) in Dr. B's life.

Again and again in Sabat's (2001) groundbreaking work, *The Experience of Alzheimer's Disease: Life Through a Tangled Veil*, the point is made that crucial to how a person reacts will be 'the effects of the social environment' (p. 111). The brain pathology will cause problems, but the social environment can either ameliorate or worsen those problems because at every turn we have the effects of our interrelationships. But these interrelationships will often be realised through sense perceptions: by the way one person approaches, talks to, touches, and listens to another. As in the conversations between Dr. B and Steven Sabat, of course, there is cognitive content, but there is also 'gestural significance' (to recall Kontos (2004)) and, therefore, an aesthetic component to our interrelatedness.

Similarly, with our interdependence, in his brilliant book *Dependence and Autonomy in Old Age: An Ethical Framework for Long-Term Care*, the geriatrician George Agich (2003) writes the following striking sentence: 'The human body is not only a vehicle for one's autonomous choice or will, but also an impediment' (p. 104). He goes on to suggest that dependence 'is an essential and ineliminable feature of human existence' (p. 104). His point is that it does not matter what age you are; we are all dependent in one way or another. Furthermore, dependence goes together with autonomy: they are different sides of the same coin. My autonomy when I choose to drive down the motorway reflects my dependence on the mechanics who built my car and on the good driving of everyone else on the motorway. I might be dependent on my walking frame to navigate the corridors of the care home, but this dependence also allows me (autonomously) to get out into the garden.

The importance of recognising our dependence is central to *Dependent Rational Animals*. Here, MacIntyre (2009) argues that in order to flourish, that is to do well as human beings, 'We need both those virtues that enable us to function as independent and accountable practical reasoners and those virtues that enable us to acknowledge the nature and extent of our dependence on others' (pp. 155–156). He further argues that in order to achieve these virtues, we must participate in social relationships. Thus, our dependence takes us straight to our interdependence and our interrelationships. And central to these constitutively human interconnections, based as they are on our nature as sentient and embodied beings, are our abilities to perceive by the senses and react accordingly. Hence, our aesthetic abilities will lead us to consider the notion of caring, not as an option for, but as a requirement of, humanity. Before we get there, however, we need to return to look a little more closely at how we are embedded in the world.

## Situated persons

Human beings are sentient, embodied, interrelated, and interdependent beings, but so too are bees and baboons. One way to mark the difference between us and other animals, even if we also need to recognise the similarities, is to focus on the multitude of ways in which we are embedded or situated as human persons. I have long argued that the best way to characterise human persons is to see us as situated embodied agents (Hughes, 2001). The key idea here is that of being situated. We are situated as bodies and as agents. But we are also situated socially, historically, physically, psychologically, spiritually, culturally, geographically, legally, ethically, and so on. Indeed, the ways in which we are situated as persons cannot be circumscribed. But our situatedness makes all the difference. I am who I am, as a person, because of where I was born, because of the family into which I was born, because I move this way, have done these things and thought these thoughts, have had these friends, have held these beliefs, and so forth.

This is very relevant to dementia because it cannot sensibly be said – although it has often been wrongly maintained (see: Hughes et al., 2006) – that I am no longer a person if my dementia means I can no longer remember certain things. Even in advanced dementia, the person can still feel and act in a human context where 'the cornerstone of meaning' (Steven Sabat's expression) can be maintained by others and where (as Pia Kontos put it) 'gestural significance' can still hold sway. In other words, this is where an aesthetic approach to people living with dementia, and an appreciation of their nature as aesthetic beings, holds sway.

It was the philosopher Ludwig Wittgenstein (1889–1951) who wrote: 'What determines our judgment, our concepts and reactions, is not what one man is doing now, an individual action, but the whole hurly-burly of human actions, the background against which we see any action' (Wittgenstein, 1967, §567). Elsewhere, he stated: 'Our talk gets its meaning from the rest of our proceedings' (Wittgenstein, 1979, §229). Both statements can be linked to his more general attitude towards meaning: 'The meaning of a word is its use in the language' (Wittgenstein, 1968, §43). In each case, Wittgenstein is pointing to the background in which our actions, our language, and our meanings gain their point and are situated. It is the background which guarantees human significance.

So, the world itself constitutes our sense of self. It is an ineluctable part of our lives as human beings. It is not us over against the world. We are made up of the world, and it is through the world that our lives are given sense. Merleau-Ponty (1962) famously wrote: 'The world is not what I think, but what I live through' (p. xviii). I can understand the world, but I must also sense it, including the meanings and actions of other people, including those of people who live with a diagnosis of dementia.

## Active agents in the world

People living with advanced dementia can show agency, as I have already discussed through the importance of 'gestural significance' (Kontos, 2004). Wim Dekkers, a clinician and ethicist, acknowledges that people living with severe dementia will eventually lose their abilities to make explicit autonomous decisions. Dekkers (2010) continues: 'This does not mean, however, that their bodily knowledge, which has been developed in the course of their lives, necessarily also disappears.

Tacit bodily knowledge is based on the sedimentation of life narratives' (p. 258). There are actions which are, as it were, stored in the body.

For instance, the person who pushes away the nasogastric tube even though he or she cannot show evidence of a rational decision made with mental capacity (sometimes called competence) might still be signifying an autonomous wish. Objecting to having a tube thrust up your nose is not *eo ipso* irrational! The person's bodily movements can remain meaningful. Certainly, they are meaningful enough to be carefully considered. But this careful consideration will not (or should not) solely be based on rational discussion, whether these discussions are with the person, with his or her family or friends, or amongst the multidisciplinary team. For one thing, although it makes perfect sense to talk to the person about your plan (in an appropriately empathic manner), if it is clear that, for a variety of reasons, they lack decision-making capacity, it is an affront to their dignity to pretend that a rational discussion about consent has occurred. Furthermore, to make some form of surrogate decision for the person still needs to take account of anything that could signify the wishes or desires of the person concerned. This will include attention to their previous inclinations and values. But the sort of careful consideration I am referring to would also include *being with* the person and taking note of their reactions. As Dekkers (2010) says, even if the body of the person living with advanced dementia has dysfunctions, 'it still remains a lived body and a body in which previous forms of autonomy have been inscribed' (p. 258).

Dekkers draws on the work of Merleau-Ponty (1962) who makes a distinction between the objective body and the phenomenal body. We might study the objective body and make predictions about it. The phenomenal body, however, is the lived body; it is the body as we experience it, not as an observed object that moves in space and time. As Merleau-Ponty (1962) wrote: 'I am not in space and time, nor do I conceive space and time; I belong to them, my body combines with them and includes them' (p. 162).

The point I am pursuing is that agency is situated and embodied. A correct understanding of this agency should show us that it is not simply the agency of the rational cognitively intact person. We have a sort of inscribed preverbal bodily agency which means that we can react to events without ratiocination. Again, this links directly to our aesthetic nature because it typically depends on perception by the senses, even if it also involves talking with and listening to all those who might be able to help. The person living with advanced dementia does not wish to have a nasogastric tube, and my task is *to be with* the person in ways which attempt to make sense of non-verbal gestures and ultimately *to be with* the person as a way to alleviate his or her condition.

## Caring aesthetic beings

We might wish to call this *being with* a type of caring. In one particular care home, I remember a daughter who would sit for long periods of time with her mother who had advanced dementia. She valued the time with her mother even though there was very little objective engagement, but every now and again her mother would respond to something; and her daughter made certain that her hair and nails were kept in a good state. The contact between them was definitely aesthetic: touch, hearing, smell, sight, and taste all played a role. In the same care home, a care assistant once took me into a room to see a bedbound, very elderly woman living with advanced dementia. The care assistant, in a very natural way, went up to her, picked up a hairbrush and started to brush her hair, whilst talking gently and affectionately to her. It seemed to me that these were examples of genuine care. Moreover, they were examples of aesthetic practice, which has 'a certain craft and involves the creation of sensory, embodied experiences' (Thompson, 2023, p. 1).

James Thompson's (2023) book, *Care Aesthetics: For Artful Care and Careful Art*, should be the *vade mecum* of all those interested in care aesthetics. It presents a detailed, layered, and nuanced account of how care can be artful, beautiful even, whilst art can be careful. In connection with dementia, Thompson (2023) writes: 'At its best, an art initiative within a care home, whether music, storytelling, movement, or visual art, is how residents with dementia have their capacities endorsed and extended, and the quality of their lives enhanced' (p. 89). He talks about the 'intensity of experience developed in a finely tuned creative act of care' (p. 89). Care aesthetics, according to Thompson, can interact with the institutions that provide care and lead to a greater awareness of how shades of care are at one with and encouraged by an aesthetic approach. There can also be moments of aesthetically rich encounter (Thompson, 2023, p. 90).

Of course, we can be mawkish about care. It can be dirty. It can be undertaken poorly or even abusively. The social standing of those who provide day-to-day, hands-on care is typically regarded as inferior and is poorly rewarded. The politics of care must inevitably note the tendency for it to reflect gendered and racist stereotypes. All of this, Thompson discusses with a good deal of insight and understanding (see, for example, Thompson, 2023, pp. 51–72). He writes: 'Care aesthetics in the everyday is saying that the moments of interhuman care or carelessness in the world … need to be analysed for their aesthetics' (Thompson, 2023, p. 153). Practices can then be considered from the perspective of their sensory qualities.

The notion of care was of central importance to the work of the philosopher Martin Heidegger (1889–1976). He used 'care' in a technical sense: the being of human beings 'is to be made visible as *care*' (Heidegger, 1962, p. 84), which is a translation of the German *Sorge*. Being-in-the-world, which is one of the ways Heidegger characterises the human existent (for which he uses the word *Dasein*), amounts to care. Our engagement with the world is a matter of care. So, this is not a psychological state (as when we say that a person is very caring), but a matter of ontology: the nature of our being-in-the-world is that we care.

This very abstract account of care (*Sorge*) dovetails with a more specific notion, that of 'taking care' (*besorgen*), more usually translated as 'concern'. Magda King (1964) put it this way: 'Since man inhabits the world by way of care, each of his fundamental relations must have a specific care-character: he is near to things by "taking care" of them … a basic way in which man inhabits his world is to reckon with things, to take account of things' (pp. 89–90). Concern, accordingly, signifies our practical relation to things.

The point of this excursion into Heideggerian philosophy is to make the point that our understanding of care moves to a more metaphysical level. I want to argue in the remainder of this chapter that the aesthetic approach starts to point us beyond the practicalities of day-to-day care to consider more deeply the nature of our place in the world. In part, we get there by seeing that Heidegger's notions of care and concern must be extended by the idea of solicitude (*Fürsorge*).

## Solicitude and authenticity

As Heidegger (1962) wrote:

> Because Being-in-the world is essentially care, Being-alongside the ready-to-hand could be taken in our previous analysis as *concern*, and Being with the Dasein-with of Others as we encounter it within-the-world could be taken as *solicitude*.
>
> *(p. 237)*

*Fürsorge* is literally translated as 'care-for', but 'solicitude' better conveys its meaning. King (1964, p. 107) suggested that 'charity' (*caritas*) might be an alternative way to render *Fürsorge*. The quotation above from Heidegger shows the movement from the general state of Being expressed by 'care' to the 'concern' we have for things around us, which then moves to solicitude: '… those entities towards which Dasein as Being-with comports itself do not have the kind of Being which belongs to equipment ready-to-hand; they are themselves Dasein. These entities are not objects of concern, but rather of *solicitude*' (Heidegger, 1962, p. 157).

'Solicitude', therefore, marks out what happens when two human beings genuinely and authentically engage in-the-world. Such engagement will include not only a cognitive and rational aspect, but also an aesthetic, sensory, and embodied reality. In this context, authenticity suggests a way of being-in-the-world in which the human being has taken hold of how his or her life will go. Rather than showing '*lostness* in the "they"' (Heidegger, 1962, p. 344), the authentic human being is willing to step forward and not to show indifference. Solicitude expresses this deep concern for other human beings as we navigate the world around us. Heidegger is driving at the idea that our genuine encounters signify a deep engagement which stems from our being beings of this sort. There is no other option at this ontological level, even if, in reality, we can choose to retreat and to hold ourselves back. Whether or not this is in Heidegger, my inclination is to interpret this sort of authentic being, which results in solicitude, as also aesthetic. Heidegger, after all, recognises the extent to which we are factually objects thrown into the world. Our embodied and situated nature as human beings means that our connections will inevitably be sentient. But solicitude, as a manifestation of our authentic being, takes us to a higher plain. The aesthetic points to something more puzzling.

Authenticity is also characterised as being true to yourself. In a project which involved an artist working in a participatory manner in a care home, we saw numerous examples of residents, who were all living with dementia, expressing themselves authentically: 'True to myself … I don't care what they think, because I'm sitting here, I'm going to have tea, I get all my washing done, what else do you want?' (Hughes et al., 2022, p. 2793). But the success of the project depended on the relationship established by the artist with the residents, staff, and research team. One member of staff put it this way: 'It's just his tone of voice and the way he asks, it didn't feel like he was interviewing them, … and he ended up building quite a good, well some of it was quite emotional, he had a really emotional bond with some of them' (Hughes et al., 2022, p. 2796).

This particular artist showed genuine solicitude. It is 'the something' in such relationships that is puzzling. His interactions with the residents were beautiful. His ability *to be with* them was apparent. The idea of charity mixes with other virtues, such as fidelity, compassion, integrity, and honesty, to produce authentic encounters based on the wholeness of our human engagement.

This sort of wholeness was of great importance to Friedrich Schiller (1759–1805). His basic idea is that, rightly understood:

> Aesthetic experience is not a matter of merely private delectation but has a civilizing function as well … The demands of specialization make it increasingly difficult to achieve a sense of wholeness in life. This is where the aesthetic comes in.
>
> *(Kimball, 2001, p. 12 of 18)*

In *On the Aesthetic Education of Man in a Series of Letters*, published in 1794, Schiller argued that aesthetic encounters would improve the moral nature of human beings. Remember, too, that Immanuel Kant (1724–1804), in *Critique of the Power of Judgment* published in 1790, had said that 'the beautiful is the symbol of the morally good' (cited by Wang, 2018, p. 854). So, Schilling and Kant take us neatly on to consider ethics and aesthetics.

## No aesthetics without ethics

On the wall of The Reina Sofía School of Music in the Plaza de Oriente in Madrid, in bold gold lettering, it is proclaimed: 'Nulla aesthetica sine ethica; nulla ethica sine aesthetica' (no aesthetics without ethics; no ethics without aesthetics). The Spanish poet and philosopher José María Valverde (1926–1996) is said to have inscribed 'no ethics without aesthetics' on his blackboard when he resigned the Aesthetics Chair at the University of Barcelona in 1964 on account of the Fascist regime, then in power in Spain, to go into exile in the United States of America. Aesthetics, therefore, can be seen as an antidote to unethical practices.

The relationship between care aesthetics and care ethics is well brought out in Chapter 2 of *Care Aesthetics: For Artful Care and Careful Art* (see: Thompson, 2023, pp. 44–72). Here, I wish to argue that because of its deep connections with how we are as persons, our aesthetic nature cannot be conceived without the context of ethics (and the reverse is also true). First, given what I have said about personhood, it is inevitable that, as persons, we are situated in the arena of ethics. But also, we are essentially aesthetic beings because of our embodiment and the sentient nature of our engagements with the world.

Second, from Heidegger, we have learned that the nature of our being is imbued with care and, in particular, when it comes to authentic engagement between human beings, solicitude. This can be directly linked to virtue ethics (Hursthouse, 1999). The correct inner dispositions to do well as human beings – in Aristotelian terms to flourish – are specified by the virtues. These include not only care and concern (in their non-technical senses), but also all the other virtues, such as fortitude, hope, humility, integrity, justice, practical wisdom, and temperance. Human beings who have the virtues (or some of them) will be more likely not only to show solicitude, but also (we would hope) to attend well.

There is, however, a problem, which is that aesthetic judgements and ethical judgements are not the same thing. Aesthetics and ethics both confront the same dilemma: how do we decide on what is good? But they are also different in that your preference for Wagner against mine for Mahler is just a matter of taste, whereas my abhorrence of assisted suicide as opposed to your support of it is a matter of deep difference that cannot be laughed off. It is perfectly possible to imagine a person of highly aesthetic sensibilities espousing a wicked morality (think of the Nazis who must have admired Bach and Beethoven).

At least the starting point to a deep solution to this problem might be if it were possible to argue for objectivity in both ethics and aesthetics. In other words, if you were able to argue that when you say 'X is good', whether in ethics or in aesthetics, objective support could be brought to bear, rather than saying that such assertions were merely subjective. Another way to put this would be to speak of moral and aesthetic realism. The objectivity of morals has long been argued for (Foot, 2001), even if ethical subjectivism is ever-present. Arguing that aesthetic judgements are also realist or objective seems harder (at least to me), but attempts have been made (Pettit, 2004). Nevertheless, and despite my sympathy with the idea that there should be some sort of realist basis to both ethics and aesthetics, the argument would still seem to require that objective goodness in both the moral and the aesthetic cases derives from the same sort of source. If we could point to some objective thing about human beings that allows us to assert that 'X is ethical' (a statement which, even if defeasible, would not be too difficult to defend) in order to say 'And therefore you should like Mahler', it would need to be true that what made X ethical also made Mahler aesthetically preferable. Or we would have to pursue an argument that because the Nazis allowed genocide, their (aesthetic) appreciation of Bach and Beethoven must have been deficient. I would love it if such arguments were true, but they seem rather too difficult. It seems easier, therefore, to stick with the idea that ethics and aesthetics just do deal with different things.

Once 'aesthetics' is linked to 'care', however, then the idea that aesthetics and ethics go hand-in-hand seems much more plausible. Hence, I think it can be argued, third, that seeing things aright, the sort of whole sight (Schiller's wholeness) that is encouraged by the careful attention that comes from a specifically *care* aesthetic approach will make it more likely that we shall make good (ethical) decisions. The temperament that understands and tolerates a care aesthetic approach, where this involves both attention to detail and an awareness of the broader social canvas, the unique situatedness of each person, will be more likely to approach ethical decisions with balance and an open mind.

My view is that the care aesthetic approach still requires more robust ethical scaffolding, which comes from consideration of the virtues. The support becomes 'more robust' simply because the virtues are broader than the idea of 'care' alone. The person who has the virtues will make decisions and choices that are rooted in our need to flourish as human beings in the community of human beings. The virtue words describe what it is to do well humanly. The person who shows good aesthetic judgement in practice is likely to care, but he or she is also likely to manifest a variety of other virtues, not solely that of being caring. You also have to be brave sometimes and honest and show practical wisdom. The caring person is likely, it seems to me, to have these inner dispositions. They are, however, different dispositions to the disposition of caring and they are not inevitable. I might be caring, but cowardly and lacking in prudence. Nevertheless, doing well humanly implies having good taste. Our aesthetic approach to a person (or lack of it) is likely to reflect the dispositions that make us good (or bad). If I have authentic (from the Greek meaning 'genuine') solicitude for other people, with all this implies in terms of my aesthetic sense and the care that I provide, my ethical decisions seem more likely to square with a view of persons that is broad and in keeping with an understanding of how we flourish together as human beings in the world. Ethical decisions, emanating from virtuous dispositions, seem likely to flow from an aesthetic approach to care.

## Friendship and love

According to the Dominican philosopher and theologian Herbert McCabe (1926–2001), 'a study of the virtues must be a study of the manifold ways in which people interact in the community of friendship' (McCabe, 2005, p. 29). Elsewhere, he wrote:

> We have … a special name for *human* living with each other: we call it friendship. Friendship is more than love. Friendship is more than people wishing well to other people. … Friendship is a matter of being *with* others.
>
> *(McCabe, 2008, p. 54)*

Care aesthetics is about practical, day-to-day things. But it is rooted in a sense of how we flourish as human beings (by living according to the virtues); and this sends us in the direction of friendship, which, in turn, points us back to the idea and possibility of *being with* others. We return, that is, to Heidegger's ontological notion of care, but specifically to his notion of *Fürsorge*: 'care-for', solicitude, or charity, which are themselves virtues. We should recall that these words were intended to tell us something about the nature of Being as such. We have seen that Being-in-the-world is a matter of our interconnections, through sensory and embodied (aesthetic) engagements, and is clearly revealed in our interactions with people living with dementia.

Another Dominican theologian, Thomas Gilby (1902–1975), in his book *Poetic Experience: An Introduction to Thomist Aesthetic*, discussed the difference between aesthetic and rational knowledge in these terms: poetic experience is 'intensely individual, not general … concrete, not abstract … real, not conceptual … complete in itself, not pedagogic … an end, not a means … a moment of unpremeditated inspiration' (Gilby, 1934, pp. 9–10). Science sees things in isolation, not as wholes, whereas the human mind is naturally disposed to grasp the whole thing. But the mind itself is not the thing that acts; it is the whole person who seeks and is sought in human interactions. Gilby (1934) writes: '*Loving draws us to things more than knowing does. ... love takes up where knowledge leaves off*' (italics in original; p. 34).

This seems highly applicable to the ideas I have been discussing in this opening chapter. At a simple (or even slightly more complicated) level, I can know all sorts of things about the person living with dementia (let us call her Felicity). I know Felicity's address, that she has a daughter, that she used to work in a pharmacy, that she had a low score on her cognitive test when last seen, that her blood sodium is slightly low, that her magnetic resonance imaging showed bilateral medial temporal lobe atrophy, and that her amyloid positron emission tomography scan was in keeping with a diagnosis of Alzheimer's disease. But I cannot yet say that I know her in any deeper sense: *loving draws us to things more than knowing does.* Remember that the revelation of Malcolm's essential self arose in the context of a loving relationship with Barbara. For all that I know about Felicity, I still need to *be with* her and her family. I need to connect. Music might help. Recall the YouTube clip in which Henry said: 'It gives me the feeling of love'. Friendship, or the love that is signified by the term *philia*, is at the heart of our authentically caring and aesthetic relationships.

Here is Gilby (1934) again:

> Love establishes a medium of experience more intimate than a notion. … the experience lies in the mind, but the instrument is the love which penetrates the object, not a notion gathered from a scientific inspection. … It is not explicitly directed on a formal truth so much as on a whole-thing … and in correspondence with our deepest and most primitive desires. In this experience love dominates.
> *(p. 81)*

The final way in which I have suggested we might flesh out the aesthetic nature of humanity emphasises the beauty of our relationships. People living with dementia, where their grip on cognitive reality is fading, will often benefit from what I have described as an aesthetic approach. Moreover, when the carapace of intellectual sophistication or social standing has slipped, something of the real person is often seen. Be that as it may, all human beings deserve to be understood in their wholeness. Where the aesthetic approach reflects genuine or authentic care, solicitude even, it will be a matter of friendship and love.

## Conclusion

We learn from our teachers, but not always from what they say. I can remember examples of people who taught me most by the way they engaged with their patients as real people, by the intensity of their gaze, by their closeness and concentration, sometimes by their touch, by their silences, by their politeness, and by their solicitude. What I saw in action in these cases were manifestations of love and friendship. Much of this connection was not a matter of intellectual communication; it was a matter of aesthetic appreciation.

Here, I have been considering the notion of aesthetics in relation to people living with a diagnosis of dementia. Dementia is a condition which requires attention to the senses in a more pronounced way than some other conditions and, importantly, people living with dementia frequently respond to artistic input in a manner that is enhancing and therapeutic. Moreover, dementia reveals the aesthetic nature of all humankind.

I have suggested that this aesthetic nature is fleshed out in nine ways. It is a matter of us (1) being sentient as well as cognitive creatures and (2) being embodied, which encompasses our mental lives too. Furthermore, (3) we interconnect by being in relationships and by being dependent. But what is required is (4) a broad view of us as situated persons, who are also (5) agents, acting in and on the world with which we engage. And part of this engagement is that (6) an essential facet of our being is to care for the world and for each other, which we do (7) by acts of solicitude. In turn, these acts reflect (8) our ethical manner of being-in-the-world as virtuous humans who aim to flourish, which we do in part (9) through friendship and love.

Even if these nine ways do not form a totally coherent argument, I hope individually they seem blatantly obvious.

## Acknowledgement

I would like to thank Anne Hughes for her valuable comments on an earlier draft of this chapter. Its deficiencies remain my own.

## Three Key Reading References

### *Reference 1*

Hughes, J.C. (2011). *Thinking Through Dementia,* Oxford: Oxford University Press.
Anyone who is really interested in the philosophical thinking being pointed at in this chapter might wish to read this book. It presents the fullest account of some of the themes discussed here. It is philosophical, but uses case histories and copious examples of poetry, as well as some references to other art forms, with some overt discussion of the idea of an aesthetic approach to people living with dementia.

### *Reference 2*

Killick, J. and Cordonnier, C. (2000). *Openings: Dementia Poems & Photographs*, London: Hawker Publications.
John Killick has inspired many of us over many years to think more deeply about the benefits of the arts for people living with dementia. His work is not represented fully enough in this chapter. But his writings are copious and innovative. This book, one of the first I owned by John, is particularly beautiful. It records the touching, happy, humorous, profound, and sad poems he co-authored with people living with dementia. The poems are perfectly complemented by the photography of Carl Cordonnier.

### *Reference 3*

Poltrum, M., Musalek, M., Galvin, K. and Saito, Y. (eds.) (2025). *The Oxford Handbook of Mental Health and Contemporary Western Aesthetics*, Oxford: Oxford University Press.
This large tome provides a broader background to the content of the present volume. Its remit is wide. It shows how the aesthetic approach or attitude is relevant and helpful in many types of mental illness. The role of aesthetics in psychiatry and psychotherapy is displayed, and the underlying conceptual issues are discussed in detail. Philosophical thought is used to shed light on the many and various ways in which aesthetics is of benefit to humanity.

## References

Agich, G.J. (2003). *Dependence and Autonomy in Old Age: An Ethical Framework for Long-Term Care*, Cambridge: Cambridge University Press.

Baumgarten, A.G. (1970). *Aesthetica*. Hildesheim and New York: G. Olms (originally published in 1750).

Beard, R.L. (2012). Art therapies and dementia care: A systematic review. *Dementia: The International Journal of Social Research and Practice*, 11 (5): 633–656. https://doi.org/10.1177/1471301211421090

Boutoleau-Bretonnière, C., Thomas-Anterion, C., Deruet, A.-L., Lamy, E. and El Haj, M. (2024). Beauty and paintings: Aesthetic experience in patients with behavioral variant frontotemporal dementia when viewing abstract and concrete paintings. *Brain Sciences*, 14 (5): 500. Available: https://doi.org/10.3390/brainsci14050500; accessed 1 March 2026.

Chauhan, S. (2020). Dementia and sculpture-making: Exploring artistic responses of people with dementia. *Dementia: The International Journal of Social Research and Practice*, 19 (2): 416–432. https://doi.org/10.1177/1471301218777446

Coaten, R. and Newman-Bluestein, D. (2013). Embodiment and dementia – Dance movement psychotherapists respond. *Dementia: The International Journal of Social Research and Practice*, 12 (6): 677–681. https://doi.org/10.1177/1471301213507033

Dalby, K., Mittner, L. and Gürgens Gjærum, R. (2024). Exploring consent as an aesthetic experience through applied theatre with people living with dementia. *Nordic Journal of Art & Research*, 13 (1): 1–21. https://doi.org/10.7577/ar.6139

Dekkers, W. (2010). Persons with severe dementia and the notion of bodily autonomy. In J.C. Hughes, M. Lloyd-Williams and G.A.Sachs (eds.) *Supportive Care for the Person with Dementia*. Oxford: Oxford University Press, pp. 253–261.

Deshmukh, S.R., Holmes, J. and Cardno, A. (2018). Art therapy for people with dementia. *Cochrane Database of Systematic Reviews*, 9 (9). Art. No. CD011073. Available: https://doi.org/10.1002/14651858.CD011073.pub2; accessed 1 March 2026.

Dooley, J., Webb, J., James, R., Davis, H. and Read, S. (2021). Everyday experiences of post-diagnosis life with dementia: A co-produced photography study. *Dementia: The International Journal of Social Research and Practice*, 20 (6): 1891–1909. https://doi.org/10.1177/1471301220973632

Dorris, J.L., Neely, S., Terhorst, L., VonVille, H.M. and Rodakowski, J. (2021). Effects of music participation for mild cognitive impairment and dementia: A systematic review and meta-analysis. *Journal of the American Geriatrics Society*, 69 (9): 2659–2667. https://doi.org/10.1111/jgs.17208

Dowlen, R., Keady, J., Milligan, C., Swarbrick, C., Ponsillo, N., Geddes, L. and Riley, B. (2018). The personal benefits of musicking for people living with dementia: A thematic synthesis of the qualitative literature. *Arts and Health: An International Journal*, 10 (3): 197–212. https://doi.org/10.1080/17533015.2017.1370718

Dowlen, R., McPherson, D.H.J., Swarbrick, C., Hoskin, L., Thompson, J. and Keady, J. (2024). Creating and reliving the moment: Using musical improvisation and care aesthetics as a lens of connection and self-expression for younger people living with dementia. *International Journal of Environmental Research and Public Health*, 21 (8): 972. Available: https://doi.org/10.3390/ijerph21080972; accessed 1 March 2026.

Foot, P. (2001). *Natural Goodness*, Clarendon Press: Oxford.

Gilby, T. (1934). *Poetic Experience: An Introduction to Thomist Aesthetic*, New York: Sheed and Ward.

Gray, J. (2019). Working within an aesthetic of relationality: Theoretical considerations of embodiment, imagination and foolishness as part of theatre making about dementia. *Ride: The Journal of Applied Theatre and Performance*, 24 (1): 6–22. https://doi.org/10.1080/13569783.2018.1535270

Gregor, M.J. (1983). Baumgarten's "Aesthetica". *The Review of Metaphysics*, 37 (2): 357–385. Available: https://maxryynanen.net/wp-content/uploads/2016/06/Mary-J.-Gregor-Baumgartens-_Aesthetica_.pdf; accessed 1 March 2026.

Guzmán, A., Freeston, M., Rochester, L., Hughes, J.C. and James, I.A. (2016). Psychomotor Dance Therapy Intervention (DANCIN) for people with dementia in care homes: A multiple-baseline single-case study. *International Psychogeriatrics*, 28 (10): 1695–1715. https://doi.org/10.1017/S104161021600051X

Guzmán-García, A., Hughes, J.C., James, I.A. and Rochester, L. (2013). Dancing as a psychosocial intervention in care homes: A systematic review of the literature. *International Journal of Geriatric Psychiatry*, 28 (9): 914–924. https://doi.org/10.1002/gps.3913

Guzmán, A., Robinson, L., Rochester, L, James, I.A. and Hughes, J.C. (2017). A process evaluation of a Psychomotor Dance Therapy Intervention (DANCIN) for behaviour change in dementia: Attitudes and beliefs of participating residents and staff. *International Psychogeriatrics*, 29 (2): 313–22. https://doi.org/10.1017/S104161021600171X

Heidegger, M. (1962). *Being and Time* (translated by J. Macquarrie and E. Robinson). Malden, Oxford and Carlton: Blackwell (first published as *Sein und Zeit* in 1927).

Hendriks, I., Meiland, F.J.M. Gerritsen, D.L. and Dröes, R.-M. (2021). Evaluation of the 'Unforgettable' art programme by people with dementia and their care-givers. *Ageing & Society*, 41 (2): 294–312. https://doi.org/10.1017/S0144686X19001089

Hughes, J.C. (2014). The aesthetic approach to people with dementia. *International Psychogeriatrics*, 26 (9): 1407–1413. https://doi.org/10.1017/S1041610214001100.

Hughes, J.C. (2001). Views of the person with dementia. *Journal of Medical Ethics*, 27 (2): 86–91. https://doi.org/10.1136/jme.27.2.86

Hughes, J.C. (2025). The aesthetics of dementia. In M. Poltrum, M. Musalek, K. Galvin and Y. Saito (eds.) *The Oxford Handbook of Mental Health and Contemporary Western Aesthetics*, Oxford: Oxford University Press, pp. 717–732.

Hughes, J.C., Baseman, J., Hearne, C., Lie, M., Smith, D. and Woods, S. (2022). Art, authenticity and citizenship for people living with dementia in a care home. *Ageing & Society*, 42 (12): 2784–2804. https://doi.org/10.1017/S0144686X21000271

Hughes, J.C., Louw, S.J. and Sabat, S.R. (2006). *Dementia: Mind, Meaning, and the Person*, Oxford: Oxford University Press.

Hursthouse, R. (1999). *On Virtue Ethics*, Oxford: Oxford University Press.

Karkou, V. and Meekums, B. (2017). Dance movement therapy for dementia. *Cochrane Database of Systematic Reviews*. 2 (2): CD011022. Available: https://doi.org/10.1002/14651858.CD011022.pub2; accessed 1 March 2026.

Kelson, E., Phinney, A. and Lowry, G. (2017). Social citizenship, public art and dementia: Walking the urban waterfront with Paul's Club. *Cogent Arts & Humanities*, 4 (1): 1354527. Available: https://doi.org/10.1080/23311983.2017.1354527; accessed 1 March 2026.

Killick, J. (2017). *Poetry and Dementia: A Practical Guide*, London: Jessica Kingsley.

Kimball, R. (2001). Schiller's "Aesthetic Education". *The New Criterion* (March). Available: https://newcriterion.com/article/schilleras-ldquoaesthetic-educationrdquo/; accessed 1 March 2026.

King, M. (1964). *Heidegger's Philosophy: A Guide to His Basic Thought*, Oxford: Basil Blackwell.

Kohler, M., Mullis, J., Karrer, M., Schwarz, J. and Saxer, S. (2021). Effectiveness of a group-walking intervention for people with dementia based on quality of life and caregivers' burden. *Nursing Open*, 8 (6): 3111–3119. https://doi.org/10.1002/nop2.1023

Kontos, P. (2004). Ethnographic reflections on selfhood, embodiment and Alzheimer's disease. *Ageing & Society*, 24 (6): 829–849. https://doi.org/10.1017/S0144686X04002375

Kontos, P. (2005). Embodied selfhood in Alzheimer's disease: Rethinking person-centred care. *Dementia: The International Journal of Social Research and Practice*, 4 (4): 553–570. https://doi.org/10.1177/1471301205058311

Kontos, P., Grigorovich, A., Kosurko, A., Bar, R.J., Herron, R.V., Menec, V.H. and Skinner, M.W. (2021). Dancing with dementia: Exploring the embodied dimensions of creativity and social engagement. *The Gerontologist*, 61 (5): 714–723. https://doi.org/10.1093/geront/gnaa129

Kontos, P., Miller, K.L., Colobong, R., Palma Lazgare, L.I., Binns, M., Low, L.F., Surr, C. and Naglie, G. (2016). Elder-clowning in long-term dementia care: Results of a pilot study. *Journal of the American Geriatric Society*, 64 (2): 347–353. https://doi.org/10.1111/jgs.13941

Li, B.Y. (2022). Cocomposing an aesthetic self through play: Toward a transformative framework for dementia care. *The Gerontologist*, 62 (3): 464–474. https://doi.org/10.1093/geront/gnab021

Li, Y., Wang, W., Zhu, L., Yang, L., Wu, H., Zhang, X., Guo, L. and Lu, C. (2023). Pet ownership, living alone, and cognitive decline among adults 50 years and older. *JAMA Network Open*, 6, (12): e2349241. Available: https://doi.org/10.1001/jamanetworkopen.2023.49241; accessed 1 March 2026.

Livingston, G., Kelly, L., Lewis-Holmes, E., Baio, G., Morris, S., Patel, N., Omar, R.Z., Katona, C. and Cooper, C. (2014). Non-pharmacological interventions for agitation in dementia: Systematic review of randomised controlled trials. *British Journal of Psychiatry*, 205 (6): 436–442. https://doi.org/10.1192/bjp.bp.113.141119

Livingston, G., Sommerlad, A., Orgeta, V., Costafreda, S.G., Huntley, J., Ames, D., Ballard, C., Banerjee, S., Burns, A., Cohen-Mansfield, J., Cooper, C., Fox, N., Gitlin, L., Howard, R., Kales, H.C., Larson, E.B., Ritchie, K., Rockwood, K., Sampson, E.L., Samus, Q., Schneider, L.S., Selbæk, G., Teri, L. and Mukadam, N. (2017). Dementia prevention, intervention, and care. *Lancet*, 390 (10113): 2673–2734. https://doi.org/10.1016/S0140-6736(17)31363-6

MacIntyre, A. (2006). *The Tasks of Philosophy: Selected Essay, Volume 1*. Cambridge: Cambridge University Press.

MacIntyre, A. (2009). *Dependent Rational Animals: Why Human Beings Need the Virtues*. London: Duckworth (first published 1999).

Manji, I. and Fallavollita, P. (2022). A brief report on reviews of existing creative art–based interventions in dementia care from 2010 to 2020. *Frontiers in Aging*, 3: 865533. Available: https://doi.org/10.3389/fragi.2022.865533; accessed 1 March 2026.

Matthews, E. (2005). *Mind: Key Concepts in Philosophy*, London and New York: Continuum.

McCabe, H. (2005). *The Good Life: Ethics and the Pursuit of Happiness*, London and New York: Continuum.

McCabe, H. (2008). *On Aquinas*, London and New York: Continuum.

Merleau-Ponty, M. (1962). *Phenomenology of Perception* (trans. C. Smith), London: Routledge. (First published as *Phénomènologie de la Perception* by Gallimard, Paris (1945)).

Murroni, V., Cavalli, R., Basso, A., Borella, E., Meneghetti, C., Melendugno, A. and Pazzaglia, F. (2021). Effectiveness of therapeutic gardens for people with dementia: A systematic review. *International Journal of Environmental Research and Public Health*, 18 (18): 9595. Available: https://doi.org/10.3390/ijerph18189595; accessed 1 March 2026.

Musalek, M. and Scheibenbogen, O. (2025). Applied social aesthetics in clinical practice: The will to beauty and its impact on mental health. In M. Poltrum, M. Musalek, K. Galvin and Y. Saito (eds.) *The Oxford Handbook of Mental Health and Contemporary Western Aesthetics*. Oxford: Oxford University Press, pp. 326–343.

Newman, A., Goulding, A., Davenport, B. and Windle, G. (2019). The role of the visual arts in the resilience of people living with dementia in care homes. *Ageing & Society*, 39 (11): 2465–2482. https://doi.org/10.1017/S0144686X18000594

Newton, R., Keady, J., Tsekleves, E. and Adams, S. (2021). 'My father is a gardener…': A systematic narrative review on access and use of the garden by people living with dementia. *Health and Place*, 68: e102516. Available: https://doi.org/10.1016/j.healthplace.2021.102516; accessed 1 March 2026.

O'Connor, C.M., Poulos, R.G., Heldon, M., Preti, C., Beattie, E. and Poulos, C.J. (2025). Implementing arts on prescription at home for people living with dementia:

A hybrid-effectiveness feasibility study. *Journal of Geriatric Psychiatry and Neurology*, 38 (2): 115–131. https://doi.org/10.1177/08919887241267335

Pettit, P. (2004). The possibility of aesthetic realism. In P. Lamarque and S. H. Olsen (eds.) *Aesthetics and the Philosophy of Art: The Analytic Tradition.* Malden, Oxford and Victoria: Blackwell, pp. 158–171.

Phinney, A. and Chesla, C.A. (2003). The lived body in dementia. *Journal of Aging Studies*, 17 (3): 283–299. https://doi.org/10.1016/S0890-4065(03)00029-X

Pointon, B. (2007). Who am i? – The search for spirituality in dementia. A family carer's perspective. In M. E. Coyte, P. Gilbert and V. Nicholls (eds.) *Spirituality, Values and Mental Health: Jewels for the Journey.* London: Jessica Kingsley, pp. 114–120.

Rollason, A., Powell, Z. and Cadet, T. (2024). Turning pages together: The power of book clubs for people living with dementia. *Australian Social Work*, 78 (3): 364–368. https://doi.org/10.1080/0312407X.2024.2430213

Sabat, S.R. (2001). *The Experience of Alzheimer's Disease: Life Through a Tangled Veil*, Oxford and Malden: Blackwell.

Shoesmith, E.K., Charura, D. and Surr, C. (2021). What are the elements needed to create an effective visual art intervention for people with dementia? A qualitative exploration. *Dementia: The International Journal of Social Research and Practice*, 20 (4): 1336–1355. https://doi.org/10.1177/1471301220938481

Sonntag, J. (2016). Atmosphere - an aesthetic concept in music therapy with dementia. *Nordic Journal of Music Therapy*, 25 (3): 216–228. https://doi.org/10.1080/08098131.2015.1056216

Taylor, C. (1995). *Philosophical Arguments,* Cambridge, MA: Harvard University Press.

Thompson, J. (2023). *Care Aesthetics: For Artful Care and Careful Art*, London: Routledge.

Twigg, J. (2000). Carework as a form of bodywork. *Ageing & Society*, 20 (4): 389–411. https://doi.org/10.1017/S0144686X99007801

Urmson, J.O. (2004). What makes a situation aesthetic? In P. Lamarque and S. H. Olsen (eds.) *Aesthetics and the Philosophy of Art: The Analytic Tradition.* Malden, Oxford and Victoria: Blackwell, pp. 19–26.

van der Steen, J.T., Smaling, H.J.A., van der Wouden, J.C., Bruinsma, M.S., Scholten, R.J.P.M. and Vink, A.C. (2018). Music-based therapeutic interventions for people with dementia. *Cochrane Database of Systematic Reviews,* 5 (5): CD003477. Available: https://doi.org/10.1002/14651858.CD003477.pub3; accessed 1 March 2026.

Vink, A.C., Bruinsma, M.S. and Scholten, R.J.P.M. (2004). Music therapy for people with dementia. *Cochrane Database of Systematic Reviews.* 3: CD003477. Available: https://doi.org/10.1002/14651858.CD003477.pub2; accessed 1 March 2026.

Walker, M. (2022). Exploring how design can support the expression of personal aesthetic preferences in dementia. *The Design Journal*, 25 (5): 887–898. https://doi.org/10.1080/14606925.2022.2088100

Wallace, J., Wright, P. C., McCarthy, J., Green, D. P., Thomas, J. and Olivier, P. (2013). A Design-led inquiry into personhood in dementia. In *Proceedings of the SIGCHI Conference on Human Factors in Computing Systems*, Association for Computing Machinery, 2617–2626. Available: https://dl.acm.org/doi/10.1145/2470654.2481363; accessed 1 March 2026.

Wang, W. (2018). Beauty as the symbol of morality: A twofold duty in kant's theory of taste. *Dialogue: Canadian Philosophical Review*, 57 (4): 853–875. https://doi.org/10.1017/S001221731800015X

Wittgenstein, L. (1967). *Zettel,* Oxford: Basil Blackwell.

Wittgenstein, L. (1968). *Philosophical Investigations* (translated by G.E.M. Anscombe), Oxford: Basil Blackwell.

Wittgenstein, L. (1979). *On Certainty,* Oxford: Basil Blackwell.

Young, R., Camic, P.M. and Tischlerb, V. (2016). The impact of community-based arts and health interventions on cognition in people with dementia: A systematic literature review. *Aging & Mental Health,* 20 (4): 337–351. https://doi.org/10.1080/13607863.2015.1011080

Zeilig, H., Killick, J. and Fox, C. (2014). The participative arts for people living with a dementia: A critical review. *International Journal of Ageing and Later Life*, 9 (1): 7–34. https://doi.org/10.3384/ijal.1652-8670.14238

# 2

# SKETCHING WITH MY MUM

## Visual autoethnographic reflections on 'care-ful' art and 'art-ful' care

*Christina Buse*

### Introduction

I began writing this chapter by returning to my sketchbooks; as Hagerty (2002) wrote about handbags, opening a sketchbook is like 'taking the cap off a whistling kettle: genies of memory escape' (p. 61). These were sketches done 'in the moment' outdoors when we were caring for my mum who is living with dementia at home. Sketching in situ etches moments into memory (Heath et al., 2018) and the sketchbooks powerfully evoke emplaced memories (Scarles, 2010), marked by splatters from the rain, smudges where my mum or I touched the paint or charcoal, or we moved on before it had dried. Revisiting the sketchbooks was not only an emotional experience which evoked joyful memories but also sadness that this time at home with my mum has ended. In this chapter, my in situ sketches provide a 'way in' to reflecting on my experiences of caring with/for my mum, organised into three broader conceptual themes: (i) sketching as a practice of 'being with', creating, and recording everyday moments; (ii) convergences and divergences in expressions of everyday creativity and identity; and (iii) bodywork, embodied adjustments, and connected/disconnected moments. These themes are situated within wider conceptual debates in care aesthetics including the connection between art and care; how 'everyday creativity' is negotiated in the context of dementia; and the tensions between care aesthetics and challenging aspects of bodywork (Thompson, 2023).

The care aesthetics framework challenges divisions between art and everyday life, and art and care, considering how creating art can be a 'careful' practice and how care involves 'craft-like' or 'artful' elements (Thompson, 2023, p. 9). This includes the crafted aspects of 'bodywork' (Twigg et al., 2011), highlighting positive sensory encounters during 'hands-on' care such as shaving and male grooming (Campbell et al., 2024) or assisting with eating and drinking (Jones et al., 2025).

DOI: 10.4324/9781003623441-4
This chapter has been made available under a (CC BY) 4.0 license.

Unpaid care was originally separated from analysis of 'bodywork', reflecting its different social, emotional, and economic positioning (Twigg et al., 2011). However, Özen (2020) highlights the bodywork and emotional labour performed by family carers. Care aesthetics creates space for embodied aspects of care which might 'elude analysis because they fall outside those that are designated or acknowledged as part of professional practice' (Campbell et al., 2024, p. 4). The care aesthetics framework contests the binary of carer/cared for, highlighting the active contribution of people living with dementia to 'caring moments' (Campbell et al., 2024). It has also been applied to exploring arts-based practices and their connection to care, for instance, music-making groups for people living with dementia (Dowlen et al., 2024). However, research on creativity and dementia has generally focused on organised group sessions in the community (Ward et al., 2021) or long-term care contexts (Kontos et al., 2020). There is scope for further exploration of how 'everyday creativity' is negotiated between people living with dementia and family members (Bellass et al., 2019), drawing on the care aesthetics framework.

This second chapter in this book considers sketching as a 'care-ful' practice (Thompson, 2023) of being with and attending 'in the moment', as well as capturing and reliving moments (Keady et al., 2022). The question of how to capture 'moments' is significant for researchers in dementia studies and for people living with dementia or carers who might want to capture 'moments' of their everyday experiences (see, for example, Fox et al., 2025). Keady et al. (2022) call for dementia studies researchers to 'embrace more confidently creative ways of getting to the (at times) fleeting and transient nature of moments' (p. 695). In their paper synthesising different studies, methods, including sensory ethnography, walking interviews, and co-produced films and video-tours, are used to record experiences 'in the moment'. This reflects an increasing use of creative methods within dementia studies (Keady et al., 2018), including the use of sketching 'in situ' (Cleeve et al., 2023; Buse et al., 2024). There is a small academic literature using autoethnographic approaches to reflect on experiences of living with dementia or caring for someone living with dementia (see, for example, Taylor, 2008; Malthouse, 2011; Bryden, 2020; Damsgaard et al., 2024). To the best of my knowledge, a visual autoethnographic approach has not been applied in this context. Capturing the moment presents a different challenge while caring for someone 'in the moment' and juggling the physical and emotional demands of caring (Herron et al., 2019). Creative practices, as discussed below, are also located within biographical and social context (Conor et al., 2015). In this chapter, I draw on autoethnographic reflections from my sketchbook and written diary, exploring not only how moments are captured but also what is absent in each representation.

## Method

Autoethnography is described as 'self-narrative that places the self in social context' (Reed-Danahey, 1997, p. 9), connecting personal reflections to a wider social and cultural context (Méndez, 2013). It is traditionally considered as a literary genre involving written narratives; however, more recently, there have been developments in 'visual autoethnography' combining written narratives with visual material such as photography (Scarles, 2010; Ownby, 2013) or artwork (Crowley, 2022). Scarles (2010) argues that the use of visuals in autoethnography can help capture multi-sensory, embodied experiences, facilitating 'moments of fleeting or extended reflection' that help the writer to 're-embody themselves in place' (p. 917). This builds on an increasing use of sensory and visual methods within ethnography more broadly to capture the multi-sensory experiences of everyday life (Pink, 2015).

Autoethnography can draw on notes made at the time or be written from memory (Ellis, 1999), while visual ethnography can use 'found images' or images made for the purpose of research (Ownby, 2013). My account draws on sketches done 'in the moment' alongside my mum from 2017 to 2022, including a more regular sketch diary kept from May 2021 to September 2022 when caring for my mum at home. These sketches are 'found images' created as part of 'being with' my mum and recording our moments together, and sometimes on my own while taking a break from caring, rather than for the purpose of research. In keeping with 'sketch journaling' practices (Heath et al., 2018) alongside sketches, I noted the date, location, who was there, and sometimes sensory experiences. From autumn 2021, I also began keeping a written journal, typed on my laptop in the evening when my parents were in bed. Again, this was not done for the purpose of research, but as a way of processing my experiences and emotions.

My analysis began with revisiting my sketchbooks – I selected images that held emotional significance, marked biographical 'turning points' (McAdams, 1993), or evoked wider themes. In analysing sketches, I paid attention to 'content' (i.e., what was depicted in the image and 'context'), who I was with, what was happening, and the embodied experience of the moment (Banks, 2001). When analysing visual images, it is important to attend to absences (Mannay, 2013; Pilcher et al., 2016) and one noticeable absence in the sketches is my mum – this is partly because she hated having her picture taken or being sketched and partly because I prefer to sketch landscapes and flowers rather than people. Yet, the sketches captured and evoked (at least for me) moments and emplaced memories of being together. Analysis of sketches was combined with a thematic analysis of my written journal, noting down initial codes or themes in comments bubbles at the side of my diary and then grouping them into overarching themes (Smith, 1995). I started writing from selected sketches, which then became 'ways into' (Scarles, 2010, p. 159) exploring broader thematic issues. Sketches are combined with written autoethnographic reflections about the images and the process of making them, as well as reflections developing the theme and describing moments beyond the sketch. Using sketches in autoethnography is argued to provide a 'snapshot' (Rambo, 2007), stepping away from more linear approaches (Crowley, 2022). However, looking through the sketchbooks evoked a sense of change over time, and I combined analysis of themes with biographical and narrative approaches paying attention to the temporal structure and storying of events (Riessman, 2008).

What is included in sketches or written diaries has ethical implications (see Buse, 2026). In telling my story, I am also telling my mum's story, and those of my family members and others involved in her care (Médez, 2013). As this chapter is based on my personal reflections and retrospective analysis of my sketches and diary, ethical approval was not required by my university ethics committee, in keeping with previous autoethnographic research on care (see, for example, Malthouse, 2011; Wilkinson and Wilkinson, 2020). However, I have sought to adhere to good ethical practice in autoethnographic research, for instance inviting my dad and brother who are mentioned in this chapter to review it before submission. My mum, at the time of writing, is in the advanced stages of dementia and does not have the capacity to review it; however, I have tried to keep in mind her preferences and also consulted family members on this. I have anonymised identifiable details in writing the autoethnography.

## Autoethnographic reflections

### *Sketching with my mum: co-creating and capturing moments*

#### *Sketching together, turning points, and change*

This section explores sketching outdoors with my mum as a way of co-creating and 'being in the moment' together (Keady et al., 2022) and an aspect of our care aesthetic. The practice of sketching is something that was present at the start of my mum's 'dementia journey', and looking through sketchbooks prompts reflections on changing experiences over time. Figure 2.1 was my first sketch outdoors with my mum in 2017. I had always enjoyed sketching and painting when I was young, but increasingly 'never had time' and lost confidence. After a sketching workshop with the artist Lynne Chapman (www.lynnechapman.net; accessed 1 March 2026), I was inspired to 'enjoy the process' and worry less about the outcome. I brought my watercolour paints on a visit to my parents at their home in North Wales and told my mum I wanted to try sketching outdoors. Initially, it felt daunting to sketch in public, but my mum happily sat with me outside while I did this sketch on a warm sunny afternoon at a local seaside resort. I can recall the sensory experience of sitting in the warm sunshine on an overturned boat as I painted, with my mum sitting nearby and chatting, making encouraging remarks while she patiently waited for me to finish. Sketching outside together therefore started as a practice of my mum showing care for me and giving me the confidence to do something creative. As Thompson (2023) has argued, art is not separate from everyday life but is intertwined with social life and practices of care.

Sketching together in the summer of 2017 also marked a turning point in our lives (McAdams, 1993), coinciding with the start of my mum's dementia journey.

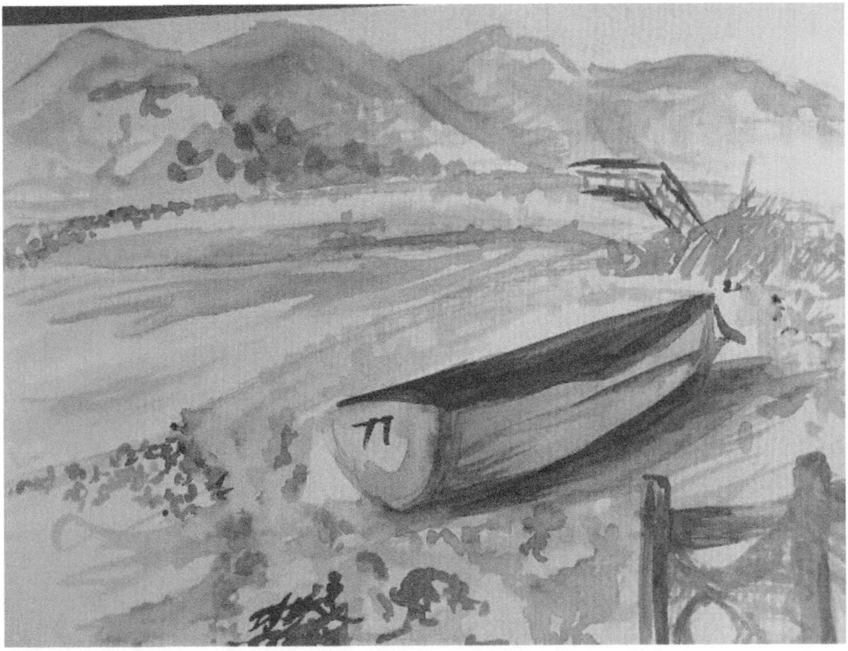


FIGURE 2.1 North Wales seaside resort, summer 2017.

It was around this time that we had started to notice early signs of memory issues with my mum, following my dad being in hospital for several weeks due to an inflammatory condition. We initially put her symptoms down to stress, but she started having tests with her general practitioner and was referred to the local memory clinic and then a specialist consultant in a different city. As is well documented, the process of diagnosis is long and complex (Hillman and Latimer, 2019), and it took until early 2019 for her to get a formal diagnosis of frontotemporal dementia. The sketch in Figure 2.2 was done in the summer of 2017 while visiting a bird reserve in [North Wales seaside area] with my mum and dad. Although the sun was shining, we could see the storm clouds gathered over the distant mountains. I later looked back and felt that it represented a sense of storm clouds beginning to gather in our lives, although, as will be discussed, moments of care, connection, and joy continued to be intertwined with challenging moments.

### *Sketching as a practice of 'being with'*

Sketching with my mum became increasingly significant as a way of 'being with' or 'caring with' (Thompson, 2023) as her dementia progressed. The sketch in Figure 2.3 was done in 2021 in my mum and dad's garden. I had returned to visit them in North Wales after we were apart for around a year due to the COVID-19 pandemic and travel restrictions, keeping in touch through Zoom and telephone calls.

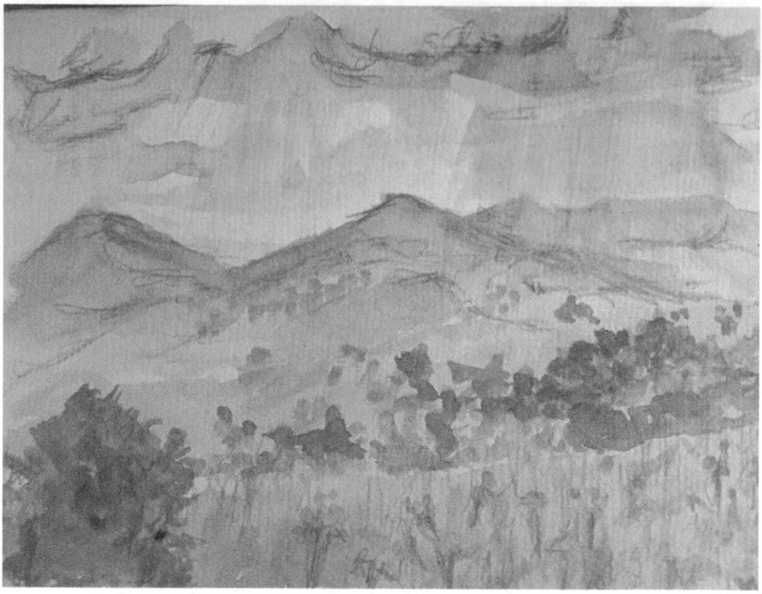

FIGURE 2.2 Storm clouds gathering, North Wales bird reserve, summer 2017.

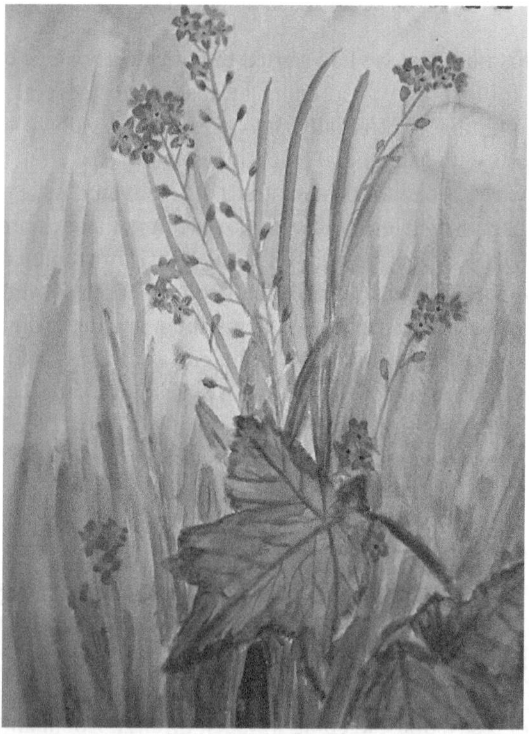

FIGURE 2.3 Forget-me-nots in the garden, 19 May 2021.

When I returned, I found that my mum's dementia had progressed significantly; she needed more help with everyday tasks, had also lost a significant amount of weight, and looked very different. Some symptoms were challenging, such as hallucinations and delusions and disrupted sleeping, and my dad was starting to find it difficult to manage. When I arrived, my mum reached out to give me a hug, but I held back because I felt worried that I might pass on COVID-19 after the long train journey. My mum looked upset and said, 'you can come near me, you know'. This illustrates the complexities of touch (Thompson, 2023), a theme I will return to. At this time, she had started needing help with using the toilet and was reluctant to let anyone but my dad assist. I felt awkward and unsure of what to do, and upset that I had got everything wrong, reflecting the emotional challenges of caring and worries about 'responding the wrong way' (Herron et al., 2019, p. 475).

I sat up much of the night worrying and crying, and the next morning I got up early and sat outside before my parents had gotten up. I started sketching some forget-me-nots in the garden – when things feel overwhelming, I find sketching something small like a flower helps. As I go on to explain in this chapter, this illustrates how sketching can be a practice of 'self-care', creating moments apart as well as moments of togetherness. While I sat sketching, my mum and dad came outside, and my mum came over to see what I was doing and remarked on how lovely it looked. My dad brought over a chair so she could sit with me. This marked the beginning of a regular practice of sketching outside in the garden with my mum as a way of being together. Sketching alongside my mum also enabled her to continue her role as a supportive mum, making encouraging comments as I sketched, which can be important to enacting selfhood and identity (Harris and Keady, 2009). This illustrates caring moments as 'co-created' (Campbell et al., 2024) and the ongoing ability of people living with dementia to engage in reciprocal care (Kontos et al., 2017).

Frontotemporal dementia affected my mum's speech and language, so verbal conversations were increasingly difficult. As discussed in Buse (2026), my mum had never been the gardener in our household, but she increasingly enjoyed sitting outside. Sketching while sitting out in the garden became important as a way of 'being alongside' (Latimer, 2013) without relying on verbal conversation (see also Cleeve et al., 2023). The garden had taken on particular significance at this time, as my mum and dad's world had shrunk – the COVID-19 pandemic was still on-going and my mum increasingly found busy places difficult. Although sketching is a visual practice, as we sat outside, we engaged with the multi-sensory experience of the garden. As noted by Taylor (2008), my mum would draw attention to small details that I had not noticed, like a robin singing, or dew on the grass, pointing out 'the sparkle'. I would sometimes record sensory details next to sketches, often ones that my mum had pointed out. For instance, next to the forget-me-nots sketch I had written, '*Painting forget-me-nots in mum and dad's garden, you can hear the river and the birds, and even a cuckoo!*' (sketch diary, 19 May 2021).

### *Sketches as a window into a 'series of moments'*

Because the sketches were often done 'in the moment' outdoors with my mum, they tended to evoke positive moments, leaving out more challenging experiences. However, sketches not only evoke vivid memories of a moment (Heath et al., 2018), but also the continuum of moments (Keady et al., 2022), or series of moments (Buse, 2026), in a single day. The sketch in Figure 2.4 captures a moment sitting with my mum painting the red roses in the garden – whenever we walked past these roses she would exclaim, 'these are my favourite' or 'I love the colour'. This illustrates the ability of people living with dementia to notice the beauty of everyday aesthetics and attend 'in the moment' (Thompson, 2023). My mum came out to join me, and I put a chair nearby where she could sit and she made encouraging comments as I painted. It was a damp, drizzly day, as I had noted next to the sketch, *'sketching in mum and dad's garden, grey and misty day, waiting for the sun but it doesn't arrive*'. In addition to the vivid colour, the smell of roses and honeysuckle wafted across the garden, brought out by the rain. I was also singing

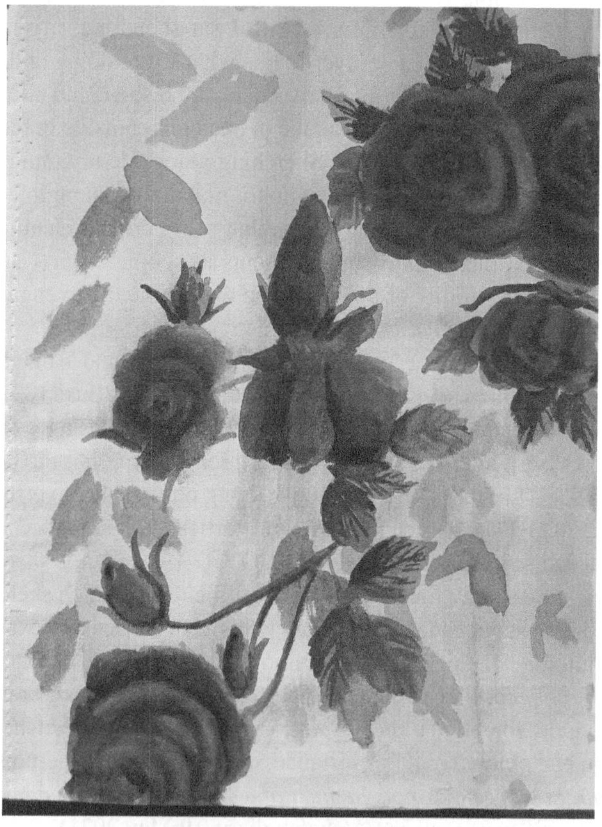

**FIGURE 2.4** 'The roses are my favourite', 1 July 2021.

with my mum. As discussed below and elsewhere (Buse, 2026), my mum enjoyed singing, and my older brother at the time was visiting from Australia and played 'The Beatles' songs for her on his guitar. I started singing a line from The Beatles song 'I am the Walrus' that mentioned an English garden and the English rain and my mum laughed.

The image also evokes the 'series of moments' beyond the sketch. While I was sketching, it started raining more heavily and we eventually came inside. As I carried on painting at the kitchen table, my mum said, 'Chrissy's very sensible', which made my dad and brother laugh and reply, 'Aren't we sensible?!' This reflected ongoing family relationships where I was the only girl (with three brothers) and my mum was normally 'in my corner'. While sitting there, my mum saw a pair of my old hiking socks on the table that were worn and bobbly. She exclaimed, 'you can't wear them, they are terrible!' I replied that they were 'fine', but she picked them up and threw them in the bin! I couldn't stop laughing – she then took me upstairs and gave me a new pair. This funny moment also has significance in terms of my mum showing care as a material practice, trying to look after me and make sure I was properly dressed, continuing her role as a supportive mum (Harris and Keady, 2009). As found in my previous research with Julia Twigg on dementia and dress (Buse and Twigg, 2014a), neatness and tidiness had been important to my mum, reflecting an emphasis on 'respectability' among working-class women (Skeggs, 1997), although maintaining neat dress and appearance became challenging as her dementia progressed (see Buse, 2026).

This funny and caring moment was then followed by a difficult moment, as we all went to [North Wales seaside resort] for my dad's optician's appointment. At this time, my mum was reluctant to be without my dad or let other people help with bodily activities like going to the toilet, so it was difficult for her to stay at home without him. However, she was very restless and struggled to sit still so it was difficult for her to go with him to the appointment. My older brother and I went for a walk on the promenade with her while he went to his appointment. My mum was very distressed and agitated and we charged up and down the promenade until my dad returned. While these difficult moments were not recorded in the sketch, they are instantly evoked when I look at it.

Sketching can therefore provide a way of being in, recording, and reliving the moment (Keady et al., 2022). Looking at the sketches reconnects me to these moments, and my mum and I would sometimes look at the sketchbooks together, and she would remark on the colours – although, perhaps, this was more about showing care and attentiveness than reliving moments from the sketches. The sketchbooks were also something physical and tangible she could hold, touch, and comment on, creating opportunities for engagement when verbal conversations were becoming difficult, and she found it difficult to perceive images on mobile phones or computer screens. As will be discussed, however, sketching does not feel comfortable to everyone (Heath et al., 2018), and 'creativity' is shaped by wider social and structural constraints (Conor et al., 2015).

## Convergences and divergences: different expressions of everyday creativity and identity

Painting with my mum, as discussed, was a way of 'being with' and demonstrating mutual care. However, my mum had other ways of expressing creativity, agency, and identity at an embodied level (Kontos, 2004; Kontos et al., 2020), which sometimes differed from my own and occurred outside the frame of the sketches. Being aware of literature on the benefits of arts-based activities for people living with dementia, including visual art (Zeilig et al., 2014), I wondered if I *should* be enabling more opportunities for my mum to practice painting herself, rather than simply observing me paint. On one occasion in the summer of 2017, inspired by Lynne Chapman's discussion of enjoying the *process* of sketching, my mum had tried painting with me in the garden and seemed to enjoy it. I was impressed with what she produced as someone who had never painted. When I was painting with her in 2021, she would occasionally say, 'maybe I'll have a go one day', but whenever I asked, 'did she want to have a go?' she would reply, 'maybe another time'. Definitions of creativity have historically been classed and gendered (Conor et al., 2015), and my mum did not define herself as a creative person, frequently saying 'I've got no imagination' and 'I can't draw'. However, she had an appreciation of art and told me that she had studied art history at a teacher training college, and we enjoyed going to see art exhibitions together. Art viewing as well as making art can represent a form of creative engagement (Ward et al., 2021) and everyday aesthetics (Thompson, 2023).

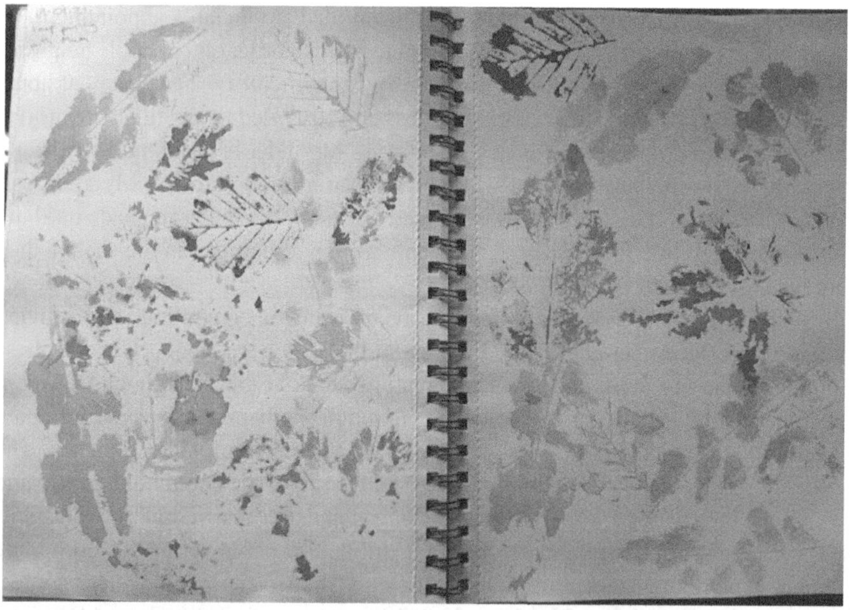

**FIGURE 2.5** Leaf printing with mum (sort of!), 19 September 2021.

I thought that doing something simple like leaf printing might break down barriers to drawing and painting (Heath et al., 2018). I suggested this to my mum, and she seemed enthusiastic about the idea and helped me find leaves in the garden. However, this enjoyment was perhaps more about 'helping out', enacting competency and agency (Hellström et al., 2015), and enjoying looking at the autumn leaves and colours. When we came indoors and I asked if she wanted to help me with the leaf printing, she walked off to do some cleaning, and I ended up finishing it myself. Research on 'everyday creativity' emphasises the importance of flexibility and recognising the varied ways people living with dementia might choose to be creative, which may differ from planned activities (Bellass et al., 2019). As a feminist and someone who is not very tidy, cleaning is not what I would see as enjoyable or creative! There are debates between feminist literature which has long highlighted women's disproportionate responsibility for domestic labour, against the revaluing of cleaning and domestic work as a form of everyday creativity and aesthetics (Besson, 2024; Casey, 2025). Cleaning was important to my mum's habitual embodied practice and identity (Kontos, 2004), situated within gendered and classed expectations about a neat and respectable home (Skeggs, 1997). She once told me she liked cleaning because she could instantly see how she had made things 'a bit better'.

Continuing household roles and rituals such as cleaning can be important to retaining a sense of competency and agency in the context of dementia and supporting selfhood (Hellström et al., 2015). Dementia altered household dynamics and my dad increasingly took on more domestic work as her dementia progressed. However, we tried to adapt creatively (Bellass et al., 2019) and find ways to involve her such as finding a cloth so she could wipe surfaces; handing her a tea towel to dry the plastic jugs when they came out of the dishwasher; or setting up the lightweight for her. Sometimes I would ask her to help me fold the towels and put them away, and she would say, 'I like doing things like this'. Cleaning became more difficult as her dementia progressed – the process remained important while the end product might be less 'helpful'; for example, sometimes she would wipe cups with a dirty handkerchief so we would discreetly rewash them afterwards. Issues with balance also began to affect her ability to clean, as I recorded in my written diary:

> We tried a bit of hoovering because she seemed to fancy it, but she started losing her balance so we stopped. She said 'you're a lovely little girl' – I'm not sure if she is seeing me as a little girl, or if it's from what she used to call me 'my lovely little girl' (even when I was far too long in the tooth!). […] [Later on that day] Listening to 'The King and I' soundtrack and walking around holding hands and singing to 'Shall we Dance?' Mum would reply saying 'yes, yes, yes' or 'no' and joining in the 'do, do, do'.
>
> *Written diary, 26 September 2022*

In this shared extract hoovering is becoming more challenging, due to issues with balance, but helping my mum is followed by a caring moment with her saying 'you're a lovely little girl' illustrating mutual care (Kontos et al., 2017). In a later moment, my mum is demonstrating everyday creativity through improvising in response to music (Dowlen et al., 2022, 2024) – saying 'yes, yes, yes' or 'no' in response to me singing 'shall we dance? As I have written about elsewhere, music, singing, and dance were important to my mum expressing creativity while living with dementia (see Buse, 2026). In the past, I had rarely heard my mum sing, and she described herself as 'tone deaf', and I had never seen her dance, describing herself as 'too shy' to dance in public. However, while living with dementia, she increasingly enjoyed singing with me while my older brother or dad played guitar. She would improvise creatively, waving her arms, making up her own lyrics, or ad-libbing in response to the emotions of the song, for instance saying, 'oh no' and pulling a sad face in response to a sad lyric (Dowlen et al., 2022). The aesthetic practices of music and dancing were woven into everyday life, and we would often sing while out on walks together. My mum's ways of being creative were therefore situated within her biography and those wider social constraints that shape our view of ourselves as creative or not. Some aspects of her creativity were in keeping with her biographical self, but others such as singing or dancing were expressed more freely (or publicly) after she was living with dementia.

My mum also found new ways of expressing everyday creativity through engagement with material objects and 'remaking' the material environment of the home (Besson, 2024). At times, these seemed unusual to us but appeared important to her. For instance, sometimes when I got up in the morning, mum had rearranged blankets, pillowcases, and handkerchiefs on the floor into a pattern. As an aspect of material culture, handkerchiefs became increasingly important to my mum. She had always carried a handkerchief with her and had lots of hankies in different colours and patterns, some with floral designs. Like other aspects of dress, such as carrying a handbag (Buse and Twigg, 2014b), the generational practice of carrying a handkerchief is perhaps comforting at an embodied as well as practical level. Handkerchiefs also took on their own aesthetic quality as a 'materiality of care' (Buse et al., 2018) and she would enjoy looking at the colours and patterns and arranging them on the table. Arranging handkerchiefs with my mum could create an enjoyable moment (Keady et al., 2022):

> When mum got distressed in the evening, I was able to calm her by setting out her hankies and she exclaimed how lovely they were with their flowers and embroidery – hankies are like a special collection that bring her joy when she looks at them…
>
> *Written diary, 30 July 2022*

This relates to consideration of the 'mundane' versus the 'exceptional' in discussions of care aesthetics (Thompson, 2023; Fox et al., 2025), and how something as mundane as a handkerchief could have special significance to my mum. Helping her maintain and engage with handkerchiefs could be a practice of care, a way to create a 'caring moment' and move beyond difficult emotions (Buse, 2026). When she first moved into a nursing home, we carefully labelled her handkerchiefs and emphasised in her care plan how having one with her at all times was important. However, the handkerchiefs were increasingly lost and left aside by my mum and, over time, became forgotten about. This illustrates the challenges of maintaining dress and material objects within the context of care (Twigg, 2010; Buse and Twigg, 2014b), but handkerchiefs also seemed less important to my mum over time, reflecting the shifting temporality of everyday aesthetics (Cribb and Pullen, 2022).

## Bodywork, care aesthetics, and embodied and sensory adjustments

### *Bodywork and connected/disconnected moments*

While my sketches normally capture positive moments, the sketch in Figure 2.6 instantly evokes memories of a difficult day, highlighting the challenges of bodywork, which can be in tension with care aesthetics (Thompson, 2023). These moments are outside of the frame of the sketch but are instantly evoked when I look at it. On that day, my mum was having bowel problems and my dad and I spent

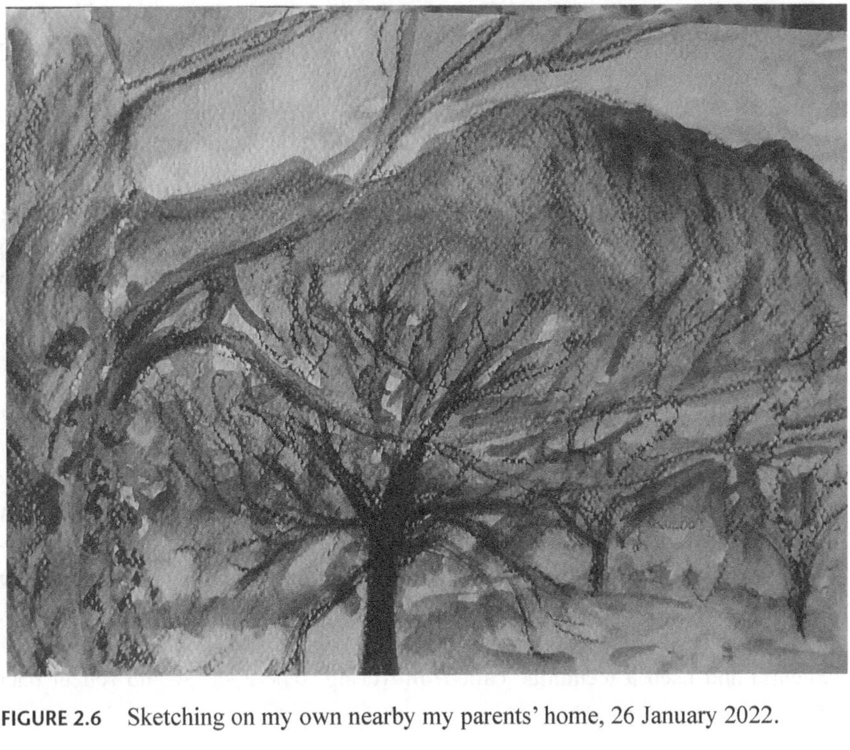

**FIGURE 2.6** Sketching on my own nearby my parents' home, 26 January 2022.

the whole day taking turns to assist her with the toilet and changing and washing clothes. Unlike other sketches that were created 'with' my mum, this sketch was done when the care worker arrived in the afternoon for their weekly visit. This illustrates sketching as a practice of self-care, creating a break from caring during a difficult day, as I noted in my sketchbook:

> Had a bit longer (around 20 minutes or so) – bit of time to myself, found a bench with a view towards the quarry…The tree nearby wrapped in ivy caught my eye, and the golden glow of light behind the mountains….
>
> *Sketch diary, 26 January 2022*

However, I did not want to be away from my mum for too long and soon hurried back. When I returned, I found out my mum had been too upset to see the care worker, so we had to take her to the doctors which she was upset and annoyed about, perhaps afraid and unsure of what was happening. This day was also recorded in my written diary, which elaborates on memories evoked by the sketch:

> Difficult day. Mum running to the toilet all day, [she was] very confused about what to do [on the toilet], getting angry and upset at times, had to take mum to the doctors which she got a bit angry about. […] Nice moment with mum at the end of the day after a very difficult time – she was waiting for dad to come to bed and didn't want to be on her own, so I pulled over a chair and held her hand while she fell asleep. Before she fell asleep, she said, 'you're a lovely, lovely person' and 'I love being with you'.
>
> *Written diary, 26 January 2022*

Here, the challenges of bodywork and moments that feel 'disconnected' exist alongside the aesthetics of care (Thompson, 2023) and are followed by a 'restorative moment' (Richardson and Campbell, 2024) at the end of the day. Holding hands is used to show mutual care and affection (Jones et al., 2025), alongside my mum's verbal expressions of love. This illustrates how people living with dementia can continue to show care and affection, even when other embodied 'activities of daily living' become more challenging (Kontos, 2004; Kontos et al., 2017).

The lens of care aesthetics creates scope for attending to embodied aspects of care that are outside the realm of bodywork (Campbell et al., 2024, p. 4). We had only just become able to leave my mum with a care worker at this time so we could take a break for a couple of hours on one day a week. My mum was very reluctant to have paid care workers visiting the home, and it took a long time to find the right care worker, and slowly introduce them, starting with ten-minute visits. After a few visits, I was surprised to come in and find my mum singing and laughing with this care worker. The care worker explained she had been reading about frontotemporal dementia and used a technique called 'mirroring' where she would reflect back what my mum said or sang because, 'imagine being in a world where no-one could understand you'. I began to try this myself, mirroring my mum's words or singing:

> Nice moments connecting with mum, I am learning that I can mirror her language, even odd sounds like 'woo-too' and 'woodi-woodi-woo'.
>
> *Written diary, 1 March 2022*

I would repeat a word like 'lovely' or 'nice' or repeat a tune my mum had hummed, and she would sometimes say 'yes', giving a sense that she had been heard and acknowledged. Mirroring is a technique used in theatre and has been written about in research on music and dementia (Dowlen et al., 2024). It became an important part of how we adjusted our embodied practices and found ways to communicate with my mum as her dementia progressed.

However, adjusting to the demands of bodywork became increasingly challenging and assisting my mum with the toilet was often one of the more stressful moments in day, disrupting enjoyable moments together. This is documented in my written diary:

> ...some difficult moments with mum, difficult getting her to sit on the toilet, and realise what she has to do in when she gets to the toilet.
>
> *Written diary, 7 August 2022*

This example highlights the challenges of assisting my mum with the toilet. While there is guidance for family carers on toilet signage and how to prompt someone with going the toilet, I could find little detailed guidance on how to support someone when they need a greater level of assistance. I found a video on the Alzheimer's and Dementia Weekly (2021) website on how to help someone living with dementia to sit down, showing an embodied technique of moving *with* the person – putting your arm around them so they feel supported, and bending your knees and going into a sitting position alongside them, encouraging their body to move with yours. My dad and I tried this technique which helped us assist my mum with sitting down but encouraging her to sit on and use the toilet was still difficult. However, even this most difficult aspect of bodywork was sometimes intertwined with moments of connection at a sensory level; for example, sometimes when I would help my mum wash her hands after going to the toilet, she would go 'oooh' and smile at the feel of the warm water. After washing her hands, my mum would often smile and wave at her reflection in the mirror. There is often a lack of mirrors in long-term care facilities and a perception that mirrors might be distressing for people living with dementia, although qualitative research suggests looking in the mirror can be a positive experience for some people (Kelsick et al., 2021). My mum seemed not to recognise herself in the mirror as her dementia progressed, but it was a positive engagement, and she appeared to enjoy waving at the person she saw and sometimes referred to her as a 'nice lady'. As someone who never liked the way she looked, she seemed to have befriended the person in the mirror.

### *Turning points, transitions, and embodied and sensory adjustments*

This is my last sketch 'with' my mum, before she moved into a nursing home. Sketching with my mum had become more difficult over time as she was increasingly restless and less able to sit still, and her balance also became impaired, so we adapted by holding her hand to support her while she was walking (see Buse, 2026). In this instance, my dad was walking with us on a local road near their home and took over holding hands with my mum so that I could sit and sketch, which I noted in my sketchbook:

> Painting on the bench on [name of local road]. I walk along holding hands with mum and then my dad takes over while I sit down to sketch. It is threatening to rain but holds off. The hedges are starting to turn to autumn colours with rusts and oranges and the leaves are starting to change.
>
> *Sketch diary, 25 September 2022*

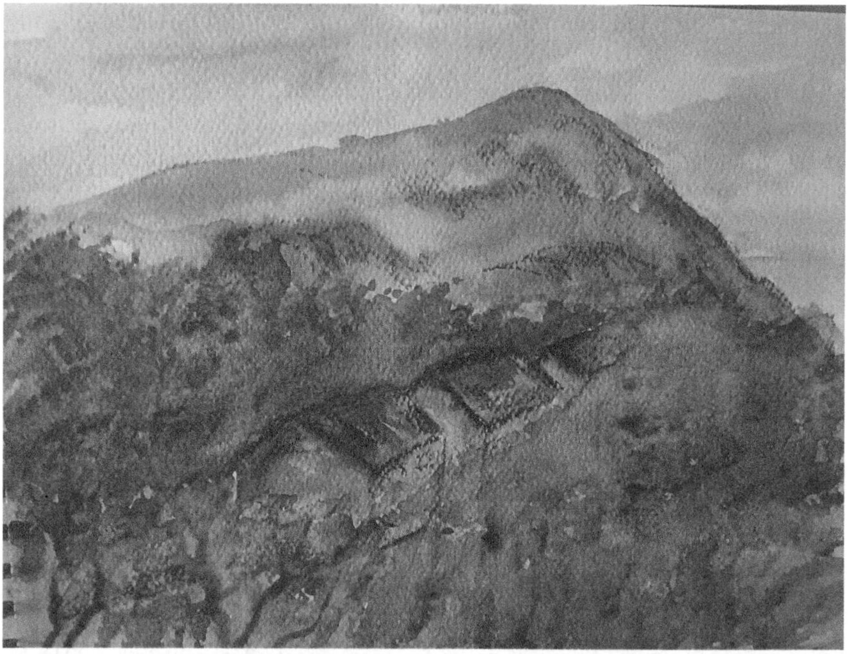

FIGURE 2.7 Sketching on the bench while my mum and dad are walking, 26 September 2022.

This extract not only captures a sense of change through the seasons but also marks a biographical turning point (McAdams, 1993) in terms of preparing for the transition to care. At this time, I had returned to work part-time which I was now juggling with 'caring at a distance' (White et al., 2020). I felt a change was coming and had been visiting and researching care homes, which I found upsetting, but I was aware that the level of 24-hour care required was becoming too much for my dad.

At this time, when my mum's dementia was progressing, sensory things, and the 'environment closest in' (Twigg, 2010, p. 223) became more important. We had some fleece blankets with animals on and she enjoyed holding them and hugging them. Sometimes she used the blankets to create a private space when she was annoyed with us, sitting on the chair in the front room and pulling a fleece blanket over her head. I wondered about buying her some soft toys but was unsure how she would respond and if it would be infantilising. As we were moving towards the transition to care, I looked into this further, thinking that it might help her feel less alone if she had a 'pet' with her. We found some 'robotic therapy cats' that mewed and purred in response to touch, by the manufacturer 'Joy for All'. I bought one and introduced it to her, not sure what she would make of it – at first she seemed a bit unsure, but holding the cat became a source of comfort:

> ...in the morning mum was in a bit of a funny mood. I gave her Ginger (the cat) to hold and it calmed her down. She started chatting while she was stroking the cat saying something about can it be done? I sang 'it can be done' (from Willy Wonka and the Chocolate Factory, a musical we had been watching) and she smiled and I went into the whole song 'I've got a golden ticket' and she was singing and laughing. Then I sung 'world of pure imagination' and she went 'ooh I know that one, where is it from?' And I said 'Willy Wonka and the Chocolate Factory' and she tapped me and said 'I like that one'. We sung a few songs and she spontaneously gave me a hug and I hugged her back – I can't remember the last time she did that.
>
> *Written diary, 15 October 2022*

In this extract, the sensory experience of stroking the cat calms my mum. There are other moments of connection throughout that day with us singing together, and my mum giving me a hug, and showing care through touch (Kontos, 2004). I was surprised and pleased at her giving me a hug spontaneously because while regular hugs were in the past an important way of us connecting, at one point whilst caring for her she 'went off' hugs. Touch in the context of care can be positive or negative and has to be carefully negotiated in keeping with different personal, biographical, and situated meanings (Thompson, 2023). At this time, I would check in with her 'do you want a hug?' and she would sometimes give firm 'no' or walk off. However, sometimes this practice returned when it was most needed.

When my mum moved into the nursing home, we brought things with her to offer comfort at a sensory level – her hankies, her blankets, her robotic cat, a compact disc (CD) player, and her favourite CDs, and recorded details of her aesthetics in her care plan. The embodied and sensory aspects of care remain important at the time of writing but are continually changing and being (re) adjusted. My mum has not said my name for some time now, but recognition is enacted at an embodied level (Taylor, 2008) – she sometimes looks at me or my dad and says 'ahh' and I stroke her hand and smile in return and say 'ahhh' and her face still sometimes 'lights up' when she sees us. There is a particular smile she gives that I had not been consciously aware of earlier, where she blinks, giving an 'eye kiss' as she smiles. I try to return the same smile, mirroring her gestures. Aesthetics like this are subtle and harder to translate into a care plan but are embodied in biographical relationships. We have to continually adjust how we position our bodies so my mum can see us – at one point her head was down a lot and we had to kneel down so that we could make eye contact. Recognition and connection come and go, appearing in fleeting moments and then disappearing. Sometimes we have a 'bad day' where my mum is asleep for the whole time when we visit, or is very restless, and it is hard to make a connection. However, those 'sparkling moments' (Damsgaard et al., 2024) of recognition and connection can still emerge and light up my day.

## Discussion

Using the care aesthetics framework as a lens, this chapter has reflected on moments of caring with/for my mum, using sketches as a 'way in' to moments and themes. Care aesthetics challenges the boundaries between art and care, exploring how art is interwoven with everyday life and care practice (Thompson, 2023). Sketching provided a care-ful way of 'being with' my mum outdoors that was not reliant on long conversations. It also provided opportunities for my mum to demonstrate mutual care (Kontos et al., 2017) and co-create caring moments (Campbell et al., 2024). Sketching 'in situ' is a practice of noticing (Heath et al., 2018; Cleeve et al., 2023) and helped us to attend to the sensory environment together. This chapter highlights not only how people living with dementia continue to express everyday creativity (Bellass et al., 2019; Kontos et al., 2020), but also how they can inspire everyday creativity in others, and how my mum inspired and gave me confidence to sketch. However, as discussed above, sketching with my mum became challenging as her condition progressed. Sketching was not only a way of 'caring with' my mum but also a practice of self-care, providing breaks from caring and illustrating potential for 'flow from one practice of care to others' (Thompson, 2023, p. 53). However, being able to take time away from caring can be challenging and requires support from a family member or care worker, which can be difficult to access in the context of constraints on social care services in the United Kingdom and elsewhere (Giebel et al., 2024).

This chapter also highlights the importance of enabling different ways of being creative and expressing identity (Bellass et al., 2019). My mum did not want to join in with visual art making but had her own ways of expressing her embodied identity, creativity, and agency (Kontos, 2004). This included practices such as cleaning, which are situated within her gendered and classed biography, and singing and dancing, which were less significant in the past but became increasingly important. This might reflect the association of frontotemporal dementia with increased musicality (Killick, 2016), but perhaps also a loss of inhibitions around feeling 'good enough', reflecting wider social divisions in creativity (Conor et al., 2015). Practices such as arranging handkerchiefs and engaging with their visual and sensory properties would not generally be seen as creative but were part of my mum's everyday aesthetics (Thompson, 2023). Helping to maintain embodied and sensory engagements with material culture can be a practice of care, although care aesthetics change over time (Cribb and Pullen, 2022).

This chapter not only considers 'care-ful art' but also 'art-ful care' (Thompson, 2023) and the crafted aspects of embodied and sensory encounters and how these are adapted over time. This included embodied practices such as hugging, holding hands, 'mirroring', and the material and sensory environment. Thompson (2023) distinguishes between the crafted aesthetics of care, and the delivery of bodywork in a way that does not feel particularly 'care-ful'. Aspects of bodywork, such as assisting with my mum to use the toilet, were extremely difficult and stressful, for us and for her. There is a need for further guidance for family carers on assisting with bodywork when caring for someone who needs a higher level of assistance. Yet, these difficult bodywork encounters were still sometimes interwoven with more positive aesthetic encounters and caring moments.

This chapter also contributes to discussions about how to record 'moments' in the context of living with dementia and the potential of creative methods for doing so (Keady et al., 2018). Considering the use of visual and sensory methods within autoethnography could bring a further element to this. Different methods not only capture different aspects of moments but also 'leave out' elements of encounters. Sketching 'fixes' moments in memory in a way that is distinct from a photograph or a written note (Heath et al., 2018, p. 722), and visual methods can help to recall 'emplaced' memories (Crowley, 2022). However, it is difficult to sketch while on the move or while carrying out physical aspects of care. There is a tendency to sketch 'special' moments, leaving more difficult ones out of the frame, and discomfort with sketching is also barrier for many people (Heath et al., 2018). Doing a written diary later in the evening helped me reflect on difficult moments alongside enjoyable ones; however, it can feel quite draining, and, unlike the sketchbook – which could be completed more collaboratively alongside my mum – it was something I did alone. This chapter also raises questions for family carers who might want to record moments with the person living with dementia. Sketching was a practice I could do with my mum, but it became more challenging as her dementia progressed and, without my dad present, I could not do this. Caring for someone living with dementia can be rewarding but is also time-intensive and can impact on physical and emotional well-being (Jones et al., 2019). For many carers, particularly those caring alone, finding the time and energy to record moments may not be possible. Further research is needed on experiences of creating, being in, and recording moments for a more diverse group of family carers and people living with dementia, which has begun to be explored in Fox et al.'s (2025) research; and see Sarah Fox's Chapter (8) in this book.

## Conclusion

This chapter has reflected on my experiences of caring with/for my mum who is living with dementia, using sketches as a 'way in' to exploring wider themes in care aesthetics. The examples highlight the ongoing ability of my mum to express identity, creativity, and care but also challenges from the perspective of a family carer. This chapter explored sketching as a care-ful way of 'being with' my mum and creating and recording everyday moments and providing opportunities for mutual care. It then explored convergences and divergences in our expressions of everyday creativity and identity, situated within biographical and social context. This includes practices such as cleaning, rearranging, and remaking the material environment, engaging with mundane materials such as handkerchiefs, as well as more conventional art forms such as music and dance. This chapter then considered embodied and sensory adaptations, and tensions between more challenging aspects of bodywork and care aesthetics. In relation to these challenges, sketching is also considered as a practice of 'self-care', providing breaks from caring. Practical implications are discussed in terms of recording moments and the need for further support for family carers around bodywork.

## Three Key Reading References

### *Reference 1*

Bellass, S., Balmer, A., May, V., Keady, J., Buse, C., Capstick, A., Burke, L., Bartlett, R. and Hodgson, J. (2019). Broadening the debate on creativity and dementia: A critical approach. *Dementia: The International Journal of Social Research and Practice*, 18 (7–8): 2799–2820. https://doi.org/10.1177/1471301218760906

This paper provides an overview of literature on creativity and dementia and considers where this could be extended further in terms of 'everyday creativity'. While there is a significant body of work on creativity in more 'formal' contexts, this paper highlights the need for more research on creativity in everyday life, as people improvise in response to the challenges of living with dementia.

### *Reference 2*

Cleeve, H., Borell, L. and Rosenberg, L. (2023). Drawing in-situ: Matters of care and representation in daily life with dementia. *Qualitative Research*, 23 (3): 782–808. https://doi.org/10.1177/14687941211049321

This paper explores the use of in situ drawing as a method for researching experiences of caring and living with dementia in a nursing home dementia unit. The method of drawing provided a way to 'be' with people living with dementia and staff without needing to talk. It also facilitated reflexive engagement through sharing drawings and recording the responses of staff and residents.

### *Reference 3*

Heath, S., Chapman, L. and Centre Sketchers, T.M. (2018). Observational sketching as method. *International Journal of Social Research Methodology*, 21 (6): 713–728. https://doi.org/10.1080/13645579.2018.1484990

This paper explores sketching as a method in sociological research, and a way of attending and 'being in the moment'. It argues for shifting the focus from the end-product to the process of sketching as a way of seeing. While not focused on dementia, this method could be applied as part of the increasing use of creative methods in dementia research.

## References


Alzheimer's and Dementia Weekly (2021). *Help someone with dementia sit down* [online]. Last updated: 6 March 2024. Available: https://alzheimersweekly.com/help-someone-with-dementia-sit-down/; accessed 1 March 2026.

Banks, M. (2001). *Visual Methods in Social Research.* London: Sage.

Bellass, S., Balmer, A., May, V., Keady, J., Buse, C., Capstick, A., Burke, L., Bartlett, R. and Hodgson, J. (2019). Broadening the debate on creativity and dementia: A critical approach. *Dementia: The International Journal of Social Research and Practice*, 18 (7–8): 2799–2820. https://doi.org/10.1177/1471301218760906

Besson, A. M. (2024). Home and beyond: Housework as aesthetic engagement with everyday environment. *European Journal of Cultural Studies*, Online first. Available: https://doi.org/10.1177/13675494241302418; accessed 1 March 2026.

Bryden, C. (2020). Challenging the discourses of loss: A continuing sense of self within the lived experience of dementia. *Dementia: The International Journal of Social Research and Practice,* 19 (1): 74–82. https://doi.org/10.1177/1471301219876711

Buse, C., Balmer, A., Keady, J., Nettleton, S. and Swift, S. (2024). 'Ways of being' in the domestic garden for people living with dementia: Doing, sensing and playing. *Ageing & Society*, 44 (11): 2351–2375. https://doi.org/10.1017/S0144686X22001489

Buse, C., Martin, D. and Nettleton, S. (eds.) (2018). *Materialities of Care: Encountering Health and Illness through Artefacts and Architecture*. Chichester: Wiley-Blackwell.

Buse, C. and Twigg, J. (2014a). Looking 'out of place': Analysing the spatial and symbolic meanings of dementia care settings through dress. *International Journal of Ageing and Later Life*, 9 (1): 69–95. https://doi.org/10.3384/ijal.1652-8670.20149169

Buse, C. and Twigg, J. (2014b). Women with dementia and their handbags: Negotiating identity, privacy and 'home' through material culture. *Journal of Aging Studies*, 30 (1): 14–22. https://doi.org/10.1016/j.jaging.2014.03.002

Buse, C.E. (2026). Singing with my mum: An autoethnography of care aesthetics and everyday moments in the context of dementia. *Ageing and Society*, 46, e35, 1–19. https://doi.org/10.1017/S0144686X26100567

Campbell, S., Dowlen, R., Keady, J. and Thompson, J. (2024). Care aesthetics and 'being in the moment' through improvised music-making and male grooming in dementia

*International Journal of Education & the Arts*, 25 (si1.13). Available: https://journals.psu.edu/ijea/article/view/63522; accessed 1 March 2026.

Casey, E. (2025). *The Return of the Housewife: Why Women are Still Cleaning Up*. Manchester: Manchester University Press.

Cleeve, H., Borell, L. and Rosenberg, L. (2023). Drawing in-situ: Matters of care and representation in daily life with dementia. *Qualitative Research*, 23 (3): 782–808. https://doi.org/10.1177/14687941211049321

Conor, B., Gill, R. and Taylor, S. (2015). Gender and creative labour. *The Sociological Review*, 63 (1_suppl): 1–22. https://doi.org/10.1111/1467-954X.12237

Cribb, A. and Pullin, G. (2022). Aesthetics for everyday quality: One way to enrich healthcare improvement debates. *Medical Humanities*, 48 (4): 480–488. https://doi.org/10.1136/medhum-2021-012330

Crowley, S. (2022). Making visible the invisible: How combining autoethnography with visual arts practice unearthed more than I imagined. *Art/Research International*, 7 (1): 156–185. https://doi.org/10.18432/ari29618

Damsgaard, J.B., Lauritzen, J., Delmar, C. and Kvande, M.E. (2024). Beyond loss: An essay about presence and sparkling moments based on observations from life coexisting with a person living with dementia. *Nursing Philosophy*, 25, e12425. Available: https://doi.org/10.1111/nup.12425; accessed 1 March 2026.

Dowlen, R., Keady, J., Milligan, C., Swarbrick, C., Ponsillo, N., Geddes, L. and Riley, B. (2022). In the moment with music: An exploration of the embodied and sensory experiences of people living with dementia during improvised music-making. *Ageing & Society*, 42 (11): 2642–2664. https://doi.org/10.1017/S0144686X21000210

Dowlen, R., McPherson, D.H.J., Swarbrick, C., Hoskin, L., Thompson, J. and Keady, J. (2024). Creating and reliving the moment: Using musical improvisation and care aesthetics as a lens of connection and self-expression for younger people living with dementia. *International Journal of Environmental Research and Public Health*, 21 (8): 972. Available: https://doi.org/10.3390/ijerph21080972; accessed 1 March 2026.

Ellis, C. (1999). Heartful autoethnography. *Qualitative Health Research*, 9 (5): 669–683. https://doi.org/10.1177/104973299129122153

Fox, S., Thompson, J. and Keady, J. (2025). Meaningful moments of connection: How people affected by dementia and their carers living at home understand, interpret and experience everyday aesthetics. *International Journal of Geriatric Psychiatry*, 40 (8): e70136. Available: https://doi.org/10.1002/gps.70136; accessed 1 March 2026.

Giebel, C., Prato, L., Metcalfe, S. and Barrow, H. (2024). Barriers to accessing and receiving mental health care for paid and unpaid carers of older adults. *Health Expectations*, 27 (2): e14029. Available: https://doi.org/10.1111/hex.14029; accessed 1 March 2026.

Hagerty, B.G.S. (2002). *Handbags: A Peek Inside a Woman's Most Trusted Accessory*. Philadelphia: Running Press.

Harris, P.B. and Keady, J. (2009). Selfhood in younger onset dementia: Transitions and testimonies. *Aging & Mental Health*, 13 (3): 437–444. https://doi.org/10.1080/13607860802534609

Heath, S., Chapman, L. and Centre Sketchers, T.M. (2018). Observational sketching as method. *International Journal of Social Research Methodology*, 21 (6): 713–728. https://doi.org/10.1080/13645579.2018.1484990

Hellström, I., Eriksson, H. and Sandberg, J. (2015). Chores and sense of self: Gendered understandings of voices of older married women with dementia. *International Journal of Older People Nursing*, 10 (2): 127–135. https://doi.org/10.1111/opn.12062

Herron, R.V., Funk, L.M. and Spencer, D. (2019). Responding the "wrong way": The emotion work of caring for a family member with dementia. *The Gerontologist*, 59 (5): e470–e478. https://doi.org/10.1093/geront/gnz047

Hillman, A. and Latimer, J. (2019). Somaticization, the making and unmaking of minded persons and the fabrication of dementia. *Social Studies of Science*, 49 (2): 208–226. https://doi.org/10.1177/0306312719834069

Jones, S.M., Killett, A. and Mioshi, E. (2019). The role of resilient coping in dementia carers' wellbeing. *British Journal of Neuroscience Nursing*, 15 (1): 6–12. https://doi.org/10.12968/bjnn.2019.15.1.6

Jones, L., Cullum, N., Watson, R., Thompson, J. and Keady, J. (2025). 'Only my family can help': The lived experience and care aesthetics of being resident on an NHS psychiatric/mental health inpatient dementia assessment ward – a single case study. *Ageing & Society*, 45 (6): 1143–1164. https://doi:10.1017/S0144686X24000096

Keady, J., Hydén, L., Johnson, A. and Swarbrick, C. (2018). Introduction. In J. Keady, L- C. Hydén, A. Johnson and C. Swarbrick (eds.) *Social Research Methods in Dementia Studies: Inclusion and Innovation*. London: Routledge, pp. 1–7.

Keady, J.D., Campbell, S., Clark, A., Dowlen, R., Elvish, R., Jones, L., Kindell, J., Swarbrick, C. and Williams, S. (2022). Re-thinking and re-positioning 'being in the moment' within a continuum of moments: Introducing a new conceptual framework for dementia studies. *Ageing & Society*, 42 (3): 681–702. https://doi.org/10.1017/S0144686X20001014

Kelsick, J.R., Freysteinson, W.M., Young, A. and Nurse, R. (2021). Experiences of viewing self in the mirror for men and women with dementia as perceived by their caregivers: A phenomenological study. *Applied Nursing Research*, 58, Article: 151398. Available: https://doi.org/10.1016/j.apnr.2021.151398; accessed 1 March 2026.

Killick, J. (2016). Creativity and dementia. In C. Clarke and E. Wolverson (eds.) *Positive Psychology Approaches to Dementia*. London: Jessica Kingsley, pp. 175–195.

Kontos, P. (2004). Ethnographic reflections on selfhood, embodiment and Alzheimer's disease. *Ageing & Society*, 24 (6): 829–849. https://doi.org/10.1017/S0144686X04002375

Kontos, P., Miller, K.L. and Kontos, A.P. (2017). Relational citizenship: Supporting embodied selfhood and relationality in dementia care. *Sociology of Health & Illness*, 39 (2): 182–198. https://doi.org/10.1111/1467-9566.12453

Kontos, P., Grigorovich, A. and Colobong, R. (2020). Towards a critical understanding of creativity and dementia: New directions for practice change. *International Practice Development Journal*, 10 (3) [online]. Available: https://doi.org/10.19043/ipdj.10Suppl.003; accessed 1 March 2026.

Latimer, J. (2013). Being alongside: Rethinking relations amongst different kinds. *Theory, Culture & Society*, 30 (7–8): 77–104. https://doi.org/10.1177/0263276413500078

Malthouse, M. (2011). An autoethnography on shifting relationships between a daughter, her mother and Alzheimer's dementia (in any order). *Dementia: The International Journal of Social Research and Practice*, 10 (2): 249–256. https://doi.org/10.1177/1471301211407626

Mannay, D. (2013). 'Who put that on there … why why why?' Power games and participatory techniques of visual data production. *Visual Studies*, 28 (2): 136–146. https://doi.org/10.1080/1472586X.2013.801635

McAdams, D.P. (1993). *The Stories We Live By*. New York: Guilford Press

Méndez, M. (2013). Autoethnography as a research method: Advantages, limitations and criticisms. *Colombian Applied Linguistics Journal*, 15 (2): 279–287. https://doi.org/10.14483/UDISTRITAL.JOUR.CALJ.2013.2.A09

Ownby, T. (2013). Critical visual methodology: Photographs and narrative text as a visual autoethnography. *Online Journal of Communication and Media Technologies*, 3: 1–24. Available: https://doi.org/10.30935/ojcmt/5707; accessed 1 March 2026.

Özen, Y. (2020). Body work and later-life care in Turkey: A qualitative study of paid and unpaid carers of older people. *Ageing & Society*, 40 (10): 2106–2127. https://doi.org/10.1017/S0144686X19000989

Pilcher, K., Martin, W. and Williams, V. (2016). Issues of collaboration, representation, meaning and emotions: Utilising participant-led visual diaries to capture the everyday lives of people in mid to later life. *International Journal of Social Research Methodology*, 19 (6): 677–692. https://doi.org/10.1080/13645579.2015.1086199

Pink, S. (2015). *Doing Sensory Ethnography*. London: Sage.

Rambo, C. (2007). Sketching as autoethnographic practice. *Symbolic Interaction*, 30 (4): 531–542. https://doi.org/10.1525/si.2007.30.4.531

Reed-Danahey, D.E. (1997). Introduction. In D. E. Reed-Danahey (ed.) *Auto/ethnography: Rewriting the Self and the Social.* Oxon: Routledge, pp.1–17.

Richardson, N. and Campbell, S. (2024). Sensory attunements of caregivers and care receivers: The value of an embodied and emplaced approach in everyday care encounters. *The Senses and Society*, 19 (3): 324–336. https://doi.org/10.1080/17458927.2024.2402965

Riessman, C.K. (2008). *Narrative Analysis*. London: Sage.

Scarles, C. (2010). Where words fail, visuals ignite: Opportunities for visual autoethnography in tourism research. *Annals of Tourism Research*, 37 (4): 905–926. https://doi.org/10.1016/j.annals.2010.02.001

Skeggs, B. (1997). *Formations of Class & Gender: Becoming Respectable*. London: Sage.

Smith, J.A. (1995). Semi-structured interviewing and qualitative analysis. In J. A Smith, R. Harré and L. Van Lagenhove (eds.) *Rethinking Methods in Psychology*. London: Sage, pp. 9–26.

Taylor, J.S. (2008). On recognition, caring, and dementia. *Medical Anthropology Quarterly*, 22 (4): 313–335. https://doi.org/10.1111/j.1548-1387.2008.00036.x

Thompson, J. (2023). *Care Aesthetics: For Artful Care and Careful Art*. London: Routledge.

Twigg, J. (2010). Clothing and dementia: A neglected dimension? *Journal of Aging Studies*, 24 (4): 223–230. https://doi.org/10.1016/j.jaging.2010.05.002

Twigg, J., Wolkowitz, C., Cohen, R.L. and Nettleton, S. (2011). Conceptualising body work in health and social care. *Sociology of Health and Illness*, 33 (2): 171–188. https://doi.org/10.1111/j.1467-9566.2010.01323.x

Ward, M.C., Milligan, C., Rose, E., Elliott, M. and Wainwright, B.R. (2021). The benefits of community-based participatory arts activities for people living with dementia: A thematic scoping review. *Arts & Health*, 13 (3): 213–239. https://doi.org/10.1080/17533015.2020.1781217

White, C., Wray, J. and Whitfield, C. (2020). 'A fifty-mile round trip to change a lightbulb': An exploratory study of carers' experiences of providing help, care and support to families and friends from a distance. *Health & Social Care in the Community*, 28 (5): 1632–1642. https://doi.org/10.1111/hsc.12988

Wilkinson, S. and Wilkinson, C. (2020). *Performing* care: Emotion work and 'dignity work' – a joint autoethnography of caring for our mum at the end of life, *Sociology of Health & Illness*, 42 (8): 1888–1901. https://doi.org/10.1111/1467-9566.13174

Zeilig, H., Killick, J. and Fox, C. (2014). The participative arts for people living with a dementia: A critical review. *International Journal of Ageing and Later Life*, 9 (1): 7–34. https://doi.org/10.3384/ijal.1652-8670.14238

# PART 2

# Care aesthetics and creative practices

# 3

# CREATING AESTHETIC OBJECTS WITH PEOPLE LIVING WITH DEMENTIA

*Henry McPherson, Rebecka Fleetwood-Smith, Robyn Dowlen, Cathy Riley, Jane Bowyer and John Keady*

## Introduction

Carrying out research with people living with dementia is a sensitive and complex undertaking. Traditional qualitative approaches which foreground recall and verbal expression are often a 'misfit' for people living with dementia (Webb et al., 2020) and can result in silencing peoples lived experiences. Research methods that are participatory and foreground embodied (including non-verbal and multisensory modes of interaction) and sensory experiences can be particularly meaningful when working with people living with dementia (see, for example, Phillipson and Hammond, 2018; Fleetwood-Smith et al., 2022; Campbell et al., 2023). Phillipson and Hammond's (2018) scoping review noted that whilst there was increased attention to the role of the arts and creativity in the lives of people living with dementia, this did not translate to the ways in which research was (or is) carried out. Historically, people living with dementia were excluded from research, and whilst from around the turn of this century there has been a shift towards the inclusion of people living with dementia (Harris, 2002; Wilkinson, 2002), there remains a need to develop approaches that are enabling, responsive, and flexible to best support people to participate in research.

Creative research methods that foreground alternative ways of knowing (e.g., tactile, non-verbal, and multisensory), and are malleable and responsive, can be well-suited to working with people living with dementia. Defining what it is to do creative research is elusive, as arguably all research endeavours involve creativity (including or outside of traditional creative practices). However, Kara's (2020) conceptualisation of creative research methods has been widely adopted within qualitative research and outlines five broad categories: (i) arts-based research; (ii) embodied research; (iii) research using technology; (iv)

DOI: 10.4324/9781003623441-6
This chapter has been made available under a (CC BY) 4.0 license.

multi-modal research; and (v) transformative research frameworks, including participatory, community-based methodologies. Creative approaches typically centre multisensory, embodied routes to meaning-making which foreground the body, challenging the traditional mind-body divide, to consider the ways in which we make sense of the world and make meaning through our bodies (Ellingson, 2017). Such approaches can be particularly powerful in the lives of people with dementia as we consider a person's actions, gestures, movements, and so forth to be expressive and meaningful (Kontos, 2015) rather than symptomatic of the condition. In dementia research, selected examples of creative research range from: sensory, visual, and material ways of carrying out interviews and observations (Richardson and Campbell, 2024), wardrobe interviews in which people living with dementia showed and discussed items of clothing (Buse and Twigg, 2016), multisensory object handing/elicitation sessions (Lee and Bartlett, 2021; Fleetwood-Smith et al., 2022) and photography (Dooley et al., 2021). There is also a growing body of co-design research, for example, the extensive work of the LAUGH project which brought together people living with dementia, their families, and those that care for them, designers, and dementia care specialists to develop prototypes designed to promote playful engagement opportunities for people living with advanced dementia (see, for example, Treadaway et al., 2019). The previous chapter in this book by Christina Buse is also an example of undertaking and reporting on creative research methods.

The use of creative research methods, in the context of dementia, is a burgeoning area. Whilst such approaches can offer exciting and innovative ways of working, there is a need to attend to the complexities of this work to ensure that approaches 'fit' and are sensitive to, or created with, the people involved in the research (Webb et al., 2020; Campbell et al., 2023). As part of this attention, there is a great opportunity to illuminate the intricacies involved and to attend to the aesthetics of this work. This involves spotlighting the processes and practices involved, moving beyond what the work looks like (and the outputs created), into what the work feels like, and the affective and relational practices at its core. This attention connects to calls within design research that advocate sharing how practices unfold and evolve to generate greater understanding around what it is to *do* co-design, beyond what may be created (see, for example, Hendriks et al., 2015). Wilkinson and Hendriks (2022) claim that relational practices are integral to co-design with people living with dementia and illuminate what it is to *be with* someone during the co-design process. Whilst Schreiber and Cürlis (2022) call for criticality around the involvement of carers in supporting people living with dementia in co-design work and acknowledge the key roles carers can play, they also highlight the challenges involved in ensuring meaningful engagement in such work. The care aesthetics lens has much to offer in examining and spotlighting the minutiae of practices involved in the *doing of* creative participatory work with people living with dementia. We propose this could lead to approaches that are, to borrow Thompson's (2023) words, 'richer, more reciprocal, nuanced in execution and respectfully crafted' (p. 156).

### *Creative 'patient and public involvement and engagement'*

In recent years, greater emphasis has been placed on the lived experience of dementia and how people living with dementia can shape the development, delivery, and dissemination of research (see, for example, Gove et al., 2018). Indeed, for many research funders, patient and public involvement and engagement (PPIE) is a mandatory prerequisite to research involving people living with dementia, and wider projects focusing on health and social care (see, for example, Keady, 2024). There are several documents that have been co-created with people living with dementia which outline best practices in working with PPIE contributors who are living with dementia (see, for example, DEEP's (2023) 'Dementia Enquirers Gold Standards for Ethical Research') but there is still a perceived gap between the requirement of researchers to engage in PPIE and meaningful, non-tokenistic (or even non-exploitative) engagement with members of the public (see, for example, Jackson et al., 2020; Islam et al., 2021).

As has already been noted, there is an overlap between creative research methods and creative approaches to PPIE. However, there is a distinction in the purpose of creative approaches in a PPIE context compared to creative research. A key purpose of using creative approaches within PPIE is to involve people meaningfully in the research process and to make research more accessible, inclusive, and responsive as it takes place. The purpose is focused on shaping processes and practices, rather than on collecting data that can be analysed. There is growing recognition that approaches that have been used in PPIE to date (group-based discussions, reviewing of ethical documents, discussion of research methods, and so on) tend to exclude those who may find verbal discussion or written feedback more challenging (Phillipson and Hammond, 2018). Having seen the benefits of creative research with people living with dementia, researchers are beginning to take note of the ways in which creative approaches can help shape research processes and involve people more meaningfully and equitably in the research process. Whilst this is an area that has been inspired by creative methods within dementia research, there is notably less reflection on what it means to use creative approaches as part of PPIE.

Although there has been less published work on the use of creative approaches to PPIE, there is a growing understanding of how creative PPIE can facilitate involvement with communities who may have previously not had their voices heard within the research process (Islam et al., 2021). Using creative approaches within PPIE aligns with developing concepts in care aesthetics in a number of ways, particularly in drawing the attentiveness of researchers to listen beyond words, to co-create spaces that afford connection, empathy, and mutual learning, as well as affording slowness and depth in working with people living with dementia (pushing back against rushed, transactional forms of involvement that are all too common). In these senses, creative approaches both enable and enact alternative, more democratised, models for sensitive and meaningful collaboration.

### *Locating ourselves in the work*

Within this chapter, we share examples from research and PPIE practice to illuminate what makes up creative work with people living with dementia – what this looks, sounds, and feels like. In sharing the 'doing of' this work, we spotlight the ways in which aesthetic sensibilities and sensitivities are inextricably intwined in our practices. We approach this by bringing together two case studies undertaken by the authorship that illustrate how care aesthetics can be both a focus of study (or project) and a way of working.

## Case Study 1: Carefully designing and facilitating object-handling sessions

**Context:** The first case study was part of Rebecka's doctoral research study (Fleetwood-Smith, 2020) that explored clothing in the everyday lives of people with dementia in a care home, and involved working with people living with dementia, care home staff, and creative practitioners. The research involved sensory, embodied, and creative methods using multisensory encounters (Pink, 2015), including object-handling sessions. The approaches foregrounded knowing 'through the body' enabling participation in the research in different forms. Recording methods reflected this focus, with video, audio recordings and fieldnotes used to explore and revisit research encounters. This work intersects with arts-based research, embodied research, and transformative research frameworks (Kara, 2020) due to the creative practice involved, the embodied focus, and the participatory way in which the research was carried out. Ethical approval for this work was granted by an NHS Research Ethics Committee [Ref: 18/LO/1707].

### What we did together

The object-handling sessions were the final cycle of study carried out in the research. The cycles of study are presented here to situate the iterative ways in which the research was carried out – each cycle informing the next.

**Cycle 1.** Multisensory research encounters to explore clothing during wear, focusing on embodied and sensory practices. This involved working with six people living with dementia and six members of care home staff.

**Cycle 2.** Translating themes into objects, materials, and images to design object-handling sessions. This involved working with six creative practitioners who specialise in creative, participatory work with people living with dementia.

**Cycle 3.** Multisensory object-handling sessions to explore clothing and textiles over three themed sessions. This involved working with five people living with dementia and supporting members of care home staff who were not research participants.

Each cycle of study was thematically analysed to inform the next. The exact approach to analysis varied according to the cycle of study and focus of the analysis. For a detailed presentation and discussion of each cycle of study, see: Fleetwood-Smith et al. (2022).

## Designing object-handling sessions

Object-handling sessions have garnered increased interest in recent years as activities for people living with dementia (D'Andrea et al., 2022). They typically involve engaging with, and exploring sensory items through, for instance, interacting with items, selecting items, discussing, critiquing, and reflecting upon the items. Those taking part in object handling can engage with the activity in different ways through, for instance, exploring the object's sensory qualities, discussing its heritage, or sharing stories relating to an item (see, for example, Thomson and Chatterjee, 2016; Camic et al., 2019; Griffiths et al., 2019). Reimagining object-handling sessions as a creative, multisensory research method to work with people living with dementia was informed not only by object-handling activities but also by creative and material research approaches (see, for example, Chamberlain and Craig, 2013; Woodward, 2020).

Designing the object-handling sessions involved working through themes from the first cycle of study with creative practitioners to explore how these may be reimagined as a series of objects, images, and materials. Due to the multisensory focus of the study, practitioners were recruited from a range of disciplinary backgrounds: visual artists, ceramicists, musicians, and designers. Practitioners took part in hour-long interviews which were analysed to identify specific materials, images, and objects and practices to design the object-handling sessions. This process was not intended to find 'things' to represent a specific theme but to identify 'things' that were inspired by the first cycle of study and shaped by practitioners' expertise. This process resulted in designing three object-handling sessions themed as follows:

**Playful object handling session** – this session was inspired by the ways in which creative practitioners suggested that objects could encourage a sense of playfulness, intrigue, and promote imaginative responses. The term 'play' can be problematic as people living with dementia are often infantilised; however, the term was used to shape a carefully designed session created to support potentially joyful moments.

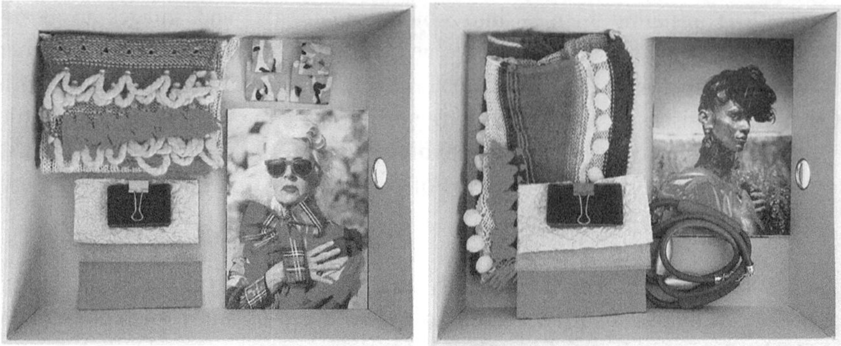

FIGURE 3.1 Examples of 'playful' object handling session boxes.

*Source:* Reproduced via Creative Commons Licence: https://doi.org/10.1080/17533015.2021.1974064

As Treadaway et al. (2019) note, there is great potential for design to promote ludic opportunities for people living with dementia. For each session, a mood board (a collection of images) was created to think through the 'essence' of the session, bringing together what creative practitioners had shared and materialising this into tangible ideas. This involved not only considering what items may be sourced and/or created for the sessions, but also how they may be presented.

For this session, participants were given a box containing six similar items (see Figure 3.1 and Fleetwood-Smith et al., 2022):

- Two handmade knitted samples containing different embellishments and different textural details using contrasting yarns and saturated colours.
- A handmade knitted pocket created with two different yarns to create a contrast in materials.
- An item of contemporary resin jewellery.
- Two tactile postcards created by hand-embroidering and collage techniques onto art/fashion imagery to create interesting surface textures.
- Swatches of contrasting textiles.

**Narrative object handling session** – this session was inspired by sentimental and emotional aspects of clothing. Creative practitioners were inspired by stories that people living with dementia shared and care home staff's awareness around the attachment people may feel to specific items of clothing and accessories. This session was designed to promote the sharing of stories and experiences. Items for the session were inspired by artist Celia Pym (https://celiapym.com/; accessed 1 March 2026) who specialises in visible mending and repair practices, and artist Grayson Perry's teddy 'Alan Measles' (for examples of Grayson Perry's work online see: https://www.royalacademy.org.uk/art-artists/name/grayson-perry-ra; accessed 1 March 2026). The session involved sourcing and creating items that showed visible signs of 'wear and tear'.

For this session, the following items were explored as a collective:

- Tactile postcards of Celia Pym's and Grayson Perry's work which contained destressed surfaces and/or hand-embroidered surfaces to highlight areas of 'wear'.
- Tactile postcards using images of clothing from 'Worn Stories' by Emily Spivack (https://wornstories.com/about/; accessed 1 March 2026) including embroidery and collage techniques.
- An Aran jumper with visible areas of repair.
- Accessories with signs of 'wear' e.g., handbag, wallet, scarf, and brooch.

**Dramatic object handling session** – this session was inspired by the theatrical aspect of clothing and the act of dressing up. It was designed to explore how clothing may be used to communicate different feelings or create a certain presence or effect. The design of this session differed as it involved using varying lengths of fabrics (e.g., velvet, silk, satin, and stiff cotton) to explore different textures, weights, and drapes, using a dressmaker's stand.

This brief presentation of the object-handling sessions seeks to contextualise the sessions and illuminate the practices involved in designing these. These practices involve a careful design and development process shaped by the research, this care-fullness (Manchester and Willatt, 2024) translated into how the items for the object-handling sessions were created and sourced and then presented to participants – all of which is an aesthetic practice. This attentive approach to developing the materials used within the research is often little explored within the literature. The following reflective note by Rebecka details some of the considerations involved in creating textile samples for the Playful session:

> I made the knitted samples on a domestic knitting machine. I wanted the samples to be robust enough to be handled, explored, and manipulated whilst also incorporating some delicate details. I added texture and interest using lace-holes, pompom embellishments, tassels, looped stiches, and through the unusual combination of different weights of yarn. The different techniques and yarn combinations meant that I had to work slowly and carefully, 'listening' to the machine to assess whether the needles could 'cope' with the materials that I was working. These considerations and the making process was an attempt to create ambiguous textile samples that were 'things' in themselves. The knitted pockets that I created brought together unexpected yarn combinations (e.g., highly textured, soft, delicate mohair with slightly lustrous smooth cotton) to create distinctions between the surfaces. The contrasting colours further added to emphasise the pocket in the knitted sample. The samples were large enough to handle and explore and, as they were abstracted, weren't immediately associated with the body. I wanted to encourage playfulness and intrigue and avoid discussions centred solely around whether someone may wear an item or not. The pieces were inspired by my work with creative practitioners and

the research to date; however, the textiles were inextricably linked to my own interests and concerns with visible making processes, unexpected textures, and bold uses of colour.

The following section explores what it is *to do* the sessions. This explores the sessions as a collective, rather than detailing individual sessions, and spotlights specific moments to share the sensory, relational, and aesthetic practices at play. As is explored also in Case Study 2 (Records of My Life), the affective aspects of research processes signify at multiple levels beyond what is made, or what is done; decisions about *how* work takes place, with what qualities of embodiment, registers of language, and in what kinds of environments, form an essential aesthetic dimension of working carefully with people living with dementia.

## Carefully carrying out the object-handling sessions

Setting up and carrying out the object-handling sessions involved creating space conducive to creativity both in a physical and intangible sense, and this was an aesthetic, embodied, and sensory practice. The creation of such space is sensitive and complex; it is physical and affective and involves multiple ongoing practices to enable, promote, and permit creative moments with people living with dementia. This is not to say that creativity is limited or contained to such spaces, but that the certain spaces can be considered enabling and potentially conducive to creative moments.

### *Inviting people into the space: physical, aesthetic, and ethical considerations*

First, it is important to reiterate that research with people living with dementia involves specific ethical practices and working in close collaboration with study sites, participants, supporting staff, and supporting family members (for a detailed discussion of such ethical complexities, see: Campbell et al., 2023). Inviting people to join the research was a lengthy undertaking that began long before the object-handling sessions took place. The focus here is on specific, slow, and careful practices involved in carrying out the sessions.

Due to carrying out research in the care home setting and the ever-changing nature of the environment, it was necessary to arrive on site hours before the sessions were scheduled. This preparation involved: (i) ensuring the room was available to host the object-handling sessions – a separate space away from communal areas was crucial due to practical and ethical reasons; (ii) revisiting the ongoing consent process with participants; (iii) confirming that the supporting member of care home staff understood the session and their role; and (iv) setting up the space. It was often at this stage that things did not go to plan; for instance, participants were sometimes unwell or did not wish to take part that day and so multiple sessions were hosted over a series of weeks to be as flexible as possible to support participation.

Prior to facilitating each session, the room was carefully set up – this typically involved tidying the space, rearranging heavy seating into a semicircle, adjusting lighting, opening curtains and windows, setting up the video camera, carefully bringing in and presenting the materials for the session, and placing signage on the door to ensure the privacy of participants. The room was quite small and so it was necessary to strike a careful balance in terms of moving furniture and introducing items into the space. The themes of the object-handling sessions guided how the space was set up. For example, the 'Playful' session involved giving participants individual boxes of items which included textile samples, textile swatches, jewellery, and tactile postcards and so small tables were placed next to each chair (see Figure 3.1 – example boxes created for the 'Playful' themed sessions). The 'narrative' session involved exploring items collectively and so items were carefully positioned on a table that was in reach so that everyone could see and access them.

Inviting people into the object handling session involved working with care home staff and typically involved supporting people to enter the space from communal areas. This movement between spaces was powerful in signifying a change and an invitation to do something different. Yet, this was also sensitive and at times disruptive to the regular routines of the care home, this at times involved navigating challenges when people who were not research participants wanted to join.

Attention to the layout of the room, the temperature of the room, how the space was lit and the transformative power of bringing unexpected 'things' into the space speaks to an attunement to the space. The careful ways in which spaces, particularly within social care settings, are reconfigured for the purpose of a creative session can be particularly important in supporting understanding and creating a sense of permission. For example, anecdotally, the process of someone rolling up their sleeves or putting on an apron can indicate the start of a creative session, whilst rearranging furniture and transforming the look of a particular area can better make room for creativity. For example, using side tables and placing objects on these meant that things were readily at hand and this promoted a sense of curiosity at the start of the playful themed object-handling sessions. Such slight changes within a space are important as it is often necessary to use the same room for multiple purposes; for instance, a dining room may also be used for creative sessions.

### *The felt space*

Attention to space was important not only in a physical sense, but also in terms of how the sessions unfolded. The 'ebb and flow' of what it is to do this work is important to acknowledge and illuminate. Within the object-handling sessions, there were often quiet moments, moments where some people were engaged, and others were not, and moments where some people took on different roles and began leading parts of the session. The purpose of the object-handling sessions was on the process of either engaging or enabling engagement with 'things'. There was not a specific outcome or end point, and this brought with it a sense of space and permission in allowing sessions to evolve gradually. There were often lulls and times when questions or prompts were not engaged with or necessary. As a researcher/facilitator, there can be a want to fill the space with words, to narrate what is happening, and to continue to offer prompts and questions to promote engagement and connection; however, adopting a quiet role meant attempting to limit verbal expression to make room for embodied and sensory practices to unfold. Knowing when to step in or hold space was a constant state of negotiation – it was improvisational and relational. This meant allowing room for disengagement, rather than always expecting continuous engagement from participants.

### *Sharing the words and experiences of participants*

Drawing on Pickering and Kara (2017), Campbell et al. (2023) note that the ways in which research is shared and presented constitute an ethical arena that must be approached sensitively. The careful practices adopted therefore extend beyond the places and spaces of *doing* research to how it is shared. This involves considering practices around, for instance, the confidentiality of participants. Within Rebecka's research, codes were used to refer to participants. The use of codes as opposed to pseudonyms was selected in an attempt to keep participants' voices and experiences their own without adding a potential layer of meaning using certain pseudonyms (see, for example, Lahman et al. 2015). Rebecka reflects in a note:

> On re-engaging with this decision, I feel a sense of uneasiness. I know that the decision was of the specific context and time in which it was made. For instance, I could not revisit participants to ask if they would like to choose a pseudonym due to the COVID-19 pandemic. This reflection speaks to the on-goingness of research and the tensions that arise as thinking and practices develop. My use of codes aligns with my doctoral thesis and the work that I have published from this, and I think it is important to retain continuity, however this is a practice that I will revisit in future work.

### *Spotlighting 'moments' from the sessions*

The following examples share specific moments from the object-handling sessions. The 'moments' focus draws on the work of Keady et al. (2022) to illuminate the aesthetic, sensory, and relational practices at play at specific points during the sessions. This is not to say that these moments were the most significant or important parts of the object-handling sessions, but that these moments are rich in what they bring to the fore.

There were powerful moments when participants (people living with dementia: PWD in the coding), researchers, and the supporting member of staff, were all together – exploring things as a collective, for instance:

P21 (PWD) picked up the 'Alan Measles' tactile postcard.
P21 (PWD): 'Ok, I am going to interview the pair of you now…' She held the card up for P22 (PWD) and me (Rebecka) to look at.
P21 (PWD): 'What does this remind you of?'
P22 (PWD) smiled: 'Cuddly teddy bears we've had'.
P21 (PWD) passed the card to P22 (PWD) – P22 (PWD) held the card out in front of her and then wrapped her arms around her body, as though cuddling a teddy bear.
P22 (PWD): 'Reminds me of my fluffy doll, it wasn't a teddy bear it was a fluffy pillowcase you zipped up … erm … but this isn't at all a doll, but it reminds me of her…'
P22 (PWD) passed the card to me and said, 'How about you?'
Rebecka: 'I didn't have a teddy bear either; I had a cuddly toy elephant'.

There were also small moments where participants engaged with items separately at the same time. P19 (PWD's) quiet interactions were missed during the live session as attention focused on P20 (PWD's) expressive actions – it was only on re-engaging with the session via videorecording that these differing concurrent moments were noticed:

> P19 (PWD) held the knitted textile sample close to her face. Leaning her chin on the pompoms, slowly she gently rubbed the pompoms back and forth under her chin [see Figure 3.2 – the knitted sample used by P19 (PWD)]. She smiled slightly, as she repeated the motion. The action seemed to be comforting/soothing. Meanwhile, P20 (PWD) immediately lifted a textile sample up and then held it out in front of her, as if analysing the piece. She was very animated and moved her arms in large, gestural, sweeping movements when talking about what the textile sample could be used for. [At this point she discussed making the textile sample into a bedspread].

There were unexpected moments that were humorous and joyful perhaps prompted by using ambiguous textiles that were not obvious in their function:

> She put her hand inside the pocket [see Figure 3.3. one of the knitted pockets used in the sessions], lifting her hand up, allowing the knit to fall around her wrist. She laughed as she did so and said: 'One of my problems is that I never understood why anybody did puppets of any kind'. She looked down at her hand inside the pocket, with her hand facing her, she waved, the textile sample dancing around her wrist. After a few moments, she removed her hand from the pocket and fiddled with the sample. I held a similar sample up for her to see and she said: 'Shit! This is all so very exciting because this looks more like a mouth than you might think!' P21 (PWD)

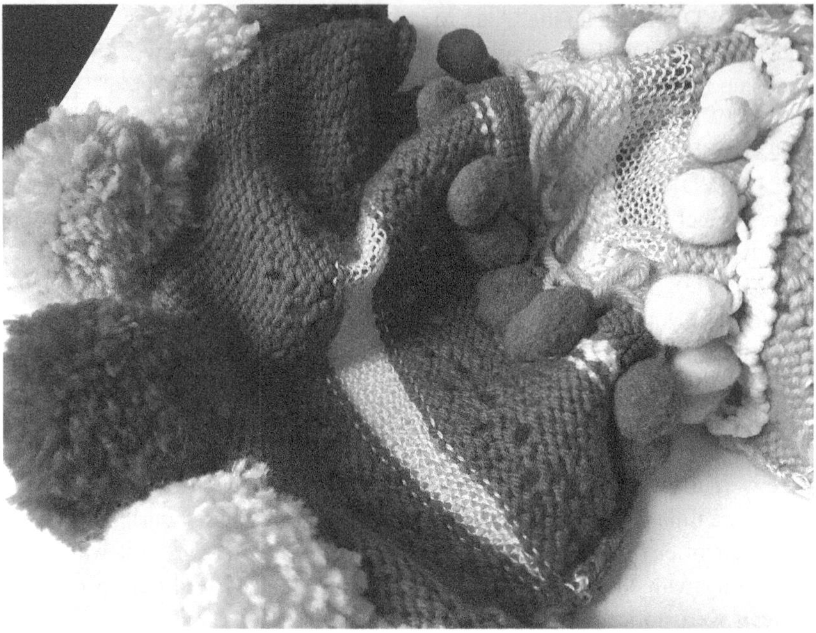

FIGURE 3.2 Example knitted textile sample.

*Source:* Created by Rebecka Fleetwood-Smith and shared with permission

These moments from the object-handling sessions reveal the intricacies involved in this way of working and what such approaches offer in terms of exploratory research with people living with dementia. The shared moments highlight people living with dementia's aesthetic sensibilities, both in terms of their physical and embodied encounters with the materials (whether overt and expressive or small and easily missed), and through their negotiation of roles and the shifting distribution within sessions. The use of ambiguous knitted textiles that were somewhat familiar (due to the knitted construction) and yet unusual, seemed to promote a sense of openness that enabled people living with dementia to explore and define the ways in which they chose to engage with the items. This permitted a sense of meaning-making together, as opposed to practices centred on determining or recognising the use of, for instance, a specific object. Attention to the unfolding of such minutiae practices, and the many things at play within such moments, brings to the fore the often unnoticed and elusive practices that are realised together 'on the ground' – from selecting, designing, and creating objects to the careful creation of spaces to explore and engage with them. This attentiveness sits at the heart of the work of researchers in both the case studies presented in this chapter (and in our Discussion section) and is a cornerstone of sensitive practice. The use of video-recording can help capture, explore, and re-engage with the embodied and sensory aspects of this work and illuminate practices easily missed within the liveliness of such workshop settings.

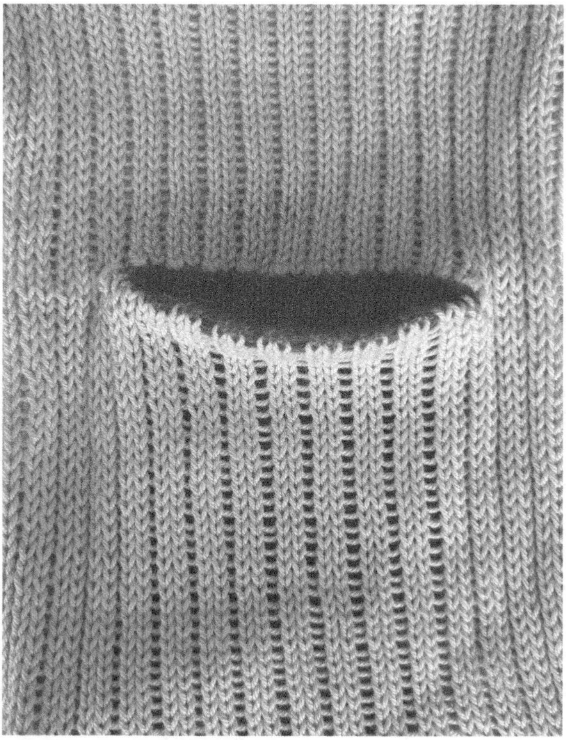

**FIGURE 3.3** Example knitted pocket sample.

*Source:* Created by Rebecka Fleetwood-Smith and shared with permission

## Case Study 2: Records of My Life – Vinyl records as artefacts

**Context:** The *Records of My Life* project involved the co-creation of a vinyl record sleeve design with the Open Doors Research Group – a self-advocacy group of people living with dementia, their families, and carers, based in Greater Manchester in the United Kingdom. Between 2023 and 2024, three half-day workshops took place at the Humphrey Booth Resource Centre in Swinton, Salford (Northwest of the city of Manchester). These creative sessions were co-facilitated by Jane and the research team (Cathy, Henry, Robyn, and John) and focused on the materiality of vinyl objects and on collective storying. The final co-designed record sleeve was installed at the entrance to an inpatient dementia assessment ward at Woodlands Hospital in Little Hulton, Salford (part of Greater Manchester Mental Health NHS Foundation Trust) and used as the cover image for this book. This project was instigated through conversations between the research team and the Open Doors Research Group during early PPIE meetings as part of a larger National Institute for Health and Care Research (NIHR) School for Social Care Research (SSCR)-funded study – a process evaluation of Manchester Camerata's *Music in Mind Training* programme (for detail of this wider study, see: McPherson et al., 2025). Ethical approval for this PPIE work was granted by The University of Manchester Research Ethics Committee (reference: 2023–15090–27165).

## What we did together

Through discussion with Robyn, Cathy, and Max Thomas (Research Assistant, Manchester Camerata) during initial PPIE sessions in 2023, Open Doors Research Group members explored the importance of music in the lives of people living with dementia and affirmed their belief in the value of programmes like Camerata's improvisation-based, group music-making programme *Music in Mind,* within residential dementia care settings. The group therefore wanted to create something tangible together to encourage more people to talk about music and dementia. They stressed that the object should advocate for embedding musical activities within care homes and community contexts, whilst also giving 'a sense of hope' to combat stigmatising societal narratives around dementia and creativity. After discussing various media (such as mixtapes, 'zines, posters), the group settled on designing and producing a vinyl record sleeve to represent the musical lives of the Open Doors Research Group members.

A commission pack was produced by the research team, and three Manchester-based designers with backgrounds in collaborative and socially engaged practice were invited to submit proposals. The commission pack emphasised an aspiration for co-created design, and for a process which would facilitate genuine collaboration between the Open Doors Research Group, the research team, and the selected creative practitioner. The Open Doors Research Group made the final decision to commission Jane Bowyer (A Studio Called Jane: https://studiocalledjane.co.uk/; accessed 1 March 2026) in September 2023. The group members were drawn to Jane's use of bold colour and shape, as well as her detailed proposal for collaborative co-design workshops to be explored in three discursive and object-handling sessions.

From the perspective of participatory research methods and project design, Vaughn and Jacquez (2020) have argued the need for criticality regarding the timing and nature of 'choice points' within ongoing activities; that is, identifying when, how, and to what effect agency for one or other party (researcher, collaborator, participant, etc.) is exercised in research activities. Whilst not a participatory research project, in the case of designing this sleeve with the Open Doors Research Group, we can also reflect on how co-creativity was manifest at such 'choice points' (understood as unfolding moments of encounter), not from a motivation of attributing degrees of authorship (thus de-emphasising process in favour of product, whilst both are important), but in order to explore how they are indicative of an aesthetics of care in our project – what they signify ethically and relationally about how we have worked together.

## Moment 1: Emotional and sensory connections to vinyl records – 6 October 2023

> It's important to hand down a physical object – something tangible, you know.
>
> *Open Doors Research Group member*

It is a wet, windy day in October. In the Humphrey Booth Resource Centre, conversations mingle with clattering plates and tea-cup clinks in the cafeteria, whilst down the corridor, Cathy and the Open Doors members have settled into the familiar room with the long table used for regular meetings. Henry, Robyn, and John join them after about ten minutes, and friendly greetings are exchanged – Offerings of tea or coffee ('oh no, hot chocolate for me!') - Looking forward to some good biscuits ('and gluten free ones too') - Introductions and compliments about a nice brooch ('very stylish'). These plenary interactions are not superficial. They are apertures through which relationships of trust and sensibilities of care can be established. They are how we begin to work together.

Today, the focus is object handling. In advance, each member has been encouraged to bring along a vinyl record that is special to them, which leads to a varied collection of musical offerings: The Moody Blues' *Days of Future Past*, a concert recording of *Godspell*, The Beatles' *Red Album 62–66* [their double-LP of classic hits], collected horn concertos by Mozart, and the Proclaimers' *Letter from America* are among the recordings shared by the group over the long table in the centre of the room. Through a series of prompts, the group are encouraged by Jane to explore the emotional and sensory connections they feel with their record (how it makes them feel 'in the moment' [i.e., today]), the imagery or memories it evokes, and who they associate with it (family members, friends, and colleagues), as well as celebrities and popular musicians from different decades in their lives. Time is taken between questions to allow for thinking, for looking, for feeling, and passing around the vinyl sleeves, and for members to respond to each other's comments. Often, one anecdote or memory leads to the sharing of another. Jane also invites attention on situated and embodied listening: 'Where do you imagine yourself when you listen to music?'; 'What kind of clothes are you wearing while you listen?'

Some pass records around the table, whilst others choose to hold and display to the group from their seat. Discussion turns to the brightness of the colours on many of the sleeves, the psychedelic imagery of the 1960s–1970s, for example:

- 'I feel like [in that era] the artwork changed and became more creative'.
- 'Sgt. Pepper's Lonely Hearts Club Band' [by The Beatles] was a revolution! It was a coming of age. You would stand in your bedroom just blasting things out!'

Several members comment that record covers are 'progressive and political', adding that vinyl artworks sometimes stick more in the memory than the music on the records. Posters and lyric inserts are unfolded and scrutinised. Records are not just products, we learn, but also objects threaded through with ritual: travel to familiar shopping outlets, curating one's own collection and musical identity, participating in cultural moments. Reflections emerge around the importance of caring for these objects ('you have to look after them and store them properly') and displaying them proudly ('my brother stuck all his records to the wall, like wallpaper. Even on the ceiling!'). Many spoke about writing their names in sleeve corners, of how one's ownership of these collections shaped musical and (sub)cultural identity. But they also emphasised the joy and importance of sharing, of passing records between friends and family, and across generations, 'My granddaughter now listens to my husband's collection of records; she's 16!'

Music is described by a member as a 'companion through life', by another as 'good for everybody', something which is, in fact, '*for* memory' which 'represents different eras of a lifetime'. Reminiscence therapy is mentioned, and the group discuss the differences between music-making 'in the moment', listening to live music, and remembering music past. It is noticeable how, as a collective, we listen closely to each other, attuning to the flow of conversation, voicing commonalities and dissonances, and collaging and layering experiences as stories are shared. Occasionally, Cathy prompts further reflections with follow-up questions, such as: 'Would you like to say any more about…'. This is afforded by her long-established and trusting relationship with the Open Doors Research Group, which is shown also in sensitivities towards the dynamics of conversation – noticing if someone seems ready to speak, but has not spoken, or gently returning to a question if the conversation diverges by a wide margin. Moving around the table, one by one, themes are voiced and collated: *being bright, being heard, capturing the personalities of the group*. The degree to which this co-created sleeve, too, might be 'progressive and political'. A keyhole (unlocking memory), and a wide-open door.

Just as is described in Rebecka's Case Study, in this project, we sought to hold space for alternative modes of knowing, expressing, and communicating beyond the verbal-textual which is ordinarily privileged in research processes. Co-facilitating these sessions required an attitude of openness, a confidence in holding space for others to reflect and share, and an attunement to the changing dynamics of interpersonal interaction – to the moment-to-moment expressions and embodiments of those in the room. But what does it really mean, in this co-creative PPIE context, to be attuned to someone 'in the moment'? We might consider it the committed cultivation and maintenance of attentiveness to the *qualities* of another's body, voice, and presence in relation to one's own. This attentiveness – in body, as much as in mind – encompasses both directed and more peripheral capacities, an awareness which extends to the person with whom you are interacting, through constellations of those sitting side-by-side, and into the dynamics of a group as a whole. Aligning with Hamington's (2020) description, across unfolding moments of improvisational encounter in making together, this attunement amounts to attending with 'head, heart, and hand' (p. 29) to another, which is really an embodiment of care.

Especially in co-creative activities where the senses are explicitly activated as domains of interaction and elicitation, for example, in passing records around a table, unfolding poster inserts, feeling the textures of paper, card, and laminate, this is a proprioceptive and somatic as much as an empathetic or cognitive experience. Attentiveness *as embodied* manifests in the qualities of our gestures and articulations (e.g., the speed and dynamic with which we move our hands when talking); in proximity and the space we afford to others (both physical, in our body language, and temporal, in 'holding space' for others to speak); in the orientations of the body and its frame (standing or sitting, leaning towards or away from, being side on or frontal); and in the sustaining or dropping of eye contact (sensing which is appropriate to provide comfort, encouragement, privacy, etc.) *as much as* in the register and content of our speech.

## Moment 2: Musical bookmarks – 3 November 2023

> Songs are bookmarks that mark the chapters of your life. There are moments in our lives that are marked by music.
>
> *Open Doors Research Group member*

The focus of this session is layout design. Emphasis returns to ensuring the design is eye-catching and bright, drawing on the psychedelic inspiration from the 1960s–1970s records from session one. Strong aesthetic preferences are voiced. A desire for colour, in contrast to entrenched narratives around dementia which accentuate mutedness, darkness, and a progressive loss of vibrancy and vitality. Cathy describes how high saturation and contrast can also help people living with dementia with visual impairments, where muted colours, creams, and whites, may be less clear or confusing. Jane offers options for different variations of sleeve design – folds, inserts, cut-out structures, concertina – and presents initial sketches of how the sleeve might look. As seen in Figure 3.4, the group are drawn to the so-called bookmarking concept – individual memories and stories being visually represented in a grid-like structure, each a 'bookmark', representing a moment in a life.

Jane asks what the Open Doors Research Group members would like to take away from the project, beyond a copy of the sleeve itself. Responses centre community and connection ('I want to learn about other people'; 'hear ideas from other people') as well as positivity ('a bit of joy and happiness'; 'enjoying myself'). There is another strong iteration of the representation of individuals and perspectives of people living with dementia ('see a bit of ourselves in the design'; 'something related to Open Doors'; 'share *our* thoughts and opinions on Music in Mind Training'). Moments of reflection and sharing as a whole group are interspersed with more localised conversations, in pairs and threes. During break periods, discussion flows freely from the importance of music in care homes, to now-closed music venues in Salford and Manchester, to challenges in

(a) (b)

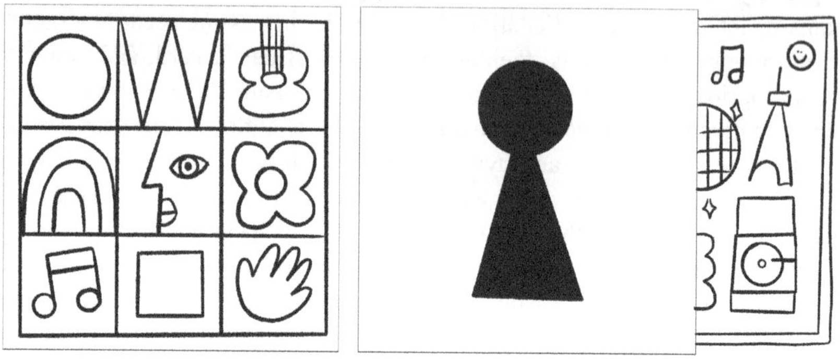

FIGURE 3.4 Developing designs. Left, bookmark concept. Right, Keyhole cut out for outer sleeve.

*Source:* Reproduced with the permission of Jane Bowyer

the dementia diagnostic pathway, to reflection on previous engagement within research projects as co-researchers. Several members speak to Jane individually, near the coffee machine, sharing their perspectives on the developing vinyl artwork, and anecdotes about their musical lives.

Through first, the process of sharing and collaging these experiences collectively and second, the resulting 'bookmark' grid and track list aspects of the sleeve design, a sense of shared ownership and of representation for the Open Doors Research Group members was afforded. Spatially, the workshops were grounded in a circular arrangement for sharing and collecting ideas in a centralised physical and interpersonal space. This was represented in tangible terms by the table, as a site for gathering both material objects and ideas, and in social and temporal terms by facilitation which opened invitations to share through reflective questions. A focus on personal stories of musical moments, allowing time for responsivity and for group members to bounce ideas off each other, formed the basis of all discussions. This was flagged early on as an important motivator for their collaboration, whilst in terms of session design, it also was a means of counteracting stigma around the creativity of people living with dementia in the design process through collective storying.

Storying, or narrating, aspects of one's life is itself a creative act, a means of rendering one's own experience within the world and in relation to the life worlds of others through verbal language, which shapes our daily life and also interprets the past (Clandinin and Connelly, 2000). The drawing together of multiple stories, and the shared identifying of themes through this process, generated a collective collage of experience which was manifest visually in the grid of bookmarks. None of this would have been possible without the generosity of the Open Doors Research Group members – a willingness to share their experiences and voice opinions – which was both acknowledged and supported through close listening and embodied attentiveness of Cathy, Jane, Henry, John, and Robyn. We consider the root of co-creativity in this context to be reciprocity, mutual respect, trust, and forthcomingness. This was enabled through a carefully held psychosocial space for listening and responding, oriented towards a common creative goal. In line with the above, Jane reflected that time allocated for comfort and access breaks was also important for precipitating less structured, 'informal' conversations with group members. Many stories and personal reflections were brought to the surface during these moments of 'softer' interaction away from the table with individuals who were less vocal during structured group discussions. Being attentive not only to the centralised or shared space, but also to peripheral and in-between spaces (between activities, between people), was therefore a central aspect of careful facilitation. In both this project and Rebecka's case study, attention to peripherality and liminality formed a fundamental aspect of the process of doing the work. As explored further in the Discussion, however, these skills are not always prioritised within institutional research environments or indeed research pedagogy.

## Moment 3: Something that looks professional – 8 December 2023

Today, Jane has brought along a series of colour swatch books – vinyl and paper stock samples for the group to handle and respond to. There are a variety of colours and textures, which are passed around the table from hand to hand. We flip open different leaves and compare the feel and look with each other ('that's quite rough, I don't like it'; 'very bright that!'; 'like my wallpaper'). Members chat over which swatches they like, surfacing memories of other vinyl, of bands and venues, and Manchester shop fronts. Conversations in pairs and threes occur naturally, and time is allowed for these to develop. Jane asks the group to share their thoughts on the material for the sleeve. There is a strong consensus that it should feel like a 'real' record sleeve: 'something professional'. Jane suggests a matte paper stock with a gloss laminate, explaining how this will closely replicate the feel of a commercial vinyl sleeve. We explore a timeline for the production stage. Cathy shares an idea to exhibit the sleeve in the corridor at the entrance to the NHS inpatient dementia assessment wards at Woodlands hospital – 'somewhere where everyone can see it' – which the group are excited by. Henry explains that when the final draft is received, he will send it on via Cathy to share with the group, so that any last amendments, tweaks, or changes can be accommodated. Jane explains how the process will work with the printer, once the design has been finalised and 'signed off' by the Open Doors Research Group.

We move from in-person gatherings to digital exchanges. Cathy collects a series of reflections from Open Doors Research Group members, which hold a range of temporalities (past and present), life experiences (partnerships, careers, and holidays), and sensibilities (reminiscent, philosophical, emotive, joyful, and identity-centred), tracing discussions and themes from the in-person sessions, for example:

> My love of music stems my former headteacher who insisted we LISTEN to the music. I found it awoke my senses, it was easy, pleasurable, I sang, I loved it, I joined a choir. As I grow older, I can lose and find myself in music. It evokes a range of my emotions, it stirs my forgotten memories, it takes away my stress, it keeps me connected to other people, it helps my wellbeing. I cannot imagine my life without it.

The vinyl record sleeve is printed, and Jane meets with Cathy to pass over the finished sleeves. Copies are given to each member of the Open Doors Research Group, to the research team, and one professionally framed to be exhibited in the Woodlands hospital at the entrance to the NHS inpatient dementia assessment wards (see Figure 3.5).

Zeilig et al. (2018) have written that in co-creative activities, 'the artists involved do not instruct but rather disperse the knowledge associated with their skills, thereby privileging the creative process' (p. 138). Although it was ultimately Jane's interpretation of the Open Doors Research Group member's stories which formed the core of the sleeve design, all creative decisions around colour, material and texture, layout, content, visual metaphors (a keyhole, an open door), track listings, as well as the naming of individuals, were made with the Open Doors Research Group themselves. Distributed decision-making was facilitated through a layering of different modalities: roundtable discussion, the passing of objects hand to hand, the displaying of personal items to the group (vinyl brought from home), intimate small group conversation, as well as one-to-one interactions during break periods away from the table. These varied types of social and sensory interaction allowed different creative apertures to open, for different voices to come to the fore in different ways. The role of the researchers, too, was more distributed in the sense that themes of the group discussions were identified by the group themselves in response to researcher prompts, noted down and collated by the researchers, and then member-checked at each session to ensure accuracy and representativeness.

In our project, it was agreed that the completed sleeve should look as close to a commercial copy as possible. This was a means of aesthetically validating the contributions of the Open Doors Research Group members, showing an endorsement of their creativity in committing to high-quality production. Ensuring that all members of the group were given a copy of the sleeve (see Figure 3.6) further invited a sense of ownership and an acknowledgement of their creative labour, whilst its public exhibition in the Woodlands hospital further legitimised the sleeve as an object not only of shared endeavour, but also of shared artistry.

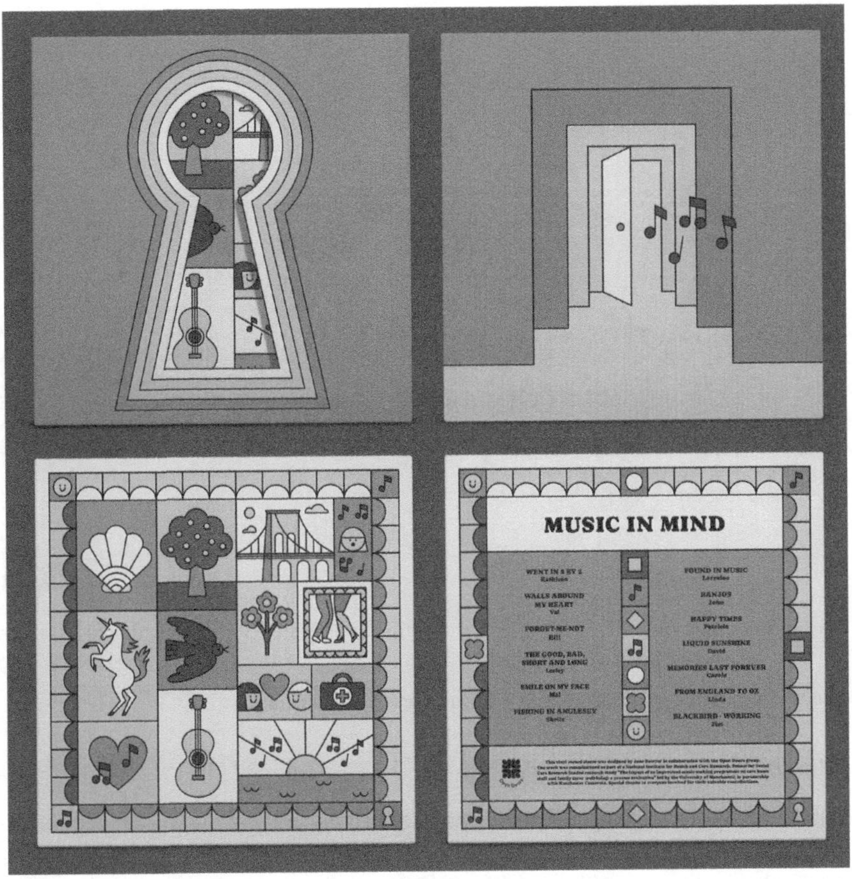


**FIGURE 3.5** Completed design. Top (outer cover). Bottom (sleeve insert).

*Source:* Reproduced with the permission of Jane Bowyer

## Discussion

The two case studies that have been presented in this chapter highlight the ways in which creative collaborations with people living with dementia can foster meaningful connection, collaboration, and support collective creativity. These reflective accounts showcase the ways in which a focus on sensory, embodied, and affective aspects of such practices can stimulate meaningful and involved contributions by people living with dementia, through researchers, artists, and facilitators co-curating spaces in which people can find voice, and in which new, more sensitive relationships can be actualised. The following section explores in more detail some common threads from the two case studies to argue the case for the ways in which a lens of care aesthetics can illuminate the small, often unnoticed moments in such projects which contribute richly to co-creative research agendas and processes.

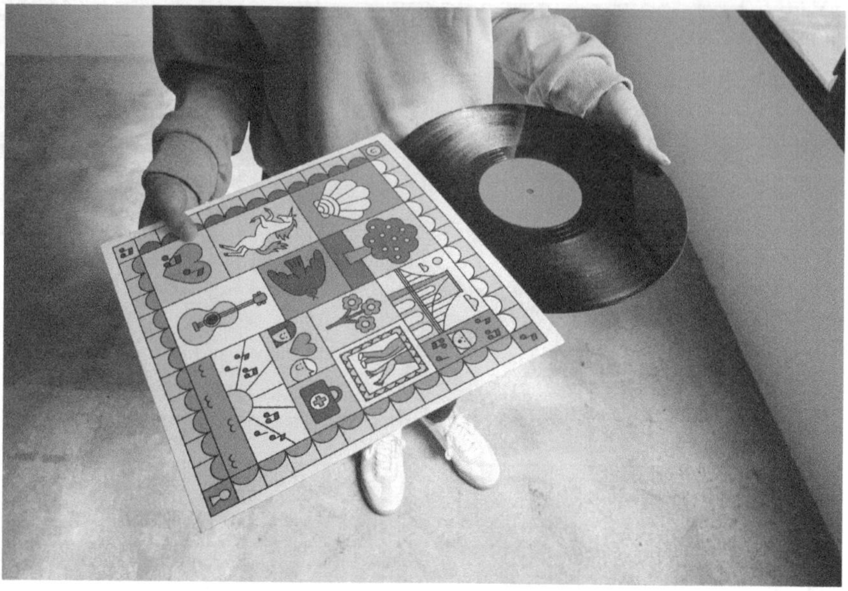

FIGURE 3.6 The Open Doors Research Groups' co-created vinyl record sleeve cover, posed with vinyl record.

*Source:* Shared with the permission of the Open Doors Research Group

### *Attuning and attending*

Both case studies highlight that working sensitively and carefully with people living with dementia is often about *noticing changes* in the tone of others' vocality or physicality, not only to mitigate distress should it arise but also to enable an authentic and relational connection with the person as they are at that precise moment. It is listening for shifts in vocal cadence and tone, for subtleties in posture or gesture which might indicate desire to contribute, or indeed to withdraw, an expression of discomfort, or the need for a change in the flow of activity. As in the situation of Cathy and John and their extensive experience with the Open Doors Research Group and other groups of people living with dementia, Robyn in her creative research methods work with people living with dementia, Rebecka and Henry as artist-researchers, and Jane as creative practitioner, this attentive sensibility is invariably conditioned by professional experience and responsibility (what we carry into the room with us); but, at the same time, to maintain attentiveness in such work is also to be flexible and responsive. It is improvisational – surfacing prior knowledge within the spontaneous moment of encounter, not getting stuck in preconceptions or anticipation at the expense of what is emerging 'in the moment'.

As Campbell et al. (2023) have proposed, for researchers, developing an awareness of the breadth of one's own sensory and embodied experience is essential to enable the effective 'multi-dimensional engagement with the experience of others from one's own body' (p. 6). In working co-creatively with people living with dementia, it is important to embody a co-presence which is empathetic, receptive, generous, and, by extension, conducive to ethical and effective collaboration. To lay the ground for this, we first must be aware of what (and how) we ourselves feel, and become aware of, how this is also at play – and in flux – within collaborative and facilitatory contexts. These felt aspects of this type of work are essential but are often underarticulated. Within the context of the Academy at large, where textual and verbal registers of language and knowledge often subsume the sensory and the embodied (see, for example, Dempster, 2018) – we must reflect on what sites of knowledge, what foci of embodied practice, might need to nourishment in order to develop what Thompson (2015) refers to as 'new virtuosities' (p. 438) of care. To enable richer, more careful relationships with our collaborators who are living with dementia, we might begin by focusing on capacities for attunement. A reaffirmation of sensing bodies (our own, our collaborators') as both present, and integral, to doing research work. A recognition of the non-verbal, the paraverbal, all that lies behind, beyond, and around the words we use, as important sites within which care is skilfully articulated and keenly felt.

### *Improvisational and relational facilitation*

Whilst we have shared some of the practical steps and skills required to work co-creatively with people living with dementia in this way, there are facilitation skills that often go unnoticed in these contexts which we believe can be illuminated further in relation to care aesthetics. Although co-creation with people living with dementia has been described as affording an inherent equality (Zeilig et al., 2018), it is perhaps more nuanced to say that co-creative activities aspire to unknit rigid hierarchies and promote alternatives within traditionally stratified spaces – to support collaborative efforts by which channels of communication, decision-making, and creative interaction can be more networked, and therefore potentially more empowering for all involved.

Irrespective of the existence of a creative 'output', the role of the creative practitioners in these contexts was not to direct but to enable the creative agency of other people. This type of practice re-renders the culturally pervasive conception of the Artist – as a figure of creative authority and autonomy whose originality both generates and legitimises aesthetic products – towards a model of one that is more of a nourisher of collective creativity. This model also sits at the heart of much participatory arts-based and creative 'action' research, in which there is increasing advocacy for methodologies which foreground intersubjective creativity, whilst allowing space to reflexively negotiate the complex questions of ethics and power imbalance which arise when working 'in community' (see, for example, Heslop et al., 2021; Nunn, 2022). In our own context, without being hyperbolic, we can consider how this pragmatic shift in rendering of the role of the artist affords a form of care. To adopt Thompson's (2015) phrasing, it 'models and exhibits the fairer and more mutually sympathetic world that is sought' (p. 439), within the microcosm of PPIE in the community centre and research in the care home, underpinned by a motivation to empower those whose creativity is often societally occluded.

### *Curating spaces for sharing*

Affirming that 'the shape and feel of the relationships at the heart of the project *are* its aesthetics' (Thompson, 2015, p. 439, emphasis added), one expression of our attentiveness is the sensitive curation of spaces in which this work can happen. As highlighted in both case studies – in Rebecka's object-handling sessions, and in the setup for the Records of My Life meetings – it matters how we construct physical and interpersonal spaces, by what sensibilities arenas for sharing and interacting are established, inhabited, and held. Thompson (2015) has proposed that decisions about accessibility, for example, 'are not mundane organisational matters, but rather crucial ethical propositions' (p. 438) through which both an aesthetics and ethics of care become actualised. We assert too that these aspects of co-creative endeavour are not only located in what is made, nor only in the act of making, but also in the framing of that process and what underpins it. In our work, decisions concerning where and for how long activity takes place, the layout of rooms and venues, the sensibility with which sessions are facilitated (register of language, degree of interactivity), and the materiality of objects used in elicitation, all are sites in which propositions are made for *how* and *with what qualities* we relate to each other – in other words, what the aesthetics of care are and how they become within our practice.

There are active decision-making processes which are acted out in the field when it comes to determining spaces which are comfortable and accessible for people living with dementia. In case study 1, Rebecka worked with care home staff to identify a quiet space away from the 'hustle and bustle' of the multifunctional communal areas. The room used was quite small; however, it contained large recliner style seating, small portable tables, and a window overlooking the care home's garden. In case study 2, sessions took place in a community centre which was known to the group, acknowledging the importance of familiarity (of spaces and routines) for people living with dementia. Members were compensated financially for their time and for transport, which indicated that their contributions were valued by the researchers and also enabled them to attend. The community centre was easily accessible by public transport links, provided an atrium space with a cafeteria and couches for socialising before the session, as well as a dedicated room at a quieter end of the building in which to conduct the PPIE activities. The choice in the spaces was therefore not only practical but also affective, rooted in an ethic of care that prioritised both the comfort and the sensory and emotional experiences of participants.

Exploring this thinking, we can consider how our activities are scaffolded to afford trust, and to support expressions of creative agency. Something as 'simple' as the provision of hot drinks and biscuits is, per Thompson's argument, not a superficial aspect of facilitation, but a means by which relational care and attentiveness are embodied (felt, expressed) and made visible (noticed). This is particularly relevant within the context of research-associated activity, including PPIE, which is fraught with complex power dynamics and imbalances. As Cathy reflects, it is these 'small things' that make a difference in making people *feel cared for*, in 'spurring a little bit of warmth' both physically and interpersonally. In many institutional and clinical contexts, which people living with dementia face regularly, Cathy reflects too that the absence of these things can have the opposite effect. Bringing food 'to the table' within the context of research work is a means of displaying thoughtfulness for the comfort and well-being of another and is a site for expressing care. Yet, rarely are such gestures of attentiveness, or the manner in which they are embodied, addressed more than superficially or anecdotally within institutional research culture, training, or design; their importance is rather felt out, learned, and replicated through practice.

Different room layouts were conducive to different kinds of careful interaction and collaboration across these two case studies. A circular layout, for example, can serve a democratising function by making each person in the circle visible. Such arrangements can also render the space in the centre as an open arena in which contributions voiced individually become held and collaged collectively. In the Humphrey Booth Resource Centre, the long table in the centre of the room became a site for both tactile and verbal mediation; it was used for displaying the vinyl record sleeves brought by the group members, for serving and sharing biscuits, for passing colour swatches and material textures for the sleeve design around the group, and for speaking across and around. In Rebecka's study, the awareness of the lighting, the atmospheres in the wider context, balanced against the need for privacy, were carefully and skilfully navigated to create a space conducive to creative exploration within the object-handling sessions. However, circular arrangements can have the potential to conduce feelings of scrutiny, of being watched, implying that each person is *expected* to speak, or indeed to speak in turn, which can prove discomforting. Session structures which are flexible and responsive and enable movement between whole-group interactions, smaller group interactions, and one-to-one interactions can help to mitigate this. In practice, fragmented pockets of interactions often occur whether they be separate discussions, or explorations of materials – these then necessitate a route by which to reconvene.

Both of our case studies highlight the need for slow and considered research in a dementia context. Cultural geographer Laura Pottinger (2021) has advocated for research methodologies rooted in 'gentleness' that are 'sensitive, collaborative, and careful' in activity 'which can attune to small-scale, mundane and non-verbal detail', often at a slower pacing (see also: Pottinger, 2025). As researchers and practitioners, we do not want to 'helicopter in' and 'helicopter out' – only engaging for a brief window of time, with little care for sustained relationship development. We need to provide time and space for interactions to develop, for relationships to deepen, over longer durations, to reveal authentic parts of ourselves to the groups that we are working with, to fulfil our aspirations for a more democratised space. For example, in the Open Doors Research Group sessions, time was taken in breaks by the members to get to know the researchers – why they were doing their work, their background, and what music and dementia meant to them. This built rapport, trust, and familiarity. Reflections from these encounters in 'informal' time became significant elements of the completed vinyl sleeve. Factoring in 'unregulated' time and space for this type of interaction outside the formalised remit of discussion or exercises, opens a sensitive, generative space for different voices and vocalities to come to the fore. But beyond access, in the context of co-creating, this provided a significant aperture for expressions of creative agency and decision-making – directly informed the co-designed objects – which might otherwise have been missed. In the case of Rebecka's study, Rebecka volunteered at the site running creative arts and textiles sessions prior to carrying out the research. This allowed her to build rapport with care home residents, staff, and families – the understandings and site-specific knowledge generated profoundly shaped how she designed and led the object-handling sessions. Despite researchers recommending 'hanging out' periods when working with people living with dementia (Fletcher et al., 2019), there is a great opportunity to attend to these practices and create space and time for such work prior to, during, and beyond the research activities.

As researchers, we often are not afforded the luxury of time when working with people living with dementia. Large chunks of the research process are often taken up by gaining ethical permissions to work creatively with these groups and so the time we have to work carefully with people living with dementia is limited. It is becoming more common for PPIE work to require full ethical approval before initiation, which can add to the timelines and limit the time researchers have to build trust and rapport with groups or individuals. There is growing recognition of the importance of 'slow' research with communities whose voices may have been marginalised through their experiences of particular health conditions, as well as those who have been excluded from dementia narratives as they are deemed 'hard to reach' (see, for example, Field et al., 2019; Jones et al., 2025). As these case studies show, there is real value and nuance afforded through working in co-creative ways with people living with dementia, and it can present opportunities for innovation within research and practice. In our research community, therefore, the ongoing critical reappraisal and, where necessary, adaptation of the formal structures and processes which underpin our work – a transparency in assessing their affordances and their limitations – is essential to ensure their efficacy and appropriacy within the expanding field of creative and participatory methodologies with people living with dementia.

## Conclusion

This chapter brings together two distinct projects, sharing examples from research and PPIE practice to illuminate what it is *to do* creative, participatory object-based work with people living with dementia. We have shared these with attention to care aesthetics, revealing the ways in which our distinct but connected practices are relational and improvisatory, necessitate attunement and attentiveness, are grounded in the creation of spaces, both physical and affective, and foreground the sensory and aesthetic. We explore our ways of working through spotlighting specific moments within our respective projects, to share the intricacies and complexities of this work. Through our sharing of specific moments, and our subsequent discussion of our work, we posit that crafting and realising such projects involves slow and careful ways of working to allow collaboration to unfold and evolve in a way which is sensitive, and which opens space for the creative agency of people living with dementia to be expressed. There is a tendency to ignore or silence the 'invisible' aspects of this work, whether that be research or PPIE practice. Through reflecting on our practice through the care aesthetics lens, we seek to illuminate the nuances involved in meaningful, creative participatory work with people living with dementia.

## Acknowledgements

We would like to thank all participants who took part in the two case studies.

## Funding

In case study 2, this work summarises research funded by the NIHR SSCR (study reference: 102645/CM/UMCR-P197). The views expressed are those of the authors and not necessarily those of the NIHR or the Department of Health and Social Care.

## Three Key Reading References

### *Reference 1*

Lee, K. and Bartlett, R. (2021). Material Citizenship: An ethnographic study exploring object–person relations in the context of people with dementia in care homes. *Sociology of Health & Illness*, 43 (6): 1471–1485. https://doi.org/10.1111/1467-9566.13321

This paper introduces the concept of material citizenship to explore how people living with dementia in care homes relate to objects as part of their sense of identity, agency, and belonging. Their ethnographic study shows how everyday and personal objects are not simply material possessions but active participants in sustaining relationships, memories, and personhood. This perspective is crucial for understanding the creation of aesthetic objects with people living with dementia, as it reframes objects as co-constructors of citizenship and care. The paper highlights how aesthetic practices can generate spaces where dignity and identity are materially and relationally upheld.

### *Reference 2*

Manchester, H. and Willatt, A. (2024). Towards care-full co-design with older adults: A feminist posthuman praxis. *Journal of Aging Studies*, 70: 101250. https://doi.org/10.1016/j.jaging.2024.101250

In this paper, Manchester and Willatt propose a feminist posthuman approach to co-design with older adults, emphasising care, and reciprocity and relationality over extractive or instrumental models. Their praxis values more-than-human entanglements, acknowledging material, spatial, and affective dimensions alongside human voices. This perspective is vital for understanding the creation of aesthetic objects with people living with dementia, as it challenges hierarchical researcher-participant dynamics and highlights the ethics of co-creation. By framing design as 'care-full', this paper underscores how collaborative aesthetic practices can honour vulnerability, foreground agency, and generate objects and environments that embody relational care as much as artistic or functional intent.

### *Reference 3*

Fleetwood-Smith, R., Tischler, V. and Robson, D. (2022). Using creative, sensory and embodied research methods when working with people with dementia: A method story. *Arts & Health*, 14 (3): 263–279. https://doi.org/10.1080/17533015.2021.1974064

This paper highlights how creative, sensory, and embodied methods enable researchers to work meaningfully with people living with dementia, offering approaches beyond conventional verbal or cognitive frameworks. Their 'method story' shows how aesthetics, touch, sound, and movement create opportunities for co-production and self-expression, emphasising relational ways of knowing. This is important for understanding the making of aesthetic objects with people living with dementia because it demonstrates how creative practices value lived experience, foster dignity, and generate new forms of knowledge rooted in embodied connection, care, and artistic collaboration.

## References

Buse, C. and Twigg, J. (2016). Materialising memories: Exploring the stories of people with dementia through dress. *Ageing & Society*, 36 (6): 1115–1135. https://doi.org/10.1017/S0144686X15000185

Camic, P.M., Hulbert, S. and Kimmel, J. (2019). Museum object handling: A health-promoting community-based activity for dementia care. *Journal of Health Psychology*, 24 (6): 787–798. https://doi.org/10.1177/1359105316685899

Campbell, S., Dowlen, R. and Fleetwood-Smith, R. (2023). Embracing complexity within creative approaches to dementia research: Ethics, reflexivity, and research practices. *International Journal of Qualitative Methods*, 22: 1–15. Available: https://doi.org/10.1177/16094069231165932; accessed 1 March 2026.

Chamberlain, P. and Craig, C. (2013). Engaging design – Methods for collective creativity. In M. Kurosu (ed.) *Human-Computer Interaction. Human-Centred Design Approaches, Methods, Tools, and Environments.* Berlin: Springer, pp. 22–31.

Clandinin, D.J. and Connelly, F. M. (2000). *Narrative Inquiry: Experience and Story in Qualitative Research.* San Francisco: Jossey-Bass.

D'Andrea, F., Dening, T. and Tischler, V. (2022). Object handling for people with dementia: A scoping review and the development of intervention guidance. *Innovation in Ageing*, 6 (5): igac043. Available: https://doi.org/10.1093/geroni/igac043; accessed 1 March 2026.

DEEP (2023). *The dementia enquirers gold standards for ethical research.* Available: https://www.dementiavoices.org.uk/wp-content/uploads/2020/07/The-DEEP-Ethics-Gold-Standards-for-Dementia-Research.pdf; accessed 1 March 2026.

Dempster, E. (2018). Undisciplined subjects, unregulated practices: Dancing in the academy. In C. Brown and A. Longley, A. (eds.) *Undisciplining Dance in Nine Movements and Eight Stumbles*. Cambridge: Cambridge Scholars Publishing, pp. 39–48.

Dooley, J., Webb, J., James, R., Davis, H. and Read, S. (2021). Everyday experiences of post-diagnosis life with dementia: A co-produced photography study. *Dementia: The International Journal of Social Research and Practice*, 20 (6): 1891–1909. https://doi.org/10.1177/1471301220973632

Ellingson, L. (2017). *Embodiment in Qualitative Research*. New York: Routledge.

Field, B., Mountain, G., Burgess, J., Di Bona, L., Kelleher, D., Mundy, J. and Wenborn, J. (2019). Recruiting hard to reach populations to studies: Breaking the silence: an example from a study that recruited people with dementia. *BMJ Open*, 9 (11): e030829. Available: https://doi.org/10.1136/bmjopen-2019-030829; accessed 1 March 2026.

Fleetwood-Smith, R. (2020). *Exploring the significance of clothing to people living with dementia using Sensory Ethnography*. PhD thesis, The University of West London. Available: https://repository.uwl.ac.uk/id/eprint/7758/1/Rebecka%20Fleetwood-Smith_Thesis_2020.pdf; accessed 1 March 2026.

Fleetwood-Smith, R., Tischler, V. and Robson, D. (2022). Using creative, sensory and embodied research methods when working with people with dementia: A method story. *Arts & Health*, 14 (3): 263–279. https://doi.org/10.1080/17533015.2021.1974064

Fletcher, J.R., Lee, K. and Snowden, S. (2019). Uncertainties when applying the mental capacity act in dementia research: A call for researcher experiences. *Ethics and Social Welfare*, 13 (2): 183–197. https://doi.org/10.1080/17496535.2019.1580302

Gove, D., Diaz-Ponce, A., Georges, J., Moniz-Cook, E., Mountain, G., Chattat, R., Øksnebjerg, L. and European Working Group of People with Dementia. (2018). Alzheimer Europe's position on involving people with dementia in research through PPI (patient and public involvement). *Aging & Mental Health*, 22 (6): 723–729. https://doi.org/10.1080/13607863.2017.1317334

Griffiths, S., Dening, T., Beer, C. and Tischler, V. (2019). Mementos from Boots multisensory boxes—qualitative evaluation of an intervention for people with dementia: Innovative practice. *Dementia: The International Journal of Social Research and Practice*, 18 (2): 793–801. https://doi.org/10.1177/1471301216672495

Hamington, M. (2020). Care ethics and improvisation: Can performance care? In A. Stuart Fisher and J. Thompson (eds.) *Performing Care: New Perspectives on Socially Engaged Performance*. Manchester: Manchester University Press, pp. 21–35. https://doi.org/10.7765/9781526146816.00009

Harris, P. B. (ed.) (2002). *The Person with Alzheimer's Disease: Pathways to Understanding the Experience*. Baltimore: The Johns Hopkins University Press.

Hendriks, N., Slegers, K. and Duysburgh, P. (2015). Codesign with people living with cognitive or sensory impairments: A case for method stories and uniqueness. *CoDesign*, 11 (1): 70–82. https://doi.org/10.1080/15710882.2015.1020316

Heslop, J., Marsden, H. and Merritt Smit, A. (2021). Social art and participatory action research in contested urban space. *AM Journal of Art and Media Studies*, 26: 115–128. https://doi.org/10.25038/am.v0i26.475

Islam, S., Joseph, O., Chaudry, A., Forde, D., Keane, A., Wilson, C., Begum, N., Parsons, S., Grey, T., Holmes, L. and Starling, B. (2021). "We are not hard to reach, but we may find it hard to trust". Involving and engaging 'seldom listened to' community voices in clinical translational health research: A social innovation approach. *Research Involvement and Engagement*, 7 (46): 1–15. https://doi.org/10.1186/s40900-021-00292-z

Jackson, T., Pinnock, H., Liew, S. M., Horne, E., Ehrlich, E., Fulton, O., Worth, A., Sheikh, A. and De Simoni, A. (2020). Patient and public involvement in research: From tokenistic box ticking to valued team members. *BMC Medicine*, 18 (79). Available: https://doi.org/10.1186/s12916-020-01544-7; accessed 1 March 2026.

Jones, L., Cullum, N., Watson, R., Thompson, J. and Keady, J. (2025). 'Only my family can help': The lived experience and care aesthetics of being resident on an NHS psychiatric/mental health inpatient dementia assessment ward – a single case study. *Ageing & Society*, 45 (6): 1143–1164. https://doi:10.1017/S0144686X24000096

Kara, H. (2020). *Creative Research Methods: A Practical Guide*. Bristol: Policy Press.

Keady, J. (ed.) (2024). *Reconsidering Neighbourhoods and Living with Dementia: Spaces, Places and People*. Maidenhead: Open University Press/McGraw-Hill.

Keady, J.D., Campbell, S., Clark, A., Dowlen, R., Elvish, R., Jones, L., Kindell, J., Swarbrick, C. and Williams, S. (2022). Re-thinking and re-positioning 'being in the moment' within a continuum of moments: Introducing a new conceptual framework for dementia studies. *Ageing & Society*, 42 (3): 681–702. https://doi.org/10.1017/S0144686X20001014

Kontos, P. (2015). Dementia and embodiment. In J. Twigg and W. Martin (eds.) *Routledge Handbook of Cultural Gerontology*. London: Routledge, pp. 173–181.

Lahman, M.K.E., Rodriguez, K.L., Moses, L., Griffin, K.M., Mendoza, B.M. and Yacoub, W. (2015). A rose by any other name is still a rose? Problematizing pseudonyms in research. *Qualitative Inquiry*, 21 (5): 445–453. https://doi.org/10.1177/1077800415572391

Lee, K. and Bartlett, R. (2021). Material Citizenship: An ethnographic study exploring object–person relations in the context of people with dementia in care homes. *Sociology of Health & Illness*, 43 (6): 1471–1485. https://doi.org/10.1111/1467-9566.13321

Manchester, H. and Willatt, A. (2024). Towards care-full co-design with older adults: A feminist posthuman praxis. *Journal of Aging Studies*, 70: 101250. Available: https://doi.org/10.1016/j.jaging.2024.101250; accessed 1 March 2026.

McPherson, D.H.J., Dowlen, R., Bithell, C., Gagatsis, A., Young, A., Hoskin, L., Thomas, M., Riley, C. and Keady, J. (2025). Music in Mind Training: Producing a theory of change model to evaluate the implementation of an improvisation-based music-making training programme for care home staff working with people with dementia. *Dementia: The International Journal of Social Research and Practice*, 24 (5): 866–883. https://doi.org/10.1177/14713012251319589

Nunn, C. (2022). The participatory arts-based research project as an exceptional sphere of belonging. *Qualitative Research*, 22 (2): 251–268. https://doi.org/10.1177/1468794120980971

Phillipson, L. and Hammond, A. (2018). More than talking: A scoping review of innovative approaches to qualitative research involving people with dementia. *International Journal of Qualitative Methods*, 17 (1): 1–13. https://doi.org/10.1177/1609406918782784

Pickering, L. and Kara, H. (2017). Presenting and representing others: Towards an ethics of engagement. *International Journal of Social Research Methodology*, 20 (3): 299–309. https://doi.org/10.1080/13645579.2017.1287875

Pink, S. (2015). *Doing Sensory Ethnography* (2nd ed.). London: Sage.

Pottinger, L. (2021). Gentle Methodologies. In A. Barron, A. L. Browne, U. Ehgartner and S. M. Hall (eds.) *Methods for Change: Impactful Social Science Methodologies for 21st Century Problems*. Manchester: ASPECT and the University of Manchester. Available: https://aspect.ac.uk/wp-content/uploads/2021/03/Laura-Pottinger-A4-Guide-1.pdf; accessed 1 March 2026.

Pottinger, L. (2025). Treading carefully through tomatoes: Embodying a gentle methodological approach. *Area*, 57 (3), e12650. Available: https://doi.org/10.1111/area.12650; accessed 1 March 2026.

Richardson, N. and Campbell, S. (2024). Sensory attunements of caregivers and care receivers: The value of an embodied and emplaced approach in everyday care encounters. *The Senses and Society*, 19 (3): 324–336. https://doi.org/10.1080/17458927.2024.2402965

Schreiber, C. and Cürlis, D. (2022). Making the fuzzy end even fuzzier: The role of the caregiving relative in participatory design processes with people living with dementia. In P. A. Rodgers (ed.) *Design for People Living with Dementia*. Milton: Taylor & Francis Group, pp. 121–132.

Thompson, J. (2015). Towards an aesthetics of care. *Research in Drama Education: The Journal of Applied Theatre and Performance*, 20 (4): 430–441. https://doi.org/10.1080/13569783.2015.1068109

Thompson, J. (2023). *Care Aesthetics: For Artful Care and Careful Art*. London: Routledge.

Thomson, L.J.M. and Chatterjee, H.J. (2016). Well-being with objects: Evaluating a museum object-handling intervention for older adults in health care settings. *Journal of Applied Gerontology*, 35 (3): 349–362. https://doi.org/10.1177/0733464814558267

Treadaway, C., Taylor, A. and Fennell, J. (2019). Compassionate design for dementia care. *International Journal of Design Creativity and Innovation*, 7 (3): 144–157. https://doi.org/10.1080/21650349.2018.1501280

Vaughn, L.M. and Jacquez, F. (2020). Participatory research methods – Choice points in the research process. *Journal of Participatory Research Methods*, 1 (1). https://doi.org/10.35844/001c.13244.

Webb, J., Williams, V., Gall, M. and Dowling, S. (2020). Misfitting the research process: Shaping qualitative research "in the field" to fit people living with dementia. *International Journal of Qualitative Methods*, 19. Available: https://doi.org/10.1177/1609406919895926; accessed 1 March 2026.

Wilkinson, A. and Hendriks, N. (2022). The emergence of empathy through designing for one. In P. A. Rodgers (ed.) *Design for People Living with Dementia*. Milton: Taylor & Francis Group, pp. 77–90

Wilkinson, H. (ed.) (2002). *The Perspectives of People with Dementia – Research Methods and Motivations*. London: Jessica Kingsley.

Woodward, S. (2020). *Material Methods: Researching and Thinking with Things*. London: Sage.

Zeilig, H., West, J. and van der Byl Williams, M. (2018). Co-creativity: Possibilities for using the arts with people with a dementia. *Quality in Ageing and Older Adults*, 19 (2): 135–145. https://doi.org/10.1108/QAOA-02-2018-0008

# 4

# CARE AESTHETICS AND THE EXPERIENCE OF LIVING WITH SEMANTIC DEMENTIA OVER TIME

*Jackie Kindell, Caroline Swarbrick, Sion Williams and John Keady*

## Introduction

Dementia is an umbrella term caused by a range of conditions, including more common dementias, such as Alzheimer's disease and vascular dementia, as well as much rarer types of dementia (Alzheimer's Society, 2014). One of these rarer conditions is semantic dementia, a condition that presents with changes in language function, rather than difficulties with memory. It is also referred to as the semantic variant of primary progressive aphasia (Gorno-Tempini et al., 2011). Semantic dementia presents with progressive and striking communication difficulties that affect both expression and understanding, arising from progressive erosion of semantic memory, the brain's store of conceptual knowledge (Snowden, 1995; Hodges and Patterson, 2007). Expressive speech in semantic dementia is described as fluent with word-finding difficulties and an increasing lack of content words (nouns and verbs) as the disease progresses (Hodges and Patterson, 2007). Alongside these expressive difficulties, there are also increasing difficulties understanding words, at first confusing words that are close in meaning (Gorno-Tempini et al., 2011). Changes in personality and behaviour are also commonly described, particularly as the condition progresses with overlap occurring with the behavioural variant of frontotemporal dementia (Kertesz et al., 2010; Rohrer and Warren, 2010). Within the literature, studies have most often concentrated on quantitative assessment of cognition and behaviour, with little research examining conversation skills in everyday life, despite people living with this condition and their family carers identifying this as the primary focus of their difficulties.

As a speech and language therapist, Jackie was interested in how communication abilities could be supported in semantic dementia to enhance participation in social interaction. One common way to do this in dementia care is through life story

DOI: 10.4324/9781003623441-7
This chapter has been made available under a (CC BY) 4.0 license.

work, for example, using life story books or memory boxes to support conversations around the person's biography (Kindell et al., 2014a; McKeown et al., 2015). In Alzheimer's disease, such resources often stimulate conversation by prompting long-term memories, which are less affected by the condition. Given that the difficulties in semantic dementia are more focused around language and communication, Jackie wanted to explore how life story work, as a widely used intervention in dementia, could be adapted to the needs of people living with semantic dementia.

At this point, it is also useful to reflect on how supporting interaction in semantic dementia at home could be informed by a care aesthetics perspective. Care aesthetics is perhaps easiest to conceptualise in terms of the delivery of important 'care tasks', such as supporting someone to wash or dress, whereby the 'care moment' requires attention to the shared experience of the senses on both bodies involved, awareness of gaze, the voice, facial expression, other features of interaction, and the relational experience of both parties (Thompson, 2023). For example, Kindell et al. (2025) noted the foundational importance of sensory, embodied, and relational practices of healthcare support staff working with people living with dementia on hospital wards. Here, the aesthetic experience exists between the member of staff and the person living with dementia. This is consistent with the view of Thompson (2022) who argues that the 'co-created experience of a caring relationship relies on embodied skills, the sensations of the moment as it is realized between people and the shape the experience takes across time' (p. 55). Care aesthetics, however, can be used to explore other encounters in care, beyond the delivery of physical care tasks, seen for example in Campbell et al.'s (2024) analysis of improvised music making that explored the use of voice, cadence, touch, and eye contact. In this chapter, we argue that engaging a person living with advanced semantic dementia in interaction is also an example of tailored and sensitive 'care' aiming to keep the person socially engaged by drawing on the skills they retain (Ryan et al., 2005). In the data that we present, the focus is particularly on facilitating the person living with dementia's embodied skills and use of voice, and how these interactions foster moments of connection that are not necessarily reliant on linguistic information exchange, but have embodied, emotional, and social importance – points that have significant overlap with the contents of Christina Buse's Chapter (2) in this book.

## Methods of data collection

Within her PhD, Jackie used a multiple case study design to explore everyday conversation at home with five individuals living with semantic dementia and their spouses. Within each case study, data was gathered through filming conversation at home (both with and without Jackie being present) alongside biographical interviewing in a longitudinal design. Video data was analysed using conversation analysis (Sidnell, 2010) and interview data via narrative analysis (Riessman, 2008). Information derived from these strands was then used to understand interaction in the home situation. Following on from this, individually tailored life story work was then carried out in collaboration with the person living with dementia and their family focusing on how this approach could be used to support interaction in each case, termed within the context of 'interaction-focused life story work' (Kindell, 2016). As we will explain, one of these case studies, Doug and Karina, offered important additional data demonstrating a longitudinal perspective, as the couple had also taken part in an earlier project. Ethical approval for this study was given from the NHS National Research Ethics Service (reference: 12/NW/0139). Pseudonyms are used in reporting this study in line with ethical permission and the supporting research protocol.

## Case study – Doug and Karina

Doug and Karina were a married couple in their 70s who had two grown-up children. Stuart, their son, lived locally and was actively involved in their lives, whilst Nicola, their daughter, lived abroad and so saw her parents less but kept in contact by telephone. Doug worked at a local engineering college as a lecturer. Doug had been diagnosed with semantic dementia four years before Jackie's first research encounter and after several years of word-finding difficulties. Doug had first noticed changes in his language abilities six years before his diagnosis, particularly in remembering people's names. Doug and Karina had taken part in an earlier study on semantic dementia which formed part of Jackie's Master's research at The University of Manchester (Kindell, 2011) which was subsequently published in two papers (Kindell et al., 2013; Kindell et al., 2014b). At this time, Doug could be described as in the 'moderate' stages of this condition, or stage four of the six stages of semantic dementia described by Hardy et al. (2024). The couple then took part in Jackie's PhD study, and this required additional ethical approval from the appropriate research governing body and agreement from the family to reveal the link between these two studies. By this point, Doug's condition had further advanced to stage 5 (Hardy et al., 2024) and whilst the PhD work initially focused on Doug's communication at home with Karina, when Doug was admitted to long-term care during the study, the focus changed to producing relevant and useable information for the nursing home, using knowledge about Doug's interaction to help staff connect with Doug and include him in the social life of the home.

We will present data from both these time points, the Master's project and then the PhD study, to illustrate Doug's changing needs, but also how, at both points, despite significant challenges with expressive language and understanding, abilities could be seen in conversation that were supported by his family. Within the data, we will also highlight issues that relate to care aesthetics, including the use of voice and embodied aspects, as well as the emotional connections created within the encounter.

## Dataset one – Master's project data

In 2010, analysis of Doug's communication indicated that he had significant expressive and receptive language difficulties, and these issues were evident in both test situations and in everyday interaction at home. Doug was video recorded in conversation with his wife and son separately (without Jackie being present) and in conversation with Jackie (total – 44 minutes). Analysis of this interaction indicated a striking ability to 'act out' scenes when talking, using body movement, facial expression, and dialogue. In the published paper, this has been termed 'enactment' (Kindell et al., 2013). Within these conversation exchanges, Doug's abilities with verbal expression were significantly compromised; however, he could still use his voice and demonstrate a broad range of his intonation. Likewise, Doug's face was highly animated, alongside his use of body movement and pointing. This enabled him to take part in the interaction and, from a care aesthetic perspective, contribute an aesthetic dimension to the encounter 'in the moment'.

The two examples presented here are from the conversation analysis in the paper (Kindell et al., 2013), but we have chosen to present this dialogue in a more accessible version – whilst retaining some of the features of conversation analytic transcription including that: all dialogue is presented, including misstarts, pauses are timed (in brackets), and very quiet speech is marked with degree signs (°quiet words°). Where Doug used direct reported speech i.e., the actual dialogue someone might say 'in the moment', this is denoted in bold text with speech marks.

## Example 1

In this first example from a conversation recorded at home, Jackie asks Doug about going to the local grocery shop, a task (at this point in time) he did every day. In his response, Doug reveals an ability to 'act out' the scene that may occur in the shop as he greets one of the staff, including, in this example, the person in the shop's response by using facial expression, and then his associated response to this, again with facial expression:

| | |
|---|---|
| *Doug:* | I went over the (0.7) *(pointing)* I zoomed out |
| *Jackie:* | you went for a walk |
| *Doug:* | *(gestures up and down)* yeah and erm then I had to go *(pointing)* and get one or two things (1.8) that I I was short of so I just walked up there *(two hands pointing)* |
| *Jackie:* | right |
| *Doug:* | and er and I know know most of the people there you see I |
| *Jackie:* | is that at the Spar shop |
| *Doug:* | yes sorry I don't say do I I keep forgetting at the Spar shop, because it's got everything that er an I I go up and say "**hello**" (*pointing*) and there's this one one wo-woman I say "**how's things?**" *(rising intonation and* |

| | |
|---|---|
| | *smiling)* and and they they just go (0.8) (*makes a face in the pause)* I said "**and I (0.6)** (*makes another face in the pause)* **for you as well"** hhhhhh (*laughing)* |
| *Jackie:* | that's nice |
| *Doug:* | oh yeah °yeah yeah° |
| *Jackie:* | pass the time of day |

In this embodied data extract, we can see that Doug uses direct reported speech to show Jackie what he says in the shop. Direct reported speech presents the actual words used in talk (Holt, 1996), for example, Doug tells us he says to the woman in the shop, 'how's things?', instead of choosing the indirect speech version, which might be something like 'I always ask the staff how they are'. Direct reported speech does not just present the words that are spoken, it also allows the speaker to present features of the delivery of the talk at the time. So, in this extract, Doug uses intonation and facial expression to depict a friendly tone and a smiling face, not just his own but also that of the woman in the shop and this demonstrates a friendly encounter. Interestingly, this example is notable for its aesthetic qualities – the use of the voice, the body, and the emotion displayed and how it allows Doug and Jackie to connect 'in the moment', consistent with Keady et al.'s (2022) description of 'being in the moment'. In addition, it also fulfils Keady et al.'s (2022) category of 'reliving the moment' in that the encounter allowed Doug to revisit a past encounter and the positive emotion contained within it.

## Example 2

In this second example, Doug and his wife Karina are talking about going to the shops, and Karina asks if there is anything in particular that they need at the shops. In his reply, Doug does not answer by saying what they might need, instead he appears to act out what he would do, and say, in the shop:

| | |
|---|---|
| *Karina:* | so is there anything in particular you can think of that we might need or |
| *Doug:* | really (at) at that at thats: (1.7) sss you cou- as y you think about (0.2) what have we got we got to take when we get there ans so we can (2.1) an an say "**oh yeah we need to get those"** (holding out two hands as if picking something up) and then "**we've got to go and get the other ones"** (*pointing to the side with the left hand*) and "**we got to go on that ways"** (*pointing to the side with the right hand*) and and (1.2) you just you walking around and making con conversations on in relation to the the actual (2.4) ◦items that are◦ (0.6) you're looking for |
| *Karina:* | mmhm (eye contact, slight nod) |

*Doug:* thing is sometimes you you go and you think "**oh blimey forgot that one!**" (*hand forward*) and you turn round (*acting out turning right*) and walk back to get it (*hand back & right*) and carry on the next bit (*body forward*)

*Karina:* mmhm, ok did ya and you've tried your (0.8) new jumper thing on haven't you that you bought

There are potentially different aspects to analyse within this segment of Doug's talk. There is, for example, a lack of specific content words, such as nouns that carry meaning, with Doug instead using words such as 'those', 'the other ones', 'that ways', and there are quite a few pauses, mild misstarts, and repetitions. These are all signs of Doug's underlying language difficulties, his disability. However, Doug does produce a significant amount of speech within his turn, and he accompanies this with several body movements that appear to support his description of walking around the shop. As he speaks, he can change the volume of his voice and use intonation; again, the segments of direct reported speech are significantly louder and animated in terms of intonation.

Within the conversation, of equal interest and importance, is Karina's reaction to Doug's communication. She does not push Doug to give a specific answer to her question or attempt to encourage him to clarify, or repair, his vague responses. Instead, she shows a remarkable acceptance of his difficulties. Indeed, Karina found a way to respond 'in the moment' ('mmhm', whilst maintaining eye contact) that kept the conversation going whilst not highlighting Doug's lack of ability. She accepted his response as a reasonable contribution to the conversation and then moved the conversation forward ('you've tried your new jumper thing on'). Interestingly, in interviews, Karina talked about prioritising the flow of the conversation, saying 'it's not a school, [as though] it has to be right! I just know there's a word in there that isn't right, but we've got the general gist of what's going on, that's fine'. Prioritising the flow of the conversation, or progressivity, and sacrificing the need for clarification in terms of information content has been noted in other conversations with people living with dementia talking with healthcare staff and family members (Pilnick et al., 2021; Slocombe et al., 2024). In these encounters, staff and family recognise that the person living with dementia would have difficulty repairing their talk, and that the disruption to the flow of the conversation would only highlight their lack of competence. There is also an additional aesthetic aspect worth noting here, in that by maintaining the progressivity of the encounter, Karina does not disrupt the overall rhythm, or the feel, of the encounter, thus allowing for the turn taking and the rhythm to continue.

Within the 44 minutes of video taken at home, Doug is observed to use 54 utterances that contain enactment with direct reported speech, whilst there is only one instance within the talk of his wife, son, and Jackie (as the researcher). Across the video-recorded conversations in the study, Doug's body movements included pointing, demonstrating the size of objects, a generic holding gesture, and demonstrating spatial representations e.g., up, down, left, and right. He could be seen to make and maintain eye contact, use facial expression, and to change his voice in terms of volume and intonation. Doug retained a sense of turn taking, and these abilities supported him to take his turn at talk. Together, this means that whilst the content of his speech is not always easy to follow, these other abilities allowed Doug to play an active part in the encounter by either depicting, or showing, what he wanted to communicate which then took the conversation forward. At its simplest level, it was easier for Doug to do conversations this way. This is consistent with their son Stuart's observation about his dad's talk: 'You start getting the hand gestures and he'll be almost...instead of using the word, he'll be describing the action of what he'd be doing, if he was doing that thing'.

Doug's wife and son also reported that he was now more animated in conversation since his dementia, with increased use of body movements, for example. This raises the question of whether this could be an adaptation to conversation on Doug's part because of his communication impairment. Such compensatory strategies have been reported in stroke aphasia (Wilkinson, 2010) but use of 'strategies' is a concept that is applied less to those with more advanced dementia, who may be thought to lack the cognitive ability to 'be strategic' within their talk. The work of Simmons-Mackie and Damico (1997) is helpful here as through case study work, including a person with a language-led dementia, they redefined compensatory strategies as:

> ...new or expanded communicative behaviour, often spontaneously acquired and systematically employed, to overcome a communicative barrier in an effort to meet both transactional and interactional communicative goals.
>
> *(p. 770)*

In this sense, then, Doug can be seen to have naturally developed this adaptation or strategy over time by making use of the abilities he does still have. In her responses, Karina clearly describes that transfer of information is perhaps less important than the interactional, or social goal, of including Doug in family conversations. From a care aesthetics lens, Karina allows and facilitates Doug to engage using a combination of language, paralinguistic features, such as intonation and stress, along with body movements and facial expression. Together, this creates rhythmic moments between them that allow for Doug's skills to be made visible, rather than press for behaviours that would display his difficulties.

## Dataset Two – PhD data

Three years later, in 2013, Doug was still living at home with Karina but there had been significant changes in his language skills and whilst he was still fit and mobile he needed his wife to help him with most activities of daily living. Video data was gathered of Doug interacting with Karina at home without Jackie (as the researcher) being present, as well as data with Doug and Karina talking together with Jackie (one hour 32 minutes). Additional audiotaped interviews were carried out with Karina, sometimes with Doug present, and analysed (eight hours). This revealed that whilst Doug was now in the advanced stages of semantic dementia, there were still striking abilities present within his interaction and Karina continued to strive to include Doug in the conversation, reporting: 'there is still a way to communicate. He's not completely cut off… You've got the body language and the facial expressions and things to go with it haven't you [turning to Doug]?' However, when asked if Doug started up conversations, Karina replied 'it depends what you mean by conversations' going on to describe his communication as:

> Interactions rather than conversations, isn't it, whether they mean something to him but don't mean anything to the other person… now, I think he does have interactions rather than conversations…because he's communicating with people and, you know, enjoying communication.

In Jackie's fieldnotes she recorded that Doug's speech now not only contained more non-English words and repetitive syllables e.g., *dadadadadad* making it harder to understand him, but also:

> He [Doug] joins in the conversation with comments like 'brilliant' or 'oh yes' and then sometimes the odd extended bit of talk. His speech is now very hard to follow but he still has good eye contact, smiles broadly and seems very sensitive to the emotion of the moment, often mirroring that.

Analysis of the data showed that Doug continued to use enactment in his talk, as described previously, but that a further decline in his language skills meant that the content of his talk was now more difficult to follow (Kindell, 2016). Doug was still observed to be animated in conversation, give extended responses with body movements and changes in facial expression, but he would now also sometimes sing lines of his talk. These sequences of talk, or performances as they appeared to be, seemed to have a structure often with a clear end, using a clap, a stamp of the foot, or a throwing gesture as the next example illustrates.

### Example 3

Here, Karina had been talking about a staff member at the nursing home where Doug goes for day care (who always hugs him). Jackie teases Doug about this and he breaks into song (singing here is in bold text) in his response although this is not a recognisable song to those present. He abruptly ends this with a clap, says *oh sorry* (spoken, not sung) and sits still with his arms folded, looking up to indicate this abrupt finish:

*Jackie:* so who's this woman you're hugging Doug?
*Doug:* hhhhh *(head back laughing)*
*Jackie:* who's that not your wife
*Doug:* no
*Karina:* no *(said at same time as Doug)*
*Doug:* **I'll see you** *(hand out shaking)* **when you're in the in the rain** *(extensive shaking all over with arms moving up over his head) (sudden clap)* oh sorry *(suddenly sits still with arms folded and looks up and stops speaking)*
*Jackie:* hhhh *(audible laughing)*

During the analysis, Jackie reported that she was not convinced that Doug knew who the person was that they were talking about, but he seemed to sense this was a jovial exchange and was responding to that emotion 'in the moment' with his singing and body movements. Again, this allowed him to take his turn at talk which he then completed with emphasis, with a clap and clear body movements showing he had finished.

As we will see in the fourth and final example, it was also remarkable that despite the advanced stage of his condition, and the presence of a severe language disorder, Doug retained the ability to act out an upper-class English accent in his talk and he often did this in sessions, as will now be illustrated.

### Example 4

Doug, Karina, and Jackie are talking, and Karina has been joking about a friend of theirs (Jim) who is 'terribly posh' (upper-class). In response to this, Doug is observed to act out a convincing upper-class accent to display the talk of what we assume is Jim. He uses extended vowel sounds (here denoted with a ':' after each vowel), with emphasis on certain syllables (underlined) along with exaggerated body movements and facial expression, including his 'nose in the air' which is a stereotypical way upper-class people are characterised in humorous encounters in the United Kingdom. Whilst as listeners, we are unsure of the content of Jim's talk (what he said), we are clear how it was delivered – in a 'posh voice' (in bold text):

*Karina:* Jim is terribly very posh
*Doug:* **there's terribly see de de very easily see ree round there I mean you can't go around not doing anything at a:ll and you need a bit mo:re you might do a little more than you're doing now** (*shrugs shoulders)* **but just go slowly round around** *(hands up and out and chin upwards*

| | |
|---|---|
| | *nose in the air)* **I'll take you around** *(leans forward)* and I'll tell you later in about yesterday I'll have more than that thank you tush tush *(throwing gesture)* |
| *Jackie:* | off you go |
| *Karina:* | was that Jim? |
| *Doug:* | yes *(sits arms folded)* |

In this sequence, Doug's behaviour is reminiscent of his previous enactment behaviours, using his voice, body movements, and facial expression, whilst the content of his talk is harder to follow. Again, he ends the turn with a definitive *thank you tush tush* and a definite throwing gesture, which Jackie summarises as *off you go,* indicating her understanding of this. This 'posh voice' (as Karina described it) represents a surprisingly high-level skill, particularly given Doug's degree of semantic dementia. Karina goes on to explain that there was a running joke in their family that Doug himself was regarded as coming from the 'upper-classes' due to the fact he went to a private school as a child, with a 'posh voice' often acted out in family jokes.

In 2010, Karina had described changes in Doug's personality and interests and by 2013, this had changed significantly. He was less serious, no longer interested in his life-long hobby of stamp collecting, and now he liked to sing and dance. As Karina now reported, this was completely out of character for Doug as he never used to enjoy dancing:

> He can't wait to dance. You know, the dance thing is just incredible… I watched him the other day [at the day centre], they were doing the conga [dancing in a line] round the room, and [another carer said] 'gosh, you know, Doug's got such good rhythm, did he always like dancing?' 'No!' But he has. And then, he will also sing songs.

Karina reported however that whilst Doug now loved to dance, it was not something that he ever talked about: 'The very favourite thing he likes doing now is the dancing, but I don't think he uses it as a topic. He doesn't talk about that'.

## Maintaining the craft of connections in long-term care

Events overtook the study in that, in the autumn of 2013, Doug was admitted to a nursing home as it was no longer possible to meet his needs at home. Thoughts therefore turned towards ways of helping the nursing home understand Doug's needs and find ways to support his interaction. Doug had a life story book, made for him at an earlier stage of his condition. However, the book and the topics within it no longer held any interest for him, and recording his responses whilst looking through the book demonstrated either a lack of recognition or that he became frustrated when asked about items on the pages. For example, Doug's life-long passion for stamp collecting held no interest and appeared to have gone. Doug's new passion for dancing had no roots in his past, and in terms of the present, it was something he loved to do but it was not a topic that prompted conversation. His love of dance, his interest in conducting to music, and his uncanny ability to do a 'posh voice' were all embodied experiences, things he liked to do which could not be displayed in picture format to stimulate conversation. Karina and Jackie decided that the best course of action was to provide simple and accessible information for the nursing home to encourage them to interact with Doug appropriately – and to focus on interaction rather than information exchange. As a result, and as seen in Figure 4.1, Karina and Jackie produced a one-page summary focused on unique ways of 'making connections' with Doug that helped to support staff to understand and value Doug's abilities with non-verbal communication and social connection. The picture of Doug is missing from Figure 4.1 as we do not have ethical permission to share it, but it was on the original as used in everyday practice.

Past interests were only included on this sheet if they were still of current relevance, e.g., Doug still liked to look at pictures of boats and aeroplanes. Karina was keen to include a line about Doug's love of carbohydrate-rich food as she had concerns about potential weight loss. Jackie made the sheet with Karina's help and then Karina took this to the nursing home. Analysing interaction and outcomes outside of the nursing home was not part of the ethical approval for the research and therefore, engaging with the care staff was beyond this study. A lack of evidence of outcomes related to the nursing home environment is a significant, yet unavoidable, limitation. However, Karina reported that she had given the sheet to the care staff and had talked them through the information, and this had been helpful to structure this process. For example, she talked them through the music Doug liked and took some of his music into the nursing home, and they agreed to play this on the compact disc player in the quiet lounge so he could dance or conduct as he wished, reporting that 'one of the girls puts his music on and they have a dance'.

## Reflections

Care aesthetics, as proposed by Thompson (2023), argues for a synthesis of the aesthetic experiences that happen within everyday life (Saito, 2008, 2017) and the aesthetic qualities that occur between human relations (Bourriaud, 2002), delivering insight and meaning for the lives of people engaged in care relationships. This chapter has explored everyday conversations at home between Doug, a gentleman living with advanced semantic dementia, and his wife Karina and within interaction with Jackie as the researcher. The data in this chapter has demonstrated the importance of 'in the moment' social and emotional connections, and how these were accepted, facilitated, and valued at a time when information exchange, or transactional abilities, had become compromised. The distinction between transaction and interaction in linguistic theory has been reported to be particularly important for the advanced stages of dementia where maintaining social connections

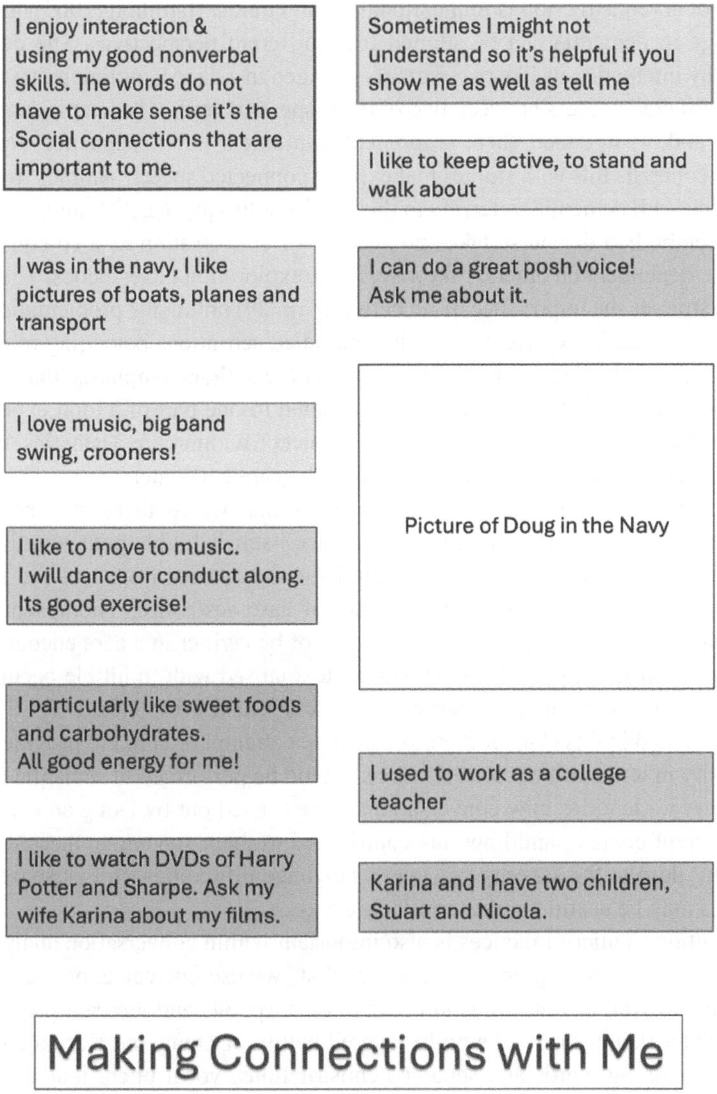


**FIGURE 4.1** Doug's A4 sheet – making connections.

may become the focus for adaptations in communication in the context of declining abilities with information exchange (Kindell et al., 2017). Karina's explanation that Doug had interactions, rather than conversations, appears to describe this issue well.

Interestingly, there is much overlap between the field of conversation analysis and the theory of care aesthetics; for example, both stress the importance of the role that both parties play to create an interactional or care encounter and this notion of co-construction is foundational to both fields. Hamilton (2005) notes that language in dementia can be studied from different perspectives. She describes everyday interaction as like two partners engaged in a dance, outlining that this is a co-constructed process between two or more speakers, rather than a product of one person and, as in dance, there is moment-to-moment interdependence. Hamilton (2005) contrasts this with studies that explore connected speech samples from people living with dementia, referring to this as 'the soliloquy' (p. 232) and argues that this disembodied discourse takes no account of conversation as a co-constructed process, dependent on others. Likewise, in his exploration of aesthetics, Thompson (2023) stresses the importance of 'in between' (p. 29) noting the problematic nature of seeing aesthetic experiences 'as the embodied sensations belonging to a single individual' and he goes on to say, maintaining the authors' emphasis, that 'there is an *in between* aesthetics, that cannot be isolated to one part of a total experience' (p. 29). Relationality, therefore, is a core concept within care aesthetics, demonstrating the interdependence of those within the care encounter.

Conversation analytical perspectives stress that whilst there may be certain conventions within interaction, the experience itself is highly contextualised and this, therefore, requires study with naturalistic data drawn from real-life settings (Sidnell, 2010). Again, in his exploration of care aesthetics, Thompson (2023) notes that whilst there may be certain norms of behaviour in a care encounter, the moment itself is a highly dynamic and contextualised with 'multiple peculiarities of skill, experience, timing, prior relations and situated knowledge' (p. 57). The data presented in this chapter therefore does not attempt or claim to provide generalisability in terms of how conversations should be performed in semantic dementia, rather it identifies how conversations were carried out by Doug and Karina in their current context, and how this contributed to them staying connected 'in the moment' despite the severity of Doug's language difficulties. In this sense, these findings may be useful to other similar contexts.

Attention to micro-practices is also important within conversation analysis and care aesthetics. Hamington (2012) argues that 'we use our voice, posture, hands, and arms as well as our minds in order to care' (p. 34) and the data presented in this chapter demonstrates the multi-layered nature of Doug and Karina's interactions, examining words and sentence constructions, vocal pitch, loudness, body movements, posture, and facial expression. Hamilton (2023) advocates that video data is critical to illuminate this multimodal analysis, and that audio-only recordings are not adequate to understand the interaction of people living with advanced dementia who communicate 'beyond words' (p. 9). There are ethical challenges in using video data to explore care with people living with advanced dementia, but we would argue data of this nature is crucial to facilitating involvement meaningful to participants whilst further exploring care aesthetics in real-life settings and, through this, lead to improved programmes of support and training for those involved in care.

Video also allows for a data-driven method, a core feature of conversation analysis (Wilkinson, 2010), and one also likely to suit the exploration of care aesthetics where use of sensory and embodied skills is highly contextualised and multilayered. This means the observable features uncovered when analysing the data drive the analysis rather than any prior hypothesis; in this way, Jackie did not set out to study enactment in semantic dementia, rather the striking nature of this became observable during detailed analysis. Care interactions, whether they be during conversation or during the delivery of care tasks, are multilayered, involving a very broad range of skills and abilities, some of which can be described but many of which are also tacit and therefore defy easy description (Thornton et al., 2017). Use of video data alongside data gathered in other ways is likely to shine a spotlight particularly on those tacit skills within care. Research of this nature, however, also requires considerable trust and commitment on behalf of participants. We are grateful to Doug and Karina for their faith in the research process and in opening their lives to this micro-scrutiny.

Within care aesthetic theory, there is also an acknowledgement that care can be refined or crafted over time (Thompson, 2023). The longitudinal data here demonstrates that this is a continuous process in family interactions in dementia. The adaptations required change over time and, as the dementia progresses, new meanings need to be found to understand experience. In the early days, Doug's difficulties were very mild with challenges in conversation relating to occasional word-finding difficulties. Earlier in his condition, looking through his life story book with him also supported topics of conversation. However, the progression of his symptoms led to increasing difficulty with verbal language and Doug adapted in conversation by using enactment or attempting to depict what he was trying to say. Within the collaborative encounter, those around him allowed, or facilitated conversations this way, with a move to focus less on the content of the words and more on the emotional and embodied aspects. At this stage, Doug's life story book was no longer a source of conversational support and many of his hobbies and interests had altered, alongside changes in his personality. Changes in interests and personality are commonly reported in the later stages of semantic dementia (Rohrer and Warren, 2010) and this presents as a challenge in the delivery of life story work (Kindell et al., 2019). The focus here as a result was less about the past and more about what encouraged interactional connections 'in the moment' (Keady et al., 2022). The life story summary sheet therefore was presented as an attempt to pass on this 'craft' of connections to the nursing home, including things that Doug liked to do now. This focused on understanding the strengths in interaction he maintained currently, rather than his deficits, as the life story summary sheet noted 'the words do not have to make sense it's the social connections that are important to me'. Supporting Doug to listen to his music and dance, or to do his 'posh voice', allowed him to relive positive moments, focusing on his strengths and facilitating quality care, or what Thompson (2023) has described as aesthetically rich moments of interaction.

## Conclusion

This chapter has outlined how adaptations within interaction occurred to keep Doug, a man living with semantic dementia, engaged in conversation at a social level. This required changes in understanding how conversation could be carried out, including an acceptance on Karina's part that information exchange was not the primary goal for interaction and facilitating Doug to draw on his abilities with body movements, facial expression, and tone of voice. This allowed Doug's participation within interaction and sustained a relational connection 'in the moment' (Keady et al., 2022). The embodied and emotional connections demonstrate the contextualised aesthetic experiences of the participants. The use of video data allowed for in-depth analysis of participant behaviours and provided a window into their everyday experiences, including analysis of micro-practices in caring conversations. Video data could be crucial to explore care aesthetics within care and interactional contexts to further understand this developing theory in practice. Lastly, whilst life story work to support interaction has commonly focused on outlining topics of interest to support talking, here the focus was on how to make embodied, sensory, and social/relational connections with an individual with dementia. This would seem to be an important focus for caring for those living with advanced dementia.

## Acknowledgements

We would like to thank Doug and Karina for inviting Jackie into their home and sharing their story at such a challenging time in their life. We would also like to thank The Dunhill Medical Trust which funded this research.

## Three Key Reading References

### *Reference 1*

Keady, J.D., Campbell, S., Clark, A., Dowlen, R., Elvish, R., Jones, L., Kindell, J., Swarbrick, C. and Williams, S. (2022). Re-thinking and re-positioning 'being in the moment' within a continuum of moments: Introducing a new conceptual framework for dementia studies. *Ageing & Society*, 42 (3): 681–702. https://doi.org/10.1017/S0144686X20001014

Drawing on several social research studies conducted by the Dementia and Ageing Research Team at The University of Manchester, this article attempts to both reframe and reposition the lived experience of dementia through a momentary conceptual framework. The authors suggest that moments experienced by people living with dementia may be fleeting or last for longer periods of time, but that all moments have significance and worth. That people living with dementia may not be able to later relive that experienced moment does not diminish its initial value, quality, or importance. The authors call for the ripple effect of such moments to be assimilated into future studies and everyday practice.

### Reference 2

Kindell, J., Wilkinson, R. and Keady, J. (2019). From conversation to connection: A cross-case analysis of life story work with five couples where one partner has semantic dementia. *Ageing & Society,* 39 (10): 2322–2345. https://doi.org/10.1017/S0144686X18000533
This paper presents the work from Jackie's PhD study with a cross-case analysis for the five couples that took part. Different life story formats are presented for each case study, for example, life story books, a music DVD, and a life story written by one man with semantic dementia on his laptop. The work responded to the needs and situation of each couple and could be conceptualised under various points of connection: interactional, emotional, new, practical, and future. This study demonstrates how life story work can foster social interaction, beyond information exchange, using both verbal and non-verbal behaviours.

### Reference 3

Hamilton, H.E. (2023). Towards a more complete picture of discourse in dementia studies. *Journal of Language and Aging Research,* 1 (1): 7–10. https://doi.org/10.15460/jlar.2023.1.1.1238
In this paper, Hamilton argues how important discourse analysis is for studying and understanding quality of life for those living with dementia. She proposes four very practical steps that researchers can take in the design of their studies to move towards a more complete picture of discourse in dementia, this is: (i) move beyond interviews and casual conversations as primary sources of data; (ii) video record activities to allow for multimodal analyses; (iii) develop sustained collaborative relationships with families, institutions, and/or individuals with dementia; and (iv) seek out partners in other disciplines.

## References

Alzheimer's Society. (2014). *Dementia UK Update.* Available: https://www.alzheimers.org.uk/sites/default/files/migrate/downloads/dementia_uk_update.pdf; accessed 1 March 2026.

Bourriaud, N. (2002). *Relational Aesthetics.* Trans. S. Pleasance and F. Woods, with M. Copeland. Dijon: Les Presses du Réel.

Campbell, S., Dowlen, R., Keady, J., and Thompson, J. (2024). Care aesthetics and 'being in the moment' through improvised music-making and male grooming in dementia care. *International Journal of Education & the Arts,* 25 (si1.13). Available: https://journals.psu.edu/ijea/article/view/63522; accessed 1 March 2026.

Gorno-Tempini, M.L., Hillis, A.E., Weintraub, S., Kertesz, A., Mendez, M., Cappa, S.F., Ogar, J.M., Rohrer, J.D., Black, S., Boeve, B.F., Manes, F., Dronkers, N.F., Vandenberghe, R., Rascovsky, K., Patterson, K., Miller, B.L., Knopman, D.S., Hodges, J.R., Mesulam, M.M. and Grossman, M. (2011). Classification of primary progressive aphasia and its variants. *Neurology,* 76 (11): 1006–1014. https://doi.org/10.1212/WNL.0b013e31821103e6

Hamilton, H.E. (2005). Epilogue: The prism, the soliloquy, the couch, and the dance - the evolving study of language and Alzheimer's disease. In B. H. Davis (ed.) *Alzheimer's Talk, Text and Context.* New York: Palgrave Macmillan, pp. 224–246.

Hamilton, H.E. (2023). Towards a more complete picture of discourse in dementia studies. *Journal of Language and Aging Research,* 1 (1): 7–10. https://doi.org/10.15460/jlar.2023.1.1.1238

Hamington, M. (2012). A performative approach to teaching care ethics: A case study. *Feminist Teacher*, 23 (1): 31–49. https://doi.org/10.5406/femteacher.23.1.0031

Hardy, C.J.D., Taylor-Rubin, C., Taylor, B., Harding, E., Gonzalez, A.S., Jiang, J., Thompson, L., Kingma, R., Chokesuwattanaskul, A., Walker, F., Barker, S., Brotherhood, E., Waddington, C., Wood, O., Zimmermann, N., Kupeli, N., Yong, K.X.X., Camic, P.M., Stott, J. and Warren, J.D. (2024). Symptom-led staging for semantic and non-fluent/agrammatic variants of primary progressive aphasia. *Alzheimer's & Dementia,* 20 (1): 195–210. https://doi.org/10.1002/alz.13415

Hodges, J. R., and Patterson, K. (2007). Semantic dementia: a unique clinicopathological syndrome. *The Lancet. Neurology*, 6 (11): 1004–1014. https://doi.org/10.1016/S1474-4422(07)70266-1

Holt, E. (1996). Reporting on talk: The use of direct reported speech in conversation. *Research on Language and Social Interaction*, 29 (3): 219–245. https://doi.org/10.1207/s15327973rlsi2903_2

Keady, J.D., Campbell, S., Clark, A., Dowlen, R., Elvish, R., Jones, L., Kindell, J., Swarbrick, C. and Williams, S. (2022). Re-thinking and re-positioning 'being in the moment' within a continuum of moments: Introducing a new conceptual framework for dementia studies. *Ageing & Society*, 42 (3): 681–702. https://doi.org/10.1017/S0144686X20001014

Kertesz, A., Jesso, S., Harciarek, M., Blair, M. and McMonagle, P. (2010). What is semantic dementia? A cohort study of diagnostic and clinical boundaries. *Archives of Neurology,* 67 (4): 483–489. https://doi.org/10.1001/archneurol.2010.55

Kindell, J. (2011). *Sustaining Conversation at Home in Semantic Dementia: A Case Study*. MClinRes Dissertation, The University of Manchester.

Kindell, J., Sage, K., Keady, J. and Wilkinson, R. (2013). Adapting to conversation with semantic dementia: Using enactment as a compensatory strategy in everyday social interaction. *International Journal of Language and Communication Disorders*, 48 (5): 497–507. https://doi.org/10.1111/1460-6984.12023

Kindell, J., Burrow, S., Wilkinson, R. and Keady, J. (2014a). Life story resources in dementia care: A review. *Quality in Ageing and Older Adults,* 15 (3): 151–161. https://doi.org/10.1108/QAOA-02-2014-0003.

Kindell, J., Sage, K., Wilkinson, R. & Keady, J. (2014b). Living with semantic dementia: A case study of one family's experience. *Qualitative Health Research*, 24 (3): 401–411. https://doi.org/10.1177/1049732314521900

Kindell, J. (2016). *Interaction-Focused Life Story Work in Semantic Dementia: A Mixed Methods Study*. PhD thesis, The University of Manchester. Available: https://pure.manchester.ac.uk/ws/portalfiles/portal/54577705/FULL_TEXT.PDF; accessed 1 March 2026.

Kindell, J., Keady, J., Sage, K. and Wilkinson, R. (2017). Everyday conversation in dementia: a review of the literature to inform research and practice. *International Journal of Language & Communication Disorders*, 52 (4): 392–406. https://doi.org/10.1111/1460-6984.12298

Kindell, J., Wilkinson, R. and Keady, J. (2019). From conversation to connection: A cross-case analysis of life story work with five couples where one partner has semantic dementia. *Ageing & Society,* 39 (10): 2322–2345. https://doi.org/10.1017/S0144686X18000533

Kindell, J.A., Harman, K., Maguire-Rosier, K., Polonyi, R., Thompson, J. and Keady, J.D. (2025). Exploring the everyday care practices of healthcare support workers when working with people with dementia admitted to National Health Service hospital wards in the United Kingdom: a qualitative systematic review of the literature. *Aging & Mental Health*, 29 (5): 915–927. https://doi.org/10.1080/13607863.2024.2447319

McKeown, J., Ryan, T. and Clarke, A. (2015). 'You have to be mindful of whose story it is': The challenges of undertaking life story work with people with dementia and their family carers. *Dementia: The International Journal of Social Research and Practice,* 14 (2): 238–256. https://doi.org/10.1177/1471301213495864

Pilnick, A., O'Brien, R., Beeke, S., Goldberg, S. and Harwood, R. (2021). Avoiding repair, maintaining face: Responding to hard-to-interpret talk from people living with dementia in the acute hospital. *Social Science & Medicine*, 282, Article 114156. Available: https://doi.org/10.1016/j.socscimed.2021.114156; accessed 1 March 2026.

Riessman, C.K. (2008). *Narrative Methods for the Human Sciences.* Thousand Oaks California: Sage.

Rohrer, J.D. and Warren, J.D. (2010). Phenomenology and anatomy of abnormal behaviours in primary progressive aphasia. *Journal of Neurological Sciences*, 293 (1–2): 35–38. https://doi.org/10.1016/j.jns.2010.03.012

Ryan, E.B., Byrne, K., Spykerman, H. and Orange, J.B. (2005). Evidencing Kitwood's personhood strategies: Conversation as care in dementia. In B. H. Davis (ed.) *Alzheimer Talk, Text and Context*. Basingstoke: Palgrave Macmillan, pp. 18–36.

Saito, Y. (2008). *Everyday Aesthetics*. Oxford: Oxford University Press.

Saito, Y. (2017). *Aesthetics of the Familiar: Everyday Life and World-Making*. Oxford: Oxford University Press.

Sidnell, J. (2010). *Conversation Analysis: An Introduction*. Chichester, West Sussex: Wiley-Blackwell.

Simmons-mackie, N.N. and Damico, J.S. (1997). Reformulating the definition of compensatory strategies in aphasia. *Aphasiology*, 11 (8): 761–781. https://doi.org/10.1080/02687039708250455

Slocombe, F., Peel, E., Pilnick, A. and Albert, S. (2024). Keeping the conversation going: How progressivity is prioritised in co-remembering talk between couples impacted by dementia. *Health: An Interdisciplinary Journal for the Social Study of Health, Illness and Medicine*, 28 (2): 272–289. https://doi.org/10.1177/13634593221127822

Snowden, J.S. (1995). Semantic dementia: A form of circumscribed cerebral atrophy. *Neurocase*, 1 (1): 39–54.

Thompson, J. (2022). Care aesthetics, coronavirus and everyday life. *Performance Research,* 27 (6–7): 54–61. https://doi.org/10.1080/13528165.2022.2197525

Thompson, J. (2023). *Care Aesthetics: For Artful Care and Careful Art*. London: Routledge.

Thornton, T., Crepaz-Keay, D., Birch, S. and Verhaegh, J. (2017). Generating nursing knowledge. In M. Chambers (ed.) *Psychiatric and Mental Health Nursing: The Craft of Caring*. London: Routledge, pp. 51–60.

Wilkinson, R. (2010). Interaction-focused intervention: A conversation analytic approach to aphasia therapy. *Journal of Interactional Research in Communication Disorders*, 1 (1): 45–68. https://doi.org/10.1558/jircd.v1i1.45

# 5

# DOING CARE AESTHETICS

## Dress, grooming, and appearance-related practices in dementia care settings

*Sarah Campbell and Rebecka Fleetwood-Smith*

### Introduction

This chapter explores what a care aesthetics lens can offer in understanding the relational, multisensory, embodied, and affective practices within dementia care. We focus specifically on dress, grooming, and other forms of appearance-related personal care to demonstrate how care aesthetics provides a framework for examining the fine-grained details within care relationships, emphasising the sensory, material, and embodied nature of these encounters (Thompson, 2023). We are interested in how care aesthetics can illuminate the micro-practices of care work that often go unrecognised, revealing the skilled, artful nature of caring practices and helping to value the complex work undertaken in social care settings.

Care aesthetics attends to process, soundscapes, touch, and visual spotlighting as dimensions through which care unfolds (Campbell et al., 2024), offering insights into the artful practices of care encounters that are often rendered invisible. Through this lens, we can examine the embodied and sensory dimensions of caring practices, identifying the intricate work involved in moments of care that other approaches may overlook. We suggest that care aesthetics brings particular value to dementia studies by moving beyond individualised care practices to consider the relational, processual, and dynamic ways in which care practices are enacted through bodies, materials, environments, and relations that extend beyond the person.

Drawing on case examples from our respective doctoral research, we explore three interconnected areas that illuminate the *doing* of care aesthetics: appearance practices that move beyond person-centred care; care enacted with, for, and through materials; and the tensions and complexities that emerge within care encounters. Through these examples, we demonstrate how a care aesthetics framework reveals

DOI: 10.4324/9781003623441-8
This chapter has been made available under a (CC BY) 4.0 license.

the intercorporeal, collaborative nature of care work whilst attending to the atmospheric, temporal, and material dimensions of caring encounters.

We also identify opportunities to further develop the care aesthetics framework, particularly around questions of material agency, expansive care practices that exceed formal care relationships, and the tensions within structural contexts within which care unfolds. Whilst care aesthetics offers valuable insights into the complexity and skilled nature of care work, we suggest there is scope to expand the framework to more fully account for the ways materials actively participate in care encounters, how people living with dementia engage in self-care practices, and how institutional and structural forces shape what kinds of care practices become possible.

Our approach draws on the recent shift towards more-than-human approaches in dementia studies, which seek to de-centre the human to recognise the interdependent things at play within care encounters. We position this exploration as contributing to ongoing conversations about how care aesthetics might be developed to encompass the entangled, relational, and emergent nature of caring practices within institutional settings. We attend throughout to the tensions between care aesthetics' emphasis on process, attunement, and embodied temporalities and the structural organisation of care work through schedules, task completion, and efficiency metrics, examining how these competing demands fundamentally shape what kinds of care practices become possible. Through examining appearance-related care in dementia settings, we hope to demonstrate both the valuable insights that care aesthetics provides and the potential for further theoretical development within this growing field.

## From person-centred to relational care in dementia studies

Nearly 30 years ago, Kitwood (1997) proposed 'person-centred care' as a corrective to the dehumanising tendencies of some treatment contexts and caregiving relationships. Whilst person-centred care has been instrumental in transforming dementia care practice, there are calls to expand the approach to address gaps in its implementation, such as the focus on the individual, and the problematic ways in which it positions people living with dementia as passive recipients of care. Further, the term is used as a catch-all, without agreement on how it should be implemented in practice, particularly when considering how it is possible to equitably provide this kind of care within collective care settings (Dewing and McCormack, 2015; Pilnick, 2022).

Critics argue that person-centred care reinforced an individualistic rather than relational understanding of care (Bellas et al., 2019). Relational approaches to dementia care emphasise how care practices manifest and are constructed between people, recognising that care emerges through relationships rather than being simply delivered to individuals. When considering bodywork specifically, as we are within this chapter, it is vital to recognise that bodies are not passive recipients; they can resist, respond, and actively participate in care encounters. A relational care approach acknowledges the importance of the quality of relational work between care worker and resident (Gurung and Chaudhury, 2025) and presents space for understanding the nuanced, intercorporeal dimensions of such encounters. Recognising the importance of embodied selfhood is essential to this, to ensure that personhood is understood beyond cognition and verbal interactions, and allows for recognition of non-verbal communications through gestures, bodily expression, and movement (Kontos, 2004).

Buse and Twigg (2015) extend this understanding of intercorporeal relations to show how identity becomes 'intertwined' not just between bodies but also through material objects and practices. In their work on appearance-related care, they demonstrate how, when people living with dementia could no longer articulate preferences, care workers engaged in 'curating identity' on their behalf, drawing on biographical knowledge to maintain what Campbell and colleagues (2015) term 'appearance signatures', distinctive aspects of dress central to someone's sense of self. This collaborative work extends beyond individual dyads; Ward et al. (2016a, 2016b) demonstrate how, in care-based hair salons, multiple bodies synchronise: hairdresser, care worker, therapeutic assistant, and person living with dementia working intercorporeally to accomplish care tasks that would be impossible individually. Ward et al. (2016b) term this 'embodied narrative support' (p. 1297), bodywork practices that simultaneously attend to physical care needs and co-construct biographical narratives.

Approaches that centre the citizenship of people living with dementia shift the discourse away from the notion that a person living with dementia is living primarily in need of care. Relational citizenship, as proposed by Kontos et al. (2017), focuses on the lived experiences of people with dementia in long-term care environments and is premised on the importance of interdependence and relational practices between people. The model recognises that 'the capacities, senses, and socio-cultural dispositions of the body are central to self-expression, interdependence, and the reciprocal nature of engagement' (Kontos et al., 2017, p. 23). Whilst relational citizenship positions people living with dementia as active, agentic citizens, we suggest the paradigm may be expanded to examine the ways in which care is co-produced between and beyond people. That is, the things that make up the space, the infrastructure, the architecture and so forth shape and make care practices, and understanding these relational practices requires attention to the structural conditions that shape care work.

## Critical perspectives on care work and structural constraints

Understanding relational approaches to care requires examining the structural conditions within which care work unfolds. Armstrong (2013) argues that care occurs within intersecting systems of inequality, where women make up most residents, workers, and care workers, with the workforce increasingly comprised of racialised women and immigrants (see also: Twigg et al., 2011). Daly (2013) explores how care practices in neoliberal contexts are constrained by an emphasis on efficiency, task completion, and measurable outcomes that override the relational and temporal qualities of care work. Drawing on her critique, we use the term 'ethos of efficiency' to describe how these priorities become embedded as a dominant value system within care settings. Lee-Treweek's (1994) concept of making residents 'lounge-ready', preparing residents with dementia for public spaces whilst potential abuse and coercion remain hidden in private spaces like bedrooms, illustrates how appearance-related care can serve institutional presentation rather than individual needs. These analyses reveal how the structural organisation of care fundamentally shapes what kinds of practices are possible, often constraining the very relational and embodied attention that residents require.

Care relationships are shaped by intersecting systems of power based on gender, race, class, age, sexuality, and disability status (Hulko, 2023). This intersectional analysis becomes particularly important when examining appearance-related care practices, as cultural differences in grooming, religious requirements around clothing and bodily care, and gendered expectations about appearance all shape how such care is provided and received (Armstrong and Day, 2020).

The concept of 'bodywork', paid work undertaken on the bodies of others, provides a lens through which to examine care practices in dementia settings (Twigg et al., 2011). Twigg and colleagues' (2011) work argues for recognising the centrality of bodily manipulation, touch, and physical intimacy in care practices, dimensions that are often downplayed or rendered invisible. This perspective is particularly relevant for appearance-related care, as it attends to the physical, tactile, and embodied dimensions of washing, dressing, and grooming which often take place in the private spaces of bathrooms and bedrooms. However, these relations unfold within troubling structural conditions. The skills and knowledge required for competent care work are systematically devalued, particularly when performed by marginalised workers (Twigg et al., 2011). Residents with dementia can resist or refuse care, yet care workers retain opportunities to exert control (Lee-Treweek, 1994), revealing how bodywork involves questions of consent, autonomy, and the potential for both care and abuse within intimate bodily encounters.

The materiality of appearance-related care extends beyond bodies to encompass the material properties of dress itself. Hayman (2009) suggests dressing involves working with 'two materialities of very different substance and in constant juxtaposition, body and cloth' (cited in Buse and Twigg, 2018, p. 343). These material constraints shape what is possible in care encounters, with fabrics and fastenings acting back on care workers and residents. Moreover, institutional laundry regimes and infection control requirements mean delicate fabrics, wool, and silk are often discouraged, fundamentally limiting the sensory and tactile dimensions that contribute to well-being (Buse and Twigg, 2018). This reveals how care practices cannot be separated from institutional infrastructures.

## Care aesthetics: theoretical framework

Care aesthetics then offers a framework for examining these embodied encounters in their complexity. Drawing upon Thompson (2020, 2023) and Saito (2017, 2022, 2023), we recognise that care is enmeshed with aesthetic sensibilities that require ethical cultivation and practice. Puig de la Bellacasa (2017) cautions that care is never neutral, rather it is both ethical and political, using the term 'as well as possible care' and considering the question of 'how to care?' (p. 11). As detailed within our presentation of dementia care models, there is often a gap in implementation, meaning the everyday, micro-practices that make up moments of care are largely ignored. We look to care aesthetics as a framework to explore care practices within dementia care settings between and beyond people.

Care aesthetics attends to process, soundscapes, touch, and visual spotlighting as dimensions through which care unfolds (Campbell et al., 2024). It illuminates the artful practices of care encounters, attending to the embodied and sensory to identify the intricate practices involved in moments of care. Campbell et al. (2023) demonstrate how creative research methods reveal these practices through what they term 'attunement and attentiveness', requiring researchers to access and engage with the senses of others by first being attuned to their own sensory perceptions. Kindell et al. (2025) demonstrate that healthcare support workers undertake this sensory attunement through 'tuning in', drawing on their full sensory perceptions during intimate care work. This 'full-bodied' approach to understanding care work foregrounds how creativity in research enables a more interconnected and multidimensional engagement with the experience of others. Thompson (2023) notes that 'good' care practices are often deemed elusive, yet there are vast opportunities to attend to the attentive, embodied, sensory, and dynamic processes at play.

This framing recognises care as fundamentally embodied performance. Hamington (2004) emphasises that all care is received and delivered through the body, with our bodies serving as the epistemological and imaginative basis for care. This extends beyond simple physical contact to encompass the use of the body, exercise of touch, tone of voice, awareness of space, and the construction of practice across time; all contributing to care aesthetics experiences. Campbell et al.'s (2024) empirical work on hairdressing in dementia care demonstrates how these dimensions operate in practice: process has pace and rhythm determined by attending to the person rather than merely completing tasks; soundscapes include the cadence of conversation, silence, and ambient sounds; touch is always bidirectional, varying from firm to gentle; and visibility involves both being witnessed and the visual presentation of care.

Time emerges as a particularly significant dimension of care aesthetics. Thompson (2023) identifies time as having an embodied, sensory aspect vital to understanding care aesthetics, noting the tension between clock-based time and task-based time. Bunting (2020) describes how carers find themselves caught between these temporal modes, where clock-based time divides experience into predictable, quantifiable portions, whilst embodied care tasks have rhythms that cannot be paced out in precise minutes. This temporal dimension shapes power dynamics within care settings, as strict time allocations can prevent the execution of quality care and create normative atmospheres that constrain rather than support caring relationships (Sumartojo and Pink, 2018; Campbell, 2019; Thompson, 2023). Yoshizaki-Gibbons (2025) demonstrates how institutional and bureaucratic time structures shape all bodily care routines in care settings, from toileting schedules to dressing times, revealing how temporal organisation fundamentally determines what kinds of care encounters become possible.

Caring is characterised as a holistic investment of thought, sensation, and emotion, resisting fragmentation inherent in purely technical approaches. Importantly, the intersection with performance philosophy suggests that caring is inherently improvisational and caregivers draw upon rehearsed skills to responsively perform care 'in the moment', with normativity emerging from relational experience rather than being imposed a priori (Hamington, 2020). This requires what Lecoq (2000) termed *disponibilité* which describes a state of openness and readiness characterised by being available, present, listening, and flexible. For people living with advanced dementia, this focus on embodied, moment-by-moment encounters aligns with Killick and Allan's (2001) emphasis on meeting people 'in the moment', repositioning dementia care from technical task completion to valuing the craft and artfulness of caring practices.

## Everyday aesthetics and the visibility problem

Attending to care aesthetics moves away from the traditional 'spectator-oriented judgemental model of aesthetics' (Saito, 2023, p. 11) to highlight the situated, embodied, and sensorial experience of being-in-the-world (and see Julian C. Hughes' opening chapter in this book, especially his eighth point 'no aesthetics without ethics'). This is significant when considering the lives of people with dementia, where someone's outward appearance is often stigmatised and judged (Twigg, 2010), leaving little room to understand the many practices and processes at play that contribute to a person's appearance (Fleetwood-Smith et al., 2022), let alone the embodied and sensory feel of appearance (Ward and Campbell, 2013).

Yet, appearance-related care in institutional settings is also subject to what might be termed a 'visibility problem', connecting directly to Lee-Treweek's (1994) concept of the 'lounge-ready' resident, where the focus falls on producing a visually presentable 'end product' rather than the relational and embodied processes of care itself. Buse and Twigg (2018) reveal how dress becomes an aesthetic indicator of care quality, with managers, families, and regulatory bodies judging care through residents' appearance. This creates tensions between care aesthetics as experienced through, for example, the feel of clothing, familiar routines, the comfort of 'worn' clothes, and care aesthetics as displayed through presentable, coordinated dress. When residents refused to change soiled clothing, care workers faced a 'catch 22': leaving someone in dirty clothes constitutes neglect, whilst forcing change violates consent (Buse and Twigg, 2018, p. 349). The emphasis on visual presentation can thus prioritise institutional aesthetics over residents' embodied comfort. Ward et al. (2014) demonstrated that appearance is as much about how it feels as how it looks, with people's sense of self tied to embodied sensations such as a clean-shaven chin or the texture of familiar fabrics. This suggests that when appearance-related care focuses only on the visual presentation, it may overlook the multi-sensory dimensions that matter most to people living with dementia.

Saito (2022) writes that care is a site where the ethical and aesthetic are deeply entrenched and posits that care for everyday 'things' involves essential but 'invisible' care practices. She draws attention to the embodied and sensory nature of everyday acts of caring for items, claiming that active engagement with 'things' through care and maintenance forms an aesthetics of care by spotlighting how practices of maintaining, cleaning, washing, and repairing are ubiquitous caring acts. Her attention to these intricacies informs our exploration of sensory experiences, materiality, and aesthetics in the context of dementia and the care home setting.

## Doing care aesthetics

Within this chapter, we attend to the 'doing of care aesthetics'. When proposing care aesthetics, Thompson (2023) suggests examining 'caring about, caring for, care-giving, care-receiving, caring-with and...witnessing care' (p. 66). We suggest that considering care aesthetics as 'doing' may be particularly important in the context of dementia studies as we attempt to move beyond positioning the person living with dementia as living in 'need' of care, or as the 'other' whom care is 'done to'. To consider a notion of 'doing', care aesthetics may be helpful in illuminating processual, dynamic, and relational practices and allow us to consider the interdependent things that make up such encounters. This may also allow room to consider how people living with dementia care for themselves (and others/things). Campbell et al. (2023) note that embracing creative approaches to understanding care requires rigorous planning, generous timelines, and interdisciplinary research teams, yet such approaches are essential to illuminate the often-invisible aspects of care work. Doing care aesthetics speaks to the liveliness of care practices and builds upon 'care aesthetics in practice' (Thompson, 2023, p. 72).

## Expanding care aesthetics – materials, expansive care, and structural contexts

Our interest in doing care aesthetics and the interdependent things at play during moments of care speaks to opportunities for further developing care aesthetics frameworks. Attention to spatialising practices reveals how carers actively assemble care environments through strategic arrangements of objects and furniture. Ward et al. (2016a, 2016b) show how care-based hairdressers transform nondescript spaces into 'knowable places' through material staging, positioning chairs, mirrors, and tools to create therapeutic 'place-events' that provide sensory cues enabling people living with dementia to enact familiar roles.

Attending to more-than-human dimensions also requires recognising that materials can be 'unruly', not simply passive or smoothly integrated into care practices. Buse and Twigg's (2014) study illustrated how handbags became too heavy or developed 'leaky' boundaries; clothing similarly resisted when residents changed out of 'appropriate' dress or tore off imposed items (Buse and Twigg, 2018). These moments of material resistance reveal care as inevitably messy and contested. Care workers sometimes responded through what Mol et al. (2010) term 'tinkering', or creative improvisation, such as buying multiple identical cardigans for a resident who wanted to 'wear the same cardigan all the time' (cited in Buse and Twigg, 2018, p. 349). Such tinkering illustrates how care aesthetics unfolds through ongoing negotiation with resistant materials, constrained resources, and competing demands to demonstrate creative, artful, and improvised care.

Recent developments in dementia studies point towards more-than-human approaches that seek to de-centre the human to recognise the interdependent things at play within care encounters (Katz and Leibing, 2023). These approaches offer possibilities for expanding care aesthetics frameworks to more fully account for material agencies, self-care practices, and the assemblages of people, objects, spaces, and policies that shape care encounters.

Having established care aesthetics as a valuable framework for illuminating the artfulness and complexity of care work, whilst identifying areas for further development, we now turn to case examples from our research.

## Situating our doctoral studies

### *'Atmospheres of dementia care: stories told through the bodies of men' – Sarah Campbell (2019)*

Sarah is a white British, cisgender woman from working-class origins and a first-generation university graduate. Her work in dementia studies began in the early 2000s, and she has first-hand experience of dementia care services through both her father and father-in-law. Her sensory and critical ethnography explored the everyday embodied lives of seven men living with dementia in residential care and a National Health Service (NHS) mental health ward for older people. Data collection used participant observation with extensive fieldnotes, attention to sensory environments, and bodily experiences, plus some video data – the methodology engaged through attuned perceptiveness to relationships between senses and environment (Abram, 1997; Ingold, 2015). Pseudonyms are used for the purpose of study reporting. NHS Research Ethics Committee approval: 11/WA/0147.

### 'Exploring the significance of clothing to people living with dementia using sensory ethnography' – Rebecka Fleetwood-Smith (2020)

Rebecka is a white British, cisgender woman, researcher, and textile artist working at the intersection of creative practice and health research. Her sensory ethnographic doctoral research explored the importance of clothing and textiles in the lives of people with early-mid-stage dementia in a care home setting. She worked with residents, staff, and creative practitioners using multisensory creative methods, including thematic elicitation cards and object handling sessions. Her research foregrounded knowing 'through the body', using audio-recording, fieldnotes, and video to capture and re-engage with encounters. Her approach was underpinned by Pink's (2015) sensory ethnography. NHS Research Ethics Committee approval: 18/LO/1707.

In the codes for Rebecka's study: P = participant (followed by their number in the study); PWD = person living with dementia; CHS = care home staff; RFS = Rebecka Fleetwood-Smith's data set.

### *Sharing case examples from our doctoral studies*

Before sharing case examples from our doctoral studies, we briefly reflect on the sharing of the words and experiences of the people that we worked with. Working with people living with dementia and care home staff is complex and involves sensitive, ethical practices (see, for instance, Campbell et al., 2023). Within our research, we adhered to practices to ensure the confidentiality of those we worked with. We did this differently. In the case of Rebecka's doctoral research, she used codes over pseudonyms due to concerns at the time around the selection of pseudonyms on behalf of the people she worked with. Whilst this was an attempt to avoid ascribing an assumed identity through using a specific pseudonym (Lahman et al., 2015), the practice of using codes in place of names can create a sense of distance when re-engaging with the words and experiences of participants. Sarah adopted carefully considered pseudonyms, selecting names that were culturally and generationally appropriate whilst acknowledging the ethical complexity of researcher-selected pseudonyms (Lahman et al., 2015). Here, we share a brief insight into the tensions and complexities involved in this work and how we both, in different ways, sought to practice careful, ethical research.

## The doing of care aesthetics

In the following section, we bring together case examples from our doctoral studies to explore three areas of interest that illuminate the *doing* of care aesthetics. We situate examples under three sections: (i) Appearance practices and care aesthetics – beyond person-centred care; (ii) Care for, with, and through materials;

and (iii) Tensions, complexities, and resistive practices. We do not formalise these areas as themes; rather, they are topics that derived iteratively through our discussions and our interest in relational care practices, care aesthetics, and our recent engagement with more-than-human centred approaches.

Within these sections, we draw on key concepts from the literature review to analyse our case examples. In examining appearance practices, we apply the lens of 'embodied narrative support' (Ward et al., 2016b, p. 1297) and intercorporeal work (Ward et al., 2016a, 2016b). When investigating care enacted through materials, we draw on spatialising practices (Ward et al., 2016b) and Saito's (2022) aesthetics of care for everyday things. In exploring tensions and resistance, we return to the visibility problem and power dynamics within bodywork (Lee-Treweek, 1994; Buse and Twigg, 2018). Throughout, we attend to the four dimensions of care aesthetics identified by Campbell et al. (2024): process, soundscapes, touch, and spotlighting. Through our case examples and intertwined discussion, we seek to expand understandings of care aesthetics in practice.

## *Appearance practices and care aesthetics – beyond person-centred care*

### *Male facial shaving as embodied narrative support*

Appearance is not simply an external signal of identity or a measure of 'good' care but something deeply felt, embodied and linked to gender, culture, age, and biographical narrative. For men living with dementia in care settings, facial shaving represents a particularly significant site where identity, masculine selfhood, and everyday care practices intersect.

For the men in Campbell's (2019) study, white British men aged 72–92, all with military service backgrounds, being clean-shaven held particular value associated with respectability and discipline. Male facial shaving is typically learned from fathers, performed in private bathroom spaces, and closely tied to masculine identity (Retallack, 1999). The deterioration of ability to shave oneself through dementia's impact thus challenges men's capacity to uphold their personal presentation of masculinity. Yet, shaving also presents practical difficulties: aged skin becomes more sensitive and craggier due to wrinkles and folds; care staff receive little formal training in wet shaving techniques; the task requires careful negotiation of mood and comfort. As one care worker noted, 'it [shaving] is very difficult. I think you have to assess what kind of mood they are in' (Campbell, 2012). Care settings for people living with dementia are gendered spaces where the predominantly female workforce navigates intimate facial touch with men. Female care workers in Campbell's (2019) study described shaving as particularly problematic, worrying about hurting men during this close bodily encounter, revealing how gender shapes the atmospherics and embodied dynamics of such care practices (see also: Sandberg, 2018).

Drawing on Sarah Campbell's (2019) PhD study data, the following encounter demonstrates how care aesthetics illuminates the intercorporeal, biographical, and sensory dimensions of this everyday care practice:

> Brigit puts a towel around Samuel's front and shoulders and sprays shaving foam, rubbing it across his face. He has his eyes closed and his mouth open. I ask Samuel if he has always been clean shaven or if he has ever had a moustache or beard and he says 'oh God no!' Brigit begins to shave, pulling the razor one way and then the other. I ask if he has always had wet shaves rather than an electric razor and he says 'oh yes'. Brigit says she has never done a wet shave before and Samuel says 'now you tell me!'
>
> Samuel says 'don't chop away' and Brigit says 'ok I'm trying not to' and begins to pull the razor for longer sweeps. Samuel has a frown on his face, and I ask him if his skin is sensitive and he says 'yes it is'. For a short time, I hear the scrapes of the razor across the skin and whiskers. Brigit moves around Samuel's face, and he keeps his eyes shut. She is on his chin and the strokes are shorter; Samuel seems to move his face with the razor pulling his mouth up to push out his chin. It is quite fast and Brigit says, 'I've done it'. I ask him how it is being shaved by someone else and he says, 'it depends on who does it, sometimes it's chop chop chop'. I ask him what having a shave is like and he says 'horrible, you want to get it out of the way quickly with as little discomfort as possible'. Then he says, 'you often don't have a lot of time before work and then away you go'. [Fieldnotes, Primrose dementia ward]

This encounter exemplifies 'intercorporeal achievement', where both bodies work together to accomplish the shaving task (Ward et al., 2016b, p. 1299). As Brigit moves the razor, 'Samuel seems to move his face with the razor pulling his mouth up to push out his chin' and this indicates how Samuel's face coordinates with her razor strokes, his body responding to and facilitating her movements. Despite Brigit's inexperience with wet shaving, they find a rhythm together through ongoing verbal negotiation: 'don't chop away' prompts responsive adjustment to 'longer sweeps', demonstrating how bodies and voices work together to shape the care encounter.

This negotiation requires what Yoshizaki-Gibbons (2025) identifies as 'giving time' to one another, both Samuel and Brigit slowing down institutional rhythms to attend to the embodied requirements of the task, creating a temporal opening within scheduled care routines. Attending to care aesthetics dimensions reveals the complexity beneath this mundane task. **Process** has particular temporal quality and Samuel notes 'you want to get it out of the way quickly' and 'you often don't have a lot of time before work', situating shaving within rhythms of his former working life. **Touch** is central, with Samuel's sensitive skin requiring careful navigation; quality depends on 'who does it, sometimes it's chop chop chop'. The **soundscape** shifts between verbal exchanges, humour ('now you tell me!'), and moments where 'I hear the scrapes of the razor across the skin and whiskers' sound providing sensory feedback about close shave quality. **Visibility** focuses on the clean-shaven result, yet what remains largely invisible is the collaborative embodied work required to achieve it, the attentiveness to facial movements, skin texture, and mood, which without this research encounter go unnoticed behind bedroom doors.

This encounter exemplifies what Ward et al. (2016b) call 'embodied narrative support' (p. 1297) which shows bodywork practices that simultaneously attend to physical care needs and co-construct biographical narratives. Samuel's emphatic responses 'oh God no!' to ever having facial hair and 'oh yes' to always preferring wet shaves assert a lifelong commitment to being clean-shaven. His reference to shaving 'before work and then away you go' connects this bodily practice to his biography as a working man with routines and standards, even though that working life belongs to his past.

A tension emerges that illuminates why embodied narrative support matters: Samuel describes shaving as 'horrible' and wanting to minimise discomfort yet maintains exacting standards about how it must be done. The discomfort is worth enduring because the identity work accomplished through being clean-shaven matters more. For Samuel and other men with military backgrounds, where clean-shaven appearance signified respectability and discipline, this daily bodily practice upholds masculine selfhood even as cognitive and physical abilities decline. Brigit's work is not simply removing facial hair but upholding Samuel's sense of himself as a respectable, well-groomed man. This demonstrates an aesthetic of care that extends beyond the visible to the felt, embodied experience of maintaining identity through everyday practice.

## *Caring with, for, and through materials*

The built environment, everyday items, and technologies shape care practices and quality of life in care settings. Drawing on Saito's (2022) aesthetics of care, we recognise material items as ever-changing as how we use and care for them alters over time, particularly in dementia care settings. Focusing on clothing and items close to hand allows us to spotlight how material objects become crucial to doing care aesthetics, shifting attention from what someone looks like to explore sensed, felt, embodied experiences of care as emplaced practice.

### *Expansive care: hidden labour behind visible appearance*

Some care home staff demonstrated expansive approaches that saw care as performed through caring for a person's clothing and appearance. The laundering process creates challenging dynamics, such as items going to laundry, being shrunk, damaged, or lost. As one participant living with dementia described in Rebecka's study: 'You have no idea when they might be taken away…they can't go on their own obviously, but they might wind up in the laundry'. To alleviate such concerns, a staff member offered to hand-wash a resident's underwear: 'Do you want me to do it for you – I can wash it if it is only knickers or brassiere or socks?' The care home resident said, 'Is it true?' 'Yeah, it is not a big deal I can do it for you' and that is when she said, 'Oh you are so nice!' (P8).

Such micro-practices exemplify what Yoshizaki-Gibbons (2025) terms 'making time' for residents, where care workers create temporal space for relational attention despite institutional pressures that render such work invisible and uncompensated. Though the staff member says, 'it is not a big deal', such instances are, in fact, of utmost importance as they demonstrate the expansive role of care work. Care home staff in Rebecka's study similarly shared how care practices extended to repairing and altering clothing: 'Yeah, if not we can get the thread or something to repair it if we got time'; 'Well, the length of her inside leg is 23 inches, and she had trousers that were 29 and 30 inches...I do them on the sewing machine, I do them quite quickly'.

This expansive care work reveals a different dimension of the visibility problem from Lee-Treweek's (1994) concept of residents being made 'lounge-ready'. Whilst that work identified how visible presentation can mask coercive care happening in private spaces, these examples demonstrate how positive, skilled care work remains invisible and undervalued too. These practices maintain the lounge-ready appearance that signals care quality to external observers, yet the actual labour involved happens behind the scenes and goes unrecognised as the artful care work it represents. They illuminate artful care practices through attentiveness, sensitivity, and skill, whilst also highlighting care done 'in spite of' task-oriented expectations (Thompson, 2023, p. 114). The unfixedness of things requires ongoing maintenance, repair, and alteration to ensure items remain usable and comfortable. Yet, such practices raise questions about care overflowing boundaries. As Puig de la Bellacasa (2017) cautions, 'too much care can be consuming' (p. 85) and 'devouring for women and other marginalised carers' (p. 167) – where do such offers end, what is a staff member's capacity, and which residents receive them? There is a tension here in considering the overflowing ways in which care is practised, and how care may be at once complex, exhausting, challenging, and rewarding. Spotlighting the minutiae of care practices involved in supporting a person's appearance illuminates the ways in which a person's outward appearance is made up of many moments of care.

### *Pockets as portable territories: spatialising practices of self-care*

Small items close to hand can be particularly meaningful in care homes where people are not surrounded by personal possessions and spontaneous engagement with things is limited. During our studies, people often carried items on or close to the body in pockets, handbags, or on walking aids. Pockets housed countless items: wallets, handkerchiefs, glasses, jewellery, and sweets. They could be rummaged in as distraction, places to discover things, habitual homes for belongings, and as spaces unseen and accessed only by the wearer.

One participant in Rebecka's study frequently expressed difficulty living in the care home, which she did not consider home, adopting strategies to demonstrate resistance. Reaching into her pocket, she said: 'Having pockets means that I can carry my business cards' (P1, PWD). Her business cards retained connection to her career, a significant and meaningful part of her life, not unlike Samuel reflecting on his biography as a working man during his shave. These echoes Ward et al.'s (2016b) concept of 'spatialising practices', where the participant transforms her pockets into knowable places holding her professional identity, creating therapeutic 'place-events' within the constraining care home environment. Her handling of the card, reading it, turning it over, and placing it securely back was important. Using pockets to carry items close to hand yet hidden from view (from staff, other residents, and visitors) acted as care for oneself, a way to move conceptually beyond the care home.

In Campbell's (2019) study, Harry always wore the same outdoor jacket. When asked about it, Harry patted his jacket pockets: 'This is the one that I stuck to actually, I quite like…I like this jacket…it's comfortable. And it's got plenty of little things where I can put my peppermint…I've got my fags [cigarettes]' (Harry, Lincoln Manor). This jacket, an important aspect of his 'appearance signature' (Ward et al., 2014), suggested gendered importance regarding pockets where Harry kept everyday things, including his valuable cigarettes. He always wore outdoor clothing, even inside, showing preparedness for going outside for a cigarette; when he returned, Harry would extract his mints from his pockets to share with his friends. As in Buse and Twigg's (2014) work on handbags, Harry's pockets held a personal world in private space.

Harry is doing care aesthetics through his preference for outdoor clothing and a jacket with pockets, care aesthetics perceived not as interaction between Harry and a care worker, but as Harry's attention to his own needs, ensuring preparedness by keeping things with him, ready to take himself for a cigarette as and when desired. Harry's patting of his jacket knowingly, feeling his things are with him, demonstrates what Saito (2022) terms care for everyday things not simply care done to objects, but also care enacted through them, creating a tactile aesthetics of self-care. This represents the inverse of the visibility problem: care aesthetics as experienced by the person themselves rather than displayed for institutional presentation, invisible to those judging care quality through appearance alone yet central to the person's embodied sense of autonomy and preparedness.

### *Tensions, complexities, and resistive practices*

Care home environments are complex settings where residents living with dementia, care staff, family members, and friends engage in ongoing, unfixed interactions centred on care. Care in relation to clothing and appearance is often, as

Thompson (2023) writes, 'visual-centric' (p. 66), bringing with it surveillance and a sense that care can be monitored and evaluated according to appearance. This is particularly powerful when considering clothing practices. People living with dementia are often reported to demonstrate challenging and difficult behaviours. It is increasingly advocated that these behaviours be reconsidered and repositioned as expressive ways in which people living with dementia communicate. In recent years, researchers have suggested the term 'post-verbal' (Quinn and Blandon, 2017; Wood, 2020) to account for the different ways in which people living with dementia communicate and to decouple sensory and embodied routes to communication from a deficiency-oriented perspective. This understanding, combined with the notion of doing care aesthetics, allows us to examine the embodied, sensory, and affective ways in which caring practices are realised when we spotlight the resistive ways that people living with dementia express themselves. We explore here how people living with dementia shape their care, considering clothing and appearance as expressive tools.

*Resistance as communication*

> Whenever somebody put on the trousers, he would undo it and then try to get it off. It took a very long time to understand the whole concept behind it because this resident wanted to go to the toilet independently.
>
> *(P7; CHS; RFS)*

This example illustrates the visibility problem we identified in our review at the start of this chapter. The man's resistance to wearing trousers was initially read through the lens of institutional concern about appropriate appearance ('lounge-ready' presentation), interpreted as sexual disinhibition (Campbell, 2012). However, the attentiveness of staff through their own sensory perceptions enabled them to engage with the senses of others, to 'tune in' (Kindell et al., 2025), revealing that this was about embodied experience: a functional need for independence in using the toilet. What appeared to be behaviour requiring management was actually sophisticated communication about care needs. Through this understanding, the man started wearing elasticated waist trousers which enabled him to continue using the toilet independently. Resistance itself becomes a communicative aesthetic practice here, expressed through the repeated process of undoing trousers and the touch-based experience of fastening mechanisms that no longer met his needs. Understanding resistance as communicative aesthetic practice reframes what is often pathologised as 'behaviour that challenges' (Dupuis et al., 2012) into embodied, sensory communication. In this example, skilled staff demonstrated attunement to bodily cues and creative interpretive capacities, drawing on their knowledge of the person to recognise that repeated undoing of trousers communicated a need for independence rather than representing problematic behaviour. Ward et al. (2008) identified a pressing need for a vocabulary to articulate these skilled interpretive practices that care workers enact, but struggle to describe, calling for 'a new lexicon of dementia care' (p. 647). Care aesthetics provides such a framework, making visible the artful, skilled work of interpreting diverse forms of embodied expression, whilst the concept of communicative aesthetic practice, in this instance, extends this lens to resistance and behaviours often dismissed as symptomatic of dementia.

As detailed earlier, one of the participants in Fleetwood-Smith's (2020) study frequently expressed how difficult she found living in the care home. During a research encounter, she spoke about the challenges and complexities that staff and care home residents navigate. The following account demonstrates challenges around bodily autonomy, agency, consent, and care practices:

> At other times they wanted to do other things really… other things that I said that they must not, could not and should not. They wanted to take my blood pressure, and I said no you can't, it is mine!
>
> *(P1, PWD)*

This participant's resistance to blood pressure monitoring reveals the power dynamics inherent in bodywork (Twigg et al., 2011). Her statement, 'it is mine' asserts bodily autonomy within institutional contexts where bodies are routinely worked upon by others. Rosendal et al. (2025) document similar resistance in long-term care, where an older woman repeatedly opposed care workers' attempts to medicalise her body and space, insisting 'I'm not ill, I'm just old'. Like the participant in Fleetwood-Smith's study, her attempts to assert control were often overruled, revealing how resistance may not translate into recognised agency when older people's self-knowledge conflicts with biomedical care regimes. Whilst this extract does not speak explicitly to clothing and appearance, it speaks to the complexity of bodywork and a person's sense of agency and autonomy (or lack of) within the setting. This account is unsurprising given the participant's feelings about the care home and sense of resistance and frustration at living there. When we think of doing care aesthetics here, we can consider this a resistive and communicative practice, one which, for this individual, was necessary to enact her agency. It was not within the remit of Fleetwood-Smith's (2020) research to explore how this may have been navigated by others involved, yet this example speaks to the complexities involved in encounters of care and how feelings of uncertainty and lack of autonomy, exacerbated by task-oriented routines and structures, and how they can permeate moments of care.

### *Atmospheres of resistance: private spaces and public soundscapes*

In Campbell's (2019) study, she describes 'atmospheres of resistance' that emerge as disruptions to the task and time-scheduled ordering of the everyday. Campbell (2019) describes 'resistance stories' that unfold and illuminate the micro-politics of 'space, gender, bodies, atmospheres and everyday life' (p. 178). Personal care and appearance-related practices scheduled to manage bodywork were tension points in the daily schedule, where a resident may, in fact, not be ready to be bathed, dressed, or shaved. To echo Lee-Treweek (1994), these activities were often not visible but took place in the private space of bedrooms and bathrooms, yet their effects spilled into public corridors through soundscapes of distress.

During a fieldwork observation on Sandbridge Ward, a mixed NHS mental health ward for older people, Sarah sat in a corridor with a participant, Larry, when cries and shouts could be heard coming from one of the bedrooms, the sounds of bodily care being enacted on someone resisting. This interaction was recorded in Sarah's fieldnotes as follows:

> Larry mimics the sounds and turns to [Sarah] and laughs, he then says 'getting killed, poor devil'.
>
> *(19 December 2011)*

Larry's mimicry creates what Campbell et al. (2024) identify as a significant soundscape dimension of care aesthetics. Here, Larry acknowledges the experience and shows empathy at the challenging sounds permeating the corridor, recognising the distress of a fellow resident. His laughter alongside his words captures the complexity of living in an environment where private struggles become public through sound, where the process of scheduled care clashes with embodied resistance.

Another resident on Sandbridge Ward, Don, regularly refused to change into his pyjamas at night or have his morning shave, and his care records noted his 'lack of compliance' around these personal care activities. Don's resistance represents a temporal disruption whereby his body's rhythm and readiness were not aligning with institutional schedules. The touch-based intimacy of changing clothes or shaving required the resident to show readiness for the activity, yet scheduled care allows little room for the improvisation that such readiness demands. The label 'lack of compliance' exemplifies how resistance is framed as deficit rather than communication (Dupuis et al., 2012), demonstrating the tension between care aesthetics as experienced by the person and care as monitored through institutional documentation focused on lounge-ready presentation over embodied comfort. This pathologising of resistance in scheduled care is not unique to acute settings. Rosendal et al. (2025) document similar dynamics in long-term care, where an older woman repeatedly refused care workers' attempts to change her clothing and body care routines. When she insisted on keeping trousers the care worker deemed 'too small', asserting 'I'll use them until I die', her resistance was interpreted as risk rather than legitimate preference. Like Don's refusal, her attempts to maintain control over her body and its temporal rhythms were positioned within institutional documentation as problematic behaviour requiring intervention rather than as expressions of bodily autonomy.

Both cases reveal how care regimes construct compliance with scheduled routines as normative, rendering any deviation, regardless of the person's own comfort or readiness, as a care deficit requiring correction rather than as communicative aesthetic practices expressing bodily autonomy and embodied needs. These cases illuminate a fundamental tension in what we consider the *doing of* care aesthetics within institutional contexts. Whilst care aesthetics attends to process, improvisatory attunement, and the sensory dimensions through which care unfolds, institutional structures demand compliance with schedules, documentation of outcomes, and risk management that prioritise efficiency over attunement. The soundscapes of resistance that permeate corridors, the temporal misalignments between bodily readiness and scheduled routines, and the documentation that frames refusal as deficit rather than communication, all reveal how aesthetic dimensions of care exist in friction with organisational imperatives. Rosendal et al. (2025) argue that care practices 'rooted in ideals of autonomy and the home as inviolable, often undermine these ideals in paradoxical ways' (p. 1). Similarly, when care aesthetics is practised within institutional rhythms that cannot accommodate meeting the person where they are at, the very attention to sensory experience and embodied readiness that such practices require may paradoxically highlight the impossibility of its full realisation. This tension suggests that care aesthetics not only offers a framework for recognising 'good' care but also serves as a critical tool for making visible the structural constraints that prevent aesthetic attunement revealing an ethos of efficiency and where embodied care ethics come into irreconcilable conflict.

## Conclusion

Through examining male facial shaving, pockets as portable territories, and resistance in scheduled care, this chapter has demonstrated how attending to situated, embodied, sensory, and material practices reveals what it means to *do* care aesthetics. Our cases illuminate care as intercorporeal where bodies synchronise. Samuel moved his face with Brigit's razor strokes, and care staff and residents worked together to accomplish intimate care tasks that would be impossible individually (Ward et al., 2016a, 2016b). They show care enacted through materials: Harry's jacket pockets holding his cigarettes and mints, business cards carried as portable connections to professional identity, and elasticated waistbands enabling continued independence in using the toilet. And they reveal care as communication, where acts of resistance convey meaning. Larry's mimicry acknowledged his fellow resident's distress, Don's refusal to change into pyjamas asserted his body's temporal rhythms, and the participant insisted 'it is mine' when claiming bodily autonomy over blood pressure monitoring.

These examples reveal multiple dimensions of what we term the visibility problem in appearance-related dementia care. Lee-Treweek's (1994) concept of 'lounge-ready' residents identified how visible presentation can mask coercive practices happening in private spaces. Our cases extend this analysis in two directions. First, they demonstrate how positive, skilled care work also remains invisible and undervalued. The handwashing of underwear, the hemming of trouser legs, and the careful navigation of sensitive aged skin during wet shaving all represent what Thompson (2023) notes as care done 'in spite of' (p. 114) task-oriented expectations, yet they occur behind closed doors, unrecognised as the artful work they represent. Second, our cases reveal care aesthetics as experienced by people living with dementia themselves rather than displayed for institutional presentation. Harry's knowing pat of his jacket pockets, checking his things are with him, demonstrates what Saito (2022) terms care for everyday things. This is not care done to objects, but care enacted through them, creating a tactile aesthetics of self-care invisible to those judging care quality through appearance alone, yet central to his embodied sense of autonomy and preparedness.

Attending to the four dimensions of care aesthetics (process, soundscapes, touch, and spotlighting) as identified by Campbell et al. (2024) revealed the complex negotiations within these encounters. Samuel's shaving demonstrated process shaped by the temporal rhythms of 'getting it out of the way quickly' before work, even though that working life belongs to his past. Soundscapes shifted between humour ('now you tell me!') and the scraping of razor across whiskers. Touch required navigation of sensitive skin where quality depends on 'who does it, sometimes it's chop chop chop'. Spotlighting focused on the clean-shaven result, whilst the collaborative embodied work remained largely invisible behind bedroom doors. Larry's mimicry of sounds emanating from private spaces created what we identify as resistive soundscapes permeating corridors, making audible the clash between scheduled care and embodied resistance. These dimensions operate not as discrete categories but as entangled elements of care encounters that cannot be separated from one another or from the materials, spaces, and institutional rhythms within which they unfold.

Yet, our cases also illuminate a fundamental tension in practising care aesthetics within institutional contexts. Whilst care aesthetics attends to process, improvisatory attunement, and the sensory dimensions through which care unfolds, institutional structures demand compliance with schedules, documentation of outcomes, and risk management that prioritise an 'ethos of efficiency' over embodied attentiveness. Don's refusal to follow nighttime and morning routines, documented as 'lack of compliance', exemplifies how resistance is framed as deficit rather than communication. Rosendal et al. (2025) show this pattern across care settings with an older woman asserting 'I'll use them until I die' about her preferred trousers, which had her resistance interpreted as risk requiring intervention rather than legitimate preference. Both cases reveal how care regimes construct compliance with scheduled routines as normative, rendering any deviation (regardless of the person's own comfort or readiness) as problematic behaviour requiring correction.

Rosendal et al. (2025) argue that care practices 'rooted in ideals of autonomy and the home as inviolable, often undermine these ideals in paradoxical ways' (p. 1). Our analysis extends this insight. When care aesthetics is practised within institutional rhythms that cannot accommodate the improvisatory attunement it requires (what theatre practitioner and educator Lecoq (2000) termed *disponibilité*, a state of openness and readiness characterised by being available, present, listening, and flexible), the very attention to sensory experience and embodied readiness that care aesthetics foregrounds may paradoxically highlight the impossibility of its full realisation. This concept of *disponibilité* is resonant with care aesthetics' roots in embodied performance practice (Thompson, 2023). This tension suggests that care aesthetics offers not only a framework for recognising 'good' care but also serves as a critical analytical tool for making visible the structural constraints that prevent aesthetic attunement, revealing how intersecting systems of inequality (Armstrong, 2013) and, what we term an 'ethos of efficiency' (drawing on Daly, 2013), come into irreconcilable conflict with embodied care ethics.

The notion of *doing* care aesthetics proves particularly valuable in addressing this tension. Rather than positioning people living with dementia solely as recipients of care, we attend to how they actively participate in appearance-related practices. Harry ensured his cigarettes and mints remained accessible; one participant transformed pockets into portable territories holding professional identity, and resistance itself operated as sophisticated communication about care needs. These reveal care as co-produced through ongoing negotiations between bodies, materials, spaces, and temporalities. This aligns with relational citizenship's recognition that agency and citizenship are processual and interdependent (Kontos et al., 2017), whilst expanding the framework through more-than-human approaches (Katz and Leibing, 2023) to encompass the material agencies at play. Handbags became too heavy, clothing resisted when torn off, elasticated waistbands enabled continued independence, and pockets created knowable places within constraining environments (Mol et al., 2010; Buse and Twigg, 2014; Ward et al., 2016a, 2016b; Buse and Twigg, 2018).

Understanding these rich, nuanced complexities through care aesthetics illuminates what Thompson (2023) identifies as the elusiveness of 'good' care practices. Our cases show such practices are not elusive because they lack skill or artfulness but because they remain invisible. They occur behind closed doors, unrecognised in documentation focused on visual presentation, undervalued when performed by marginalised care workers, and existing in friction with institutional structures that cannot accommodate their improvisatory, relational, and temporal requirements. Attending to the fine-grained details of embodied narrative support, intercorporeal synchronisation, and material tinkering makes visible the skilled, artful nature of these practices whilst simultaneously revealing the structural impossibilities care workers navigate daily.

This represents a radical shift from deficit-oriented models focused on 'maintaining' and 'preserving' towards understanding that we are all in a constant state of becoming. Samuel maintained masculine selfhood through the daily practice of being clean-shaven despite cognitive and physical decline (Ward et al., 2014; Buse and Twigg, 2015). Harry's jacket enabled preparedness for the cigarette breaks that structured his day. Participants transformed constraining spaces through material practices of self-care. This is no less true for people living with dementia than for anyone else. Foregrounding the entangled, relational, and emergent nature of caring practices through a care aesthetics lens that attends to process, soundscapes, touch, and spotlighting offers a potentially radical route to exploring futures of dementia care that move beyond individualised, deficit-focused approaches towards recognition of care as lively, co-produced, and fundamentally more-than-human.

As we are developing our engagement with approaches that de-centre the human whilst recognising the interdependent things at play within care encounters (Katz and Leibing, 2023), we anticipate that this emerging area holds significant potential for radically reimagining dementia care. We see value in continuing to develop thinking around *doing* care aesthetics through moment-based approaches that attend to the sensory, material, and structural dimensions of care practices. This will require innovative research methods that can access and illuminate these often-invisible dimensions. As Campbell et al. (2023) note, embracing creative approaches to understanding care requires rigorous planning, generous timelines, and interdisciplinary collaboration. We hope to draw on our knowledge and engagement with co-creative, sensory, and material-based approaches to develop our work within this expanding area of research and practice, attending to how care aesthetics might be practised differently when institutional structures are reimagined to accommodate the improvisatory attunement, temporal flexibility, and relational attention that aesthetic care encounters require.

## Three Key Reading References

### *Reference 1*

Hulko, W. (2023). Revolutionising dementia policy and practice: Guidance from 'the memory girl', an accomplice. In R. Ward and L. J. Sandberg (eds.) *Critical Dementia Studies: An Introduction.* London: Routledge, chapter 16. Available: https://www.taylorfrancis.com/chapters/oa-edit/10.4324/9781003221982-21/revolutionising-dementia-policy-practice-wendy-hulko?context=ubx&refId=9a5c7e53-ae8b-4411-807c-457da8753800; accessed 1 March 2026.

This chapter is pivotal in shifting dementia research and practice towards a more inclusive, justice-oriented future. Hulko offers a radical reimagining of dementia care through anti-oppression gerontology, integrating intersectional feminist, queer, critical race, and disability perspectives. Her concept of the 'accomplice' resonates strongly with our own ethical and political stance throughout this chapter, where we foreground the systemic inequalities shaping care work and the lived experiences of people with dementia. Hulko's emphasis on counter-storytelling, cultural safety, and the destabilisation of dominant discourses aligns with our use of care aesthetics not only as a framework for recognising relational, sensory, and embodied practices, but also as a critical tool for making visible the institutional constraints that inhibit aesthetic attunement. We see this chapter by scholar Wendy Hulko as foundational to our thinking and as a key text for readers seeking to understand how care aesthetics can be mobilised in solidarity with diverse lived experiences and structural critique.

### *Reference 2*

Fleetwood-Smith, R., Tischler, V. and Robson, D. (2022). Aesthetics and dementia: Exploring the role of everyday aesthetics in dementia care settings. *Design for Health*, 6 (1): 91–113. https://doi.org/10.1080/24735132.2022.2074207

This paper positions the importance of everyday aesthetics within dementia care settings, identifying the ways in which aesthetics permeates everything – from the design and use of everyday items to the provision of activities, to opportunities for engagement, and relational approaches to care. Through a series of creative, sensory, and embodied approaches to working with people living with dementia, this paper reveals the ways in which people living with dementia engage with everyday aesthetics and express their aesthetic preferences. Whilst this paper predominantly focuses on engagement with materials and objects, it does explore the ways in which foregrounding aesthetic experiences promotes opportunities for relational care practices. Implicitly, this paper invites us to explore what dementia care could look and feel if rich aesthetic experiences were privileged. This chapter builds upon this emergent thinking, to attend to the material, sensory, and relational dimensions that shape moments of care.

### *Reference 3*

Campbell, S., Buse, C., Twigg, J., Keady, J. and Ward, R. (2015). Appearance matters: It's integral to our sense of self. *Journal of Dementia Care*, 23 (2): 20–23.

This practice-oriented article introduces the concept of multi-sensory appearance biographies, offering a method for bringing embodied and sensory dimensions into life story work in dementia care. It foregrounds the significance of appearance in maintaining identity and personhood and highlights how everyday routines, objects, and tactile experiences can support more relational and person-centred care. Although written some years ago, this piece laid the groundwork for our current chapter's development of 'doing care aesthetics' – not as a fixed framework, but as a dynamic, relational, and critical practice. It reflects our longstanding commitment to recognising the artfulness and complexity of appearance-related care, and our desire to build theory that remains deeply applicable to practice. The article's emphasis on attunement, sensory engagement, and ethical reflection continues to shape our thinking, and we see this chapter as an extension of that work – one that contributes to the growing field of critical dementia studies by making visible the structural and aesthetic dimensions of care and moving beyond the limits of person-centred approaches.

## References

Abram, D. (1997). *The Spell of the Sensuous: Perception and Language in a More-than-Human World*. New York: Vintage Books.

Armstrong, P. (2013). A gendered analysis of long-term residential care. In P. Armstrong and S. Braedley (eds.) *Troubling care: Critical Perspectives on Research and Practices*. Toronto: Canadian Scholars, pp. 59–70.

Armstrong, P. and Day, S. (2020). Clothing matters: Locating wash, wear, and care. *Studies in Political Economy/Recherches en économie politique*, 101 (1): 1–16. https://doi.org/10.1080/07078552.2020.1738777

Bellass, S., Balmer, A., May, V., Keady, J., Buse, C., Capstick, A., Burke, L., Bartlett, R. and Hodgson, J. (2019). Broadening the debate on creativity and dementia: A critical approach. *Dementia: The International Journal of Social Research and Practice*, 18 (7–8): 2799–2820. https://doi.org/10.1177/1471301218760906

Bunting, M. (2020). *Labours of Love: The Crisis of Care*. London: Granta Books.

Buse, C. and Twigg, J. (2014). Women with dementia and their handbags: Negotiating identity, privacy and 'home' through material culture. *Journal of Aging Studies*, 30 (1): 14–22. https://doi.org/10.1016/j.jaging.2014.03.002

Buse, C.E. and Twigg, J. (2015). Clothing, embodied identity and dementia: Maintaining the self through dress. *Age, Culture, Humanities*, No. 2. Available: https://ageculturehumanities.org/WP/clothing-embodied-identity-and-dementia-maintaining-the-self-through-dress/; accessed 1 March 2026.

Buse, C. and Twigg, J. (2018). Dressing disrupted: Negotiating care through the materiality of dress in the context of dementia. *Sociology of Health & Illness*, 40 (2): 340–352. https://doi.org/10.1111/1467-9566.12575

Campbell, S. (2012). A close shave: Masculinity and bodywork in dementia care. *Graduate Journal of Social Science*, 9 (3): 87–95.

Campbell, S. (2019). *Atmospheres of Dementia Care: Stories told through the bodies of men*. PhD thesis, The University of Manchester. Available: https://core.ac.uk/reader/365179054; accessed 1 March 2026.

Campbell, S., Buse, C., Twigg, J., Keady, J. and Ward, R. (2015). Appearance matters: It's integral to our sense of self. *Journal of Dementia Care*, 23 (2): 20–23.

Campbell, S., Dowlen, R. and Fleetwood-Smith, R. (2023). Embracing complexity within creative approaches to dementia research: Ethics, reflexivity, and research practices. *International Journal of Qualitative Methods*, 22: 1–15. Available: https://doi.org/10.1177/16094069231165932; accessed 1 March 2026.

Campbell, S., Dowlen, R., Keady, J., and Thompson, J. (2024). Care aesthetics and 'being in the moment' through improvised music-making and male grooming in dementia care. *International Journal of Education & the Arts*, 25 (si1.13). Available: https://journals.psu.edu/ijea/article/view/63522; accessed 1 March 2026.

Daly, T. (2013). Imagining an ethos of care in policies, practices and philosophy. In P. Armstrong and S. Braedley (eds.) *Troubling Care: Critical Perspectives on Research and Practices*. Toronto: Canadian Scholars' Press, pp. 33–46.

Dewing, J. and McCormack, B. (2015). Engagement: A critique of the concept and its application to person-centred care. *International Practice Development Journal*, 5 (Suppl 6): 1–8. Available: https://www.fons.org/wp-content/uploads/2024/03/IPDJ_05suppl_06.pdf; accessed 1 March 2026.

Dupuis, S.L., Wiersma, E. and Loiselle, L. (2012). Pathologizing behavior: Meanings of behaviors in dementia care. *Journal of Aging Studies*, 26 (2): 162–173. https://doi.org/10.1016/j.jaging.2011.12.001

Fleetwood-Smith, R. (2020). *Exploring the significance of clothing to people living with dementia using Sensory Ethnography*. PhD thesis, The University of West London. Available: https://repository.uwl.ac.uk/id/eprint/7758/1/Rebecka%20Fleetwood-Smith_Thesis_2020.pdf; accessed 1 March 2026.

Fleetwood-Smith, R., Tischler, V. and Robson, D. (2022). Aesthetics and dementia: Exploring the role of everyday aesthetics in dementia care settings. *Design for Health*, 6 (1): 91–113. https://doi.org/10.1080/24735132.2022.2074207

Gurung, S. and Chaudhury, H. (2025). Relationship-centered care for older adults in long-term care homes: A scoping review. *Journal of Applied Gerontology*, 44 (9): 1513–1532. https://doi.org/10.1177/07334648241309761

Hamington, M. (2004). *Embodied Care: Jane Addams, Maurice Merleau-Ponty, and Feminist Ethics*. Chicago: University of Illinois Press.

Hamington, M. (2020). Care ethics and improvisation: Can performance care? In A. Stuart Fisher and J. Thompson (eds.) *Performing Care: New Perspectives on Socially Engaged Performance*. Manchester: Manchester University Press, pp. 21–35. https://doi.org/10.7765/9781526146816.00009

Hayman, E. (2009). Dressing made tangible: Disability perspectives. In E. Rouse. (ed.) *Conference Proceedings 2009 Fashion & Well-Being?* International Foundation of Fashion Technology Institutes. London: The Centre for Learning and Teaching in Art and Design. Available: https://opus.lib.uts.edu.au/handle/10453/11285; accessed 1 March 2026.

Hulko, W. (2023). Revolutionising dementia policy and practice: Guidance from 'the memory girl', an accomplice. In R. Ward and L. J. Sandberg (eds.) *Critical Dementia Studies: An Introduction*. London: Routledge, chapter 16. Available: https://www.taylorfrancis.com/chapters/oa-edit/10.4324/9781003221982-21/revolutionising-dementia-policy-practice-wendy-hulko?context=ubx&refId=9a5c7e53-ae8b-4411-807c-457da8753800; accessed 1 March 2026.

Ingold, T. (2015). *The Life of Lines*. London: Routledge.

Katz, S. and Leibing, A. (2023). 'Lost in time like tears in rain': Critical perspectives on personhood and dementia. In R. Ward and L. J. Sandberg (eds.) *Critical Dementia Studies: An Introduction*. London: Routledge, chapter 6. Available at: https://www.taylorfrancis.com/books/oa-edit/10.4324/9781003221982/critical-dementia-studies-richard-ward-linn-sandberg?refId=11c60a23-97d4-4a27-b200-1ff68986d09d&context=ubx; accessed 1 March 2026.

Killick, J. and Allan, K. (2001). *Communication and the Care of People with Dementia*. Buckingham: Open University Press.

Kindell, J., Maguire-Rosier, K., Polonyi, R., Thompson, J., Cleasby, R., Watson, R. and Keady, J.D. (2025). Healthcare support workers working with people with dementia on mental health wards: A practice model informed by care aesthetics. *Qualitative Health Research*, 1–14. Online First (December). Available: https://doi.org/10.1177/10497323251393890; accessed 1 March 2026.

Kitwood, T. (1997). *Dementia Reconsidered: The Person Comes First*. Buckingham: Open University Press.

Kontos, P. (2004). Ethnographic reflections on selfhood, embodiment and Alzheimer's disease. *Ageing & Society*, 24 (6): 829–849. https://doi.org/10.1017/S0144686X04002375

Kontos, P., Miller, K.L. and Kontos, A.P. (2017). Relational citizenship: Supporting embodied selfhood and relationality in dementia care. *Sociology of Health & Illness*, 39 (2): 182–198. https://doi.org/10.1111/1467-9566.12453

Lahman, M.K.E., Rodriguez, K.L., Moses, L., Griffin, K.M., Mendoza, B.M. Yacoub, W. (2015). A rose by any other name is still a rose? problematizing pseudonyms in research. *Qualitative Inquiry*, 21 (5): 445–453. https://doi.org/10.1177/1077800415572391

Lecoq, J. (2000). *The Moving Body: Teaching Creative Theatre*. London: Methuen Drama.

Lee-Treweek, G. (1994). Bedroom Abuse: The hidden work in a nursing home. *Generations Review*. Available: https://pureportal.bcu.ac.uk/en/publications/bedroom-abuse-the-hidden-work-in-a-nursing-home; accessed 1 March 2026.

Mol, A., Moser, I. and Pols, J. (2010). *Care in Practice: On Tinkering in Clinics, Homes and Farms*. London: Transaction Publishers.

Pilnick, A. (2022). *Reconsidering Patient Centred Care: Between Autonomy and Abandonment*. Leeds: Emerald Publishing Limited.

Pink, S. (2015). *Doing Sensory Ethnography*. London: Sage.

Puig de la Bellacasa, M. (2017). *Matters of Care: Speculative Ethics in More than Human Worlds*. Minnesota: University of Minnesota Press.

Quinn, C. and Blandon, C. (2017). The potential for lifelong learning in dementia: A posthumanist exploration. *International Journal of Lifelong Education*, 36 (5): 578–594. https://doi.org/10.1080/02601370.2017.1345994

Retallack, G.B. (1999). Razors, shaving and gender construction: An inquiry into the material culture of shaving. *Material Culture Review*, 49 (Spring): 1–15. Available: https://journals.lib.unb.ca/index.php/MCR/article/view/17782; accessed 1 March 2026.

Rosendal, K.A., Langstrup, H. and Krøll, V. (2025). The choreographies of the elimination of faeces: An ethnographic study of the institutionalized body care practices of older people in different health care settings. *Journal of Advanced Nursing*, 80 (3): 1004–1017. https://doi.org/10.1111/jan.15864

Saito, Y. (2017). *Aesthetics of the Familiar: Everyday Life and World-Making*. Oxford: Oxford University Press.

Saito, Y. (2022). *Aesthetics of Care: Practice in Everyday Life*. Bloomsbury Academic Collections. Available: https://www.bloomsbury.com/uk/aesthetics-of-care-9781350134218/; accessed 1 March 2026.

Saito, Y. (2023). Living with everyday objects: Aesthetic and ethical practice. In E. K. W. Man and J. Petts (eds.) *Comparative Everyday Aesthetics: East-West Studies in Contemporary Living*. Amsterdam: Amsterdam University Press, pp.9–20. Available: https://assets.ctfassets.net/4wrp2um278k7/eZ4rfIbpAGnYepOPclR9x/1e5ccd60dccf13beaa5253e3784a80da/TOC_INTRO_9789048554508.pdf; accessed 1 March 2026.

Sandberg, L. (2018). Dementia and the gender trouble? Theorising dementia, gendered subjectivity and embodiment. *Journal of Aging Studies*, 45 (6): 25–31. https://doi.org/10.1016/j.jaging.2018.01.004

Sumartojo, S. and Pink, S. (2018). *Atmospheres and the Experiential World: Theory and Methods*. London: Routledge.

Thompson, J. (2020). Towards an aesthetics of care. In A. Stuart Fisher and J. Thompson (eds.) *Performing Care: New Perspectives on Socially Engaged Performance*. Manchester: Manchester University Press, pp. 36–38.

Thompson, J. (2023). *Care Aesthetics: For Artful Care and Careful art*. London: Routledge.

Twigg, J. (2010). Clothing and dementia: A neglected dimension? *Journal of Aging Studies*, 24 (4): 223–230. https://doi.org/10.1016/j.jaging.2010.05.002

Twigg, J., Wolkowitz, C., Cohen, R.L. and Nettleton, S. (2011). Conceptualising body work in health and social care. *Sociology of Health and Illness*, 33 (2): 171–188. https://doi.org/10.1111/j.1467-9566.2010.01323.x

Ward, R. and Campbell, S. (2013). Mixing methods to explore appearance in dementia care. *Dementia: The International Journal of Social Research and Practice*, 12 (3): 337–347. https://doi.org/10.1177/1471301213477412

Ward, R., Campbell, S. and Keady, J. (2014). 'Once I had money in my pocket, I was every colour under the sun': Using appearance biographies to explore the meanings of appearance for people with dementia. *Journal of Aging Studies*, 30: 64–72. https://doi.org/10.1016/j.jaging.2014.03.006

Ward, R., Campbell, S. and Keady, J. (2016a). 'Gonna make yer gorgeous': Everyday transformation, resistance and belonging in the care-based hair salon. *Dementia: The International Journal of Social Research and Practice*, 15 (3): 395–413. https://doi.org/10.1177/1471301216638969

Ward, R., Campbell, S. and Keady, J. (2016b). Assembling the salon: Learning from alternative forms of body work in dementia care. *Sociology of Health & Illness*, 38 (8): 1287–1302. https://doi.org/10.1111/1467-9566.12461

Ward, R., Vass, A.A., Aggarwal, N., Garfield, C. and Cybyk, B. (2008). A different story: Exploring patterns of communication in residential dementia care. *Ageing & Society*, 28 (5): 629–651. https://doi.org/10.1017/S0144686X07006927

Wood, S. (2020). Beyond Messiaen's birds: The post-verbal world of dementia. *Medical Humanities*, 46 (1): 73–83. https://doi.org/10.1136/medhum-2018-011616

Yoshizaki-Gibbons, H. (2025). *Gifts of time: Disrupting dominant temporalities in the dementia unit*. Hastings Center Report, 55 (Supplement 1): S105–S110. Available: https://doi.org/10.1002/hast.5000; accessed 1 March 2026.

# 6

# EXCHANGING MOMENTS

## What happens if we integrate language describing the 'care work' of artists with that of healthcare support workers?

*Kate Maguire-Rosier and Réka Polonyi*

### Introduction

Dementia studies show that aesthetic care is not necessarily about doing art. An aged care facility like a care home or hospital ward may have arts activities with and for people living with dementia (for a sample review see: Zeilig et al., 2014) but aesthetic care is not limited to the explicit engagement in arts and craft activities like clowning (Hendriks, 2017) or storytelling (Basting, 2020). While many studies focus on the embodied communication practices of people living with dementia, particularly advanced dementia (see, for example, Campbell et al., 2024), no study on such everyday dementia care has been considered as already, always, and fundamentally, aesthetic (for an exception, see: Fleetwood-Smith et al., 2022). Given the more conventional framing of aesthetics as arts, very few studies seek to expand the term to encompass everyday acts in dementia care (for an exception and example, see: Gibson, 2020). The purpose of this chapter is therefore to reframe care from (only) clinical to (also) aesthetic. Certainly, this reframing is a key objective of this edited collection, and our fellow authors are seeking to develop this as well. However, in this chapter, we juxtapose moments identified in the Care Aesthetics Research Exploration (CARE) project that will be more fully addressed in the next section. Indeed, the word 'moment' is deliberately chosen to build on the work of John Keady et al. (2022) and other colleagues, especially Sarah Campbell et al. (2024), Robyn Dowlen et al. (2024), Henry McPherson et al. (2025), and Sarah Fox et al. (2025).

**We ask:** What might we learn from two different case studies of dementia care – one performed by artists skilled and experienced in working with people living with dementia in care homes, and another performed by healthcare support

DOI: 10.4324/9781003623441-9
This chapter has been made available under a (CC BY) 4.0 license.

workers (HCSWs) also skilled and experienced in working in dementia settings? What knowledge might we gain by juxtaposing these practices and these different 'languages' of care: one from the arts, one from healthcare?

## Research context

### *Case studies*

The two case studies constitute part of the CARE project funded by the Arts and Humanities Research Council at The University of Manchester, led by a cross-disciplinary team in the performing arts (Principal Investigator James Thompson in Applied Theatre; Research Associates Kate Maguire-Rosier and Réka Polonyi), academic-clinicians specialised in dementia care and National Health Service (NHS) mental health wards for older people (Jacqueline Kindell and John Keady), a feminist education scholar (Kerry Harman), a cultural anthropologist (Elise Imray-Papineau), and a lead theatre artist experienced in working with people living with dementia (Jenny Harris). As also shared in the Introduction to this book, the CARE project ran over three years (2022–2025) with the aim of developing a theoretical framework for the study of the aesthetic dimension of care practices, drawing on scholarship from feminist care ethics, socially engaged theatre studies, social sciences, and health studies. The two case studies that will be focused on in this chapter (out of four in the CARE project) comprised the following:

1 HCSWs working with people living with dementia in three NHS mental health wards for older people across two NHS sites over 20 weeks from February through to June 2024 (hereafter the 'NHS Case Study'); and
2 Two experienced artists, Jenny Harris and Sara Cocker, delivering their project 'Beautiful Feast' with people living with dementia in a care home, over ten weeks from April to June 2024 (hereafter, the 'Arts Case Study').

For readers unfamiliar with the United Kingdom (UK) NHS mental health wards for older people, it is important to note that these locations admit and care for people living with dementia who are sectioned under the UK's Mental Health Act (1983). This smaller number of people living with dementia are compulsorily admitted into NHS mental health wards for older people, often under a section of the Mental Health Act (1983), for an assessment of their dementia because of the complexity of its presentation and the potential risk to the person him or herself, or to others (Jones et al., 2025).

Participants in the NHS Case Study were exclusively HCSWs with active support worker roles, including nursing assistants, occupational therapy assistants, and activity coordinators. The reasons for selecting this specific cohort were twofold. First, the participants from the NHS Case Study comprise a substantive proportion of the NHS workforce and yet little research has been undertaken in relation to their practice or by means of involving them in the research process (for discussion, see: Kindell et al., 2025a). Furthermore, HCSWs are amongst the lowest paid within the NHS, often migrant workers, women, and have limited recourse to professional opportunities. And yet, what was perhaps most telling and most interesting for our research team was that – and here is the second arguably more important reason – these employees worked the closest in terms of everyday physical proximity to, and thus of daily care for, the bodies and minds of people living with dementia. This meant that their experiences, thoughts, and interpretations of everyday care were deemed essential to the project's ability to capture potentially less recognised, and less studied, instances of relational practices.

### *Methodology*

As our research involved people living with dementia without capacity, an appropriate, and extensive, range of ethical permissions were needed to undertake the study, including clearance through the Health Research Authority (HRA) Research Ethics Committee for the NHS Case Study (approval reference: AH/W003104/1) and, separately, the HRA Social Care Research Ethics Committee for the Arts Case Study (approval reference: 23/IEC08/0040). Therefore, once approval was given for work to be undertaken in both these settings, Kate and Réka began gathering data using mixed qualitative methods. These included ethnographic observations (in both case studies), in-depth semi-structured interviews with the artists, photography, researchers' reflective notes, snapshot ('in the moment') interviews with HCSWs to complement observations, and six collaborative learning groups (CLGs) (Clarke et al., 2011) with consenting HCSW participants in the NHS Case Study. The purpose of the CLGs was to collectively explore, in more detail, how care aesthetics looked, felt, and were experienced in practice and how staff processed these practices. In total, we conducted 56 hours of observations on the NHS Case Study (not including the six hours of CLGs (x2)), and 20 hours of observations on the Arts Case Study.

Collected data was then analysed using qualitative methods of thematic analysis (Braun and Clarke, 2022) through interdisciplinary team meetings, which meant leaning on the different lenses of each team member's expertise to uncover a complex, dynamic, and nuanced understanding of aesthetic elements in care practices. Of interest to us was what we noticed as performance artists and scholars and what we might productively cross-pollinate from both settings to extrapolate meaningful moments of aesthetic care. In other words, our inquiry was not only related to an understanding of care aesthetics across disciplines, but also across sectors. So, what happens if we borrow the language we use to describe the 'care work' of artists in a dementia setting to understand that of HCSWs in another (and vice versa)?

### *Researchers' positionality*

Importantly, we both entered these two case study sites fully disclosing that neither of us were clinicians nor health or social care academics. We are, respectively, a dance and a performance scholar. Sending the two of us to these sites was a deliberate choice by the wider research team as our disciplinary backgrounds have trained us to notice the subtle practices of the body: its gestures, movements, touch, alterations in the voice and tone, and the gaze, as well as embodied interactions in space, whether deliberate or not, fleeting or held. In short, our 'artists' gaze' was a key part of our methodology.

To develop the preceding point further, Kate is a dance artist with 20 years formation classical ballet, specifically, Australian Dance Vision, culminating in a vocational Diploma in Performance. She is trained in, and also performed, folkloric dance (traditional and social dances from various parts of the world), some favourites being the Armenian dance *Shalaho*, Filipino scarf dance or *Kadtendung,* and 'Balalaika' Russian dance. Kate is also a Sabar or Senegalese traditional dancer, training in Sydney, Australia and Dakar, Senegal and performing with *Sama Sabar* group. As a dance theatre maker, Kate has directed an Aboriginal Australian 'Dreaming' story called 'Wonga Pigeon and the White Waratah' and 'Mediating Weeping Woman' inspired by the desensitisation of images of war and suffering when mediated via screens. In the latter, she tested performance theories of presence and liveness, affirming the theory that the liveness of a human actor is enhanced when accompanied by mediatised images in the form of video projections (for further information, see: Maguire-Rosier, 2013). Working at Jacob's Pillow Dance Festival, a dance work by Groupe Emile Dubois entitled 'Des Gens Qui Dansent' (People Dancing), particularly motivated her to explore everyday movement by, and with, disabled and older bodies. Kate worked as a support artist for the poet and performing artist Georgia Rose Cranko, learning her bespoke fingerspelling alphabet and becoming her 'voice' interpreting for her throughout the creative development of 'Second Skin' created by Australian choreographers Philip Channels, Sue Healey, and Dean Walsh. Her interest in older, disabled, and untrained movement aesthetics, eventually led her complete a doctoral project (Maguire-Rosier, 2018) focused on disability and Deaf aesthetic dance with Force Majeure, Dance Integrated Australia, and dance partners Diane Reid and Mel Smith (Maguire-Rosier, 2016) wherein she observed acts of and tensions inherent to care between performance makers.

Along parallel lines, Réka is a researcher and trained artist in the field of socially engaged theatre, often referred to (in predominantly Anglophone academia) as Applied Theatre. Embedded in specific sites outside traditional venues and harnessed with participatory methods of working with audiences and communities, Applied Theatre seeks to directly engage with societal issues and communities, and develops an analytical narrative to examine the 'micro' scales of performance within the 'macro' levels of societal interactions, expanding a reading of performance as one that moves beyond the stage and enters everyday life (Fischer-Lichte, 2008). In this manner, Réka has worked for over a decade with groups of people often seen as socially 'vulnerable' in collaboration with arts and civic organisations that promote the rights of immigrants. She has worked in prisons, refugee camps, immigration and community centres, and in public spaces, in Europe, the Middle East, and in Ecuador and Colombia. She is also a trained clown, originally working as a clown doctor in hospital wards, a practice that involved bringing 'laughter therapy' to people living with dementia. Réka's clowning has widely influenced her general work as a practitioner and researcher, as her practice and academic work often focus on play and playfulness, on spontaneity and creative improvisation, and imaginative connections people experience in settings where playfulness is not traditionally expected (see: Polonyi, 2023).

## Findings

The wider objective of the case studies under discussion in this chapter aimed to identify and describe acts of aesthetic care taking place in each case study setting. This chapter, however, focuses on only two themes: the care skill of (1) 'stepping into their world', and that of (2) 'clinical attitude disguised as chummy'. These two themes were co-produced with HCSWs and 'clinical attitude disguised as chummy' is a direct, verbatim title from one participant. This co-production was part of the CARE project's research design whereby as arts researchers, Kate and Réka would be learning about the practice and experience of HCSWs through both observation and CLGs. In the two following sections named accordingly, we describe two moments of care (one from each case study) that reflect this theme to extrapolate what we might learn about aesthetic care from these dementia care settings.

In the next section, we attend to the recurring act of 'stepping into their world', an act we observed almost continuously being done by both artists and HCSWs with people living with dementia during our time at both sites. We define this theme as recognising and acknowledging a world created by a person living with dementia and then finding an entry point. In the following section, we explore what is meant by the phrase 'clinical attitude disguised as chummy'. We define this theme as approaching a person living with dementia with an ethos of safeguarding their health and well-being but, at the same time, portraying this as overt/covert friendliness. The ethical implications of this terminology (such as the use of the word 'disguise') are further discussed in relation to the two examples in this section to highlight the complex interplay between 'pretend' and so-called 'authentic' acts of care.

For both themes, we draw on one example from each case study to elaborate, cross-pollinate, and expand our understanding of care aesthetic dimensions. Our analysis is a selective one that uses specific examples to demonstrate what we are calling 'the care act'. We argue that this is not only a clinical practice of care but also an aesthetic expression of it; that an act of care is also one that holds performative, *enacted* qualities which, once acknowledged, have the potential to be further refined through practice.

## Theme 1: Care practised as 'stepping into their world'

The idea of 'stepping into' a world is borrowed from a theatrical understanding of imagination, role play, and improvisation. The concept is familiar amongst performers, whether jazz musicians, ensemble group actors, or dancers: we watch, listen, wait for the right 'cue', and then place ourselves within that particular, imaginary frame that has presented itself onstage. In order to do this, a performer first acknowledges the other's 'game', accepts the offer, and then adds to it – this is often referred to informally as the moment of 'Yes, and' (Barker, 1977; Johnstone, 1981). The purpose of accepting an invitation to improvise is to *meet* the other on their own terms – for a jazz improviser, that might be responding to the same harmonic key and working along the same chord changes. The 'cue' to enter depends on how we might read the other performers and/or the audience in that given moment. In other words, 'stepping into the world' of someone requires three steps: first, recognising that there *is,* in fact, another world playing out in this moment; second, acknowledging that this other world has the right to exist; and finally, being attentive for the right 'cue' to enter this world in a way that is respectful of the other's world and personal dignity. This last step acknowledges that improvising is a deeply relational act that holds a responsibility towards the other's lived moment. 'The improviser', writes improv expert Keith Johnstone (1981), has to 'understand that his first skill lies in releasing his partner's imagination' (p. 93). We would also add a fourth step: recognising when (and how) to exit that world, equally respectfully.

We will now focus on two key moments which pinpoint this theme across both case studies. Please note that fieldnote extracts throughout this chapter have been both pseudonymised (for consenting participants) and anonymised (for others observed on site) to adhere to our research ethics permissions.

> Moment One
>
> … On the other side of the space, someone else is fishing, winding the mechanism back, reigning in his catch. [The HCSW] walks past and steps over the invisible line, in one smooth and nonchalant move … in the CLG that follows, I pick up on this moment. [The HCSW] explains that this person living with dementia would shout angrily at anyone who walked through their line, so staff had learnt to simply step over. It's not really there, but 'for them, it's serious, it's real', they say. During the same session, another HCSW, Daniel, gave another example of a person living with dementia on the ward handing them (Daniel) a fish while the person living with dementia was 'fishing' by embodying those actions as if he were sitting on a riverbank casting off. In our reality, it was an

> invisible fish that he [the person living with dementia] handed to Daniel, but the important point was that the person living with dementia then expected Daniel to do something with that invisible fish. But the person living with dementia made sure Daniel didn't just throw the invisible fish away … Daniel then had to interact and improvise a performance with them, with this little invisible fish in their hands.
>
> *NHS Case Study (Fieldnote, 22 May 2024)*

Moment Two

> The group is sitting around a table, busy decorating wooden, cut-out muffins with colourful, soft pompons, glitter stickers, thick markers, glue sticks … I note different ways people work together: one staff member Martin hovers next to a participant, marker poised over the muffin: 'How many shapes you want on your muffin, darlin'? And diamonds?' Second, there's Jenny, who goes around commenting, 'Mary that's great, love the pom poms. Do you want another pom pom? There's no right or wrong, do what you like, you're an artist!' She proceeds to give stickers to the resident, inviting her to stick them anywhere. And finally, there's staff member Elana who is with another resident, her head bent down close to hers. They silently work together, the resident seemingly pointing her finger to a spot, Elana gently placing tiny stickers wherever the resident places her finger. This starts on the muffin, but then slowly the stickers move on to the table, the chair, Dorry's hand … like a meticulously mastered game, that they're both in on and mischievously complicit in.
>
> *Arts Case Study (Observation 22 April 2024)*

In Moment Two, we paid particular attention to the contrasting forms of interactions between staff/artist and residents. Martin is focused on the task at hand – decorating the cut-out muffins – asking for the residents' input but ultimately taking charge and handling it on their own. Jenny (the leading artist) walks around the space shouting encouragement, compliments, and generally handing out the resource (pom poms) for the resident to have free reign and express themselves however they want to ('you're an artist!', otherwise saying 'your choices are legitimate'). Elena, however, holds the most engaging moment with a resident: they are both 'in on it' together, apparently enjoying this complicity. The rules have not been imposed (the stickers have travelled beyond the confines of the muffin), and Elena gently follows wherever the resident goes next – meeting her where she is, finger tap by finger tap. Both of these instances demonstrate a particular skill set, from the part of the 'carer' that requires the improvisational and performative ability to observe, acknowledge, and meet the person living with dementia 'in the moment', based on their own terms, for the purpose of making a meaningful, albeit fleeting, connection.

In Moment One, the world of a person living with dementia is identified by HCSWs (they are fishing), acknowledged as important, and responded to accordingly. The seemingly extra effort of lifting a leg when passing this person living with dementia in the hall may seem, at first glance, irrelevant in the overall care practices of the HCSW. Similarly, staff member Daniel did not have to stop and interact with the imaginary fish. And yet, staff acknowledged that this enactment of fishing, or of passing the fish to Daniel, was meaningful enough (for the person living with dementia) to warrant their attention. They responded, improvising, meeting the person living with dementia 'in the moment', in an embodied and wordless exchange that signalled to the person living with dementia that they were being seen.

An interesting discussion emerged within our team in relation to the 'fish' moment captured in the NHS Case Study. Was the act of stepping over an imaginary fishing line one that qualified as 'therapeutic lying'? The term 'therapeutic lying' was first encountered by us when used by HCSWs to describe the practice of make-believe with people living with dementia in order to avoid 'agitation'. Interestingly, for our cross-disciplinary team – James Thompson, John Keady, and Jacqueline Kindell, as well as Kate and Réka – the term carries variegated connotations. These ranged from a seemingly negative valency of lying to a more positive association with performance as playful pretence. Scholarship on therapeutic lying reveals difficulties in setting clear, defining parameters for this practice (Long et al., 2024; Murray et al., 2024) which can range from anything like concealing the truth and 'white lies' (see, for example, Blum, 1994) to 'purposeful deception' (Williamson and Kirtley, 2016) and 'treachery' used to 'force [the person living with dementia] into compliance' (Kitwood, 1997, p. 46). A recent publication by Murray et al. (2024) proposed a taxonomy of lies in dementia care that, perhaps surprisingly, includes the use of banter (and jokes) as well as the use of 'familiarity' in verbal language. Nevertheless, some of the literature expands the definition of lying in dementia care towards a form of positive, 'creative' interaction between the carer and the person living with dementia (see: Kitwood, 1997) that can be a gentle practice of acknowledging the person's momentary reality (James et al., 2006). Long et al. (2024), in fact, call for a less stigmatised understanding of this practice and for recognising the required skills, when conducted ethically, as a 'highly skilled empathic, self-aware carer has a greater ability to come up with creative alternatives to a lie' (p. 525). This recognition, however, is apparently limited to brief, verbal exchanges with the person living with dementia. What our research team eventually agreed on, however, was the evident inadequacy of the term 'therapeutic lying' to capture what was unfolding in moments such as these. The observed care practice of 'stepping into their world' contributes to the ongoing discussion on therapeutic lying by complementing the carer's creative skill with one that points to an *embodied* ability to 'step' alongside the person living with dementia and join them in their reality. The instances we caught are not only verbal, but also gestural, relying on sensorial interactions (seeing the fishing line or fish, feeling it on the hand, and communicating through touch in the muffin decoration task) and a quiet commitment to staying with the moment.

Both moments explicitly feature elements of improvisation: recognising a scene, accepting its legitimacy as a person's 'in the moment' reality, responding to cues with a 'yes, and' approach in order to step into it, and being 'co-present' (see: Kindell et al., 2025b) with the other person. Describing these two instances side by side exposes the deeply creative, imaginative, and playful abilities of carers in both situations – regardless of whether they have prior training in creative improvisation – to apply such skills when engaging with people living with dementia. It does not take an artist to tap into creative ways of connecting with a person living with dementia; similarly, an artist can also spend time caring for a resident without performing clinical duties. The aesthetic nature of care, in both instances, resides in carers' respective recognitions of a fishing line or a trail made by fingers, and in the resulting decision to either step over it or stick a sticker in the trace of those fingers, while proactively legitimising the person living with dementia and their own aesthetic acts.

## Theme 2: Care practised as 'clinical attitude disguised as chummy'

As shared earlier, the title of this theme refers to the words of an HCSW during a CLG session when asked to define everyday care on the NHS mental health wards for older people/people living with dementia. The sentence struck us as revealing various layered complexities around care practices. 'Clinical attitude', in this case, was referring to task-based care work, or the labour-efficient and sometimes mechanical attitude of 'tick box' routines relating to basic personal care and safety of a person living with dementia. The work needs to be done, this staff member was saying, and it is easier to do this when the person living with dementia is willing and cooperative, which requires being friendly. The word 'disguise', however, is both a theatrical term and one colloquially used to describe deception and its potentially unethical implications in healthcare; for instance, a masking of 'true' character (the care worker). In theatrical usage, a disguise (such as a mask) is not necessarily a (material) concealment, but can also be a means to heighten and support the character/role being played. Did this render the staff member's 'chumminess' inauthentic, or simply part of the job and therefore embedded and validated in the care act itself? And what might this approach reveal about artists working in a care setting, for whom the idea of playful 'pretend' is at the core of their artform?

> Moment One
>
> During the CLG, HCSW Bill tells us about a time he noticed a person living with dementia refusing to go to bed. This person liked to take a whisky nightcap [which was not permitted on the ward]. Bill explained that he'd 'hang out' with them in the lounge, sitting 'at the bar' with two cups of orange juice. They'd

> have a good banter and sip their drinks. The person living with dementia seemed to respond positively. They did this regularly for some time, until the person's state deteriorated.
>
> *NHS Case Study (CLG 3 April 2024)*

Moment Two

> Jenny Harris: [Bringing up the example of Talia, a partially speaking resident who participates in a wheelchair and responds predominantly to one-on-one support with eye contact, touch, and sometimes facial expressions. At each session, she has her fingernails painted different colours]. Today, Talia actually smiled at me! First response! … So I now do my fingernails in a different colour each time before [our weekly sessions on] Mondays, as a way to connect with her. But I don't know if this is meaningful at all for her. The fingernails are a way in. Or, at least, that's *my* way in, you know what I mean? And I say 'Hi' and have a bit of 'Ah, ooh look, we've got matching colours today' kinda thing. [...] Entering a person's space is about *you making an offer* and seeing *what they have to offer* ... and working with that, going with that. We're like magpies … we notice nuggets of creativity that we pick up on, and then respond to, as maybe *a way in* … Often what we do is banal and silly, it's not about the activity, or what we're pretending to do, but about being together.
>
> *Arts Case Study (interview with artists, 8 April 2024)*

In the first moment, Bill's imaginative exchange with the person living with dementia (having a regular nightcap) started from having noticed that the person refused to go to bed. Recovering a ritual, in the form of a small drink and chat, seemed to this carer as the most efficient solution – not just in terms of the task at hand (going to bed), but also in relation to the well-being of the person living with dementia. Perhaps, it was felt that they needed reassuring through something familiar, rather than relying on a forceful removal to their bedroom. In the Arts Case Study, Jenny's connection with resident Talia is framed by her excitement at having 'gotten through' to her, even in the smallest exchange. The 'clinical' attitude here is, arguably, in checking for, and actively seeking out, a physical or verbal response or engagement from Talia. The 'disguised' endeavour to bring about this response was through Jenny's insistence on painting her fingernails like Talia's. Although this gesture of attention to Talia – a small act of 'I see you' to the other – might seem trivial to an observer or seem insignificantly minor in the overall care of the resident, Jenny demonstrates a commitment to seeking moments of connection with her. What the artists in the Arts Case Study refer to as 'magpie moments' in which one finds opportunities to connect, and what the HCSW in the NHS Case Study calls 'clinical attitude disguised as chummy', equally cultivate a sense of continuity for people living with dementia which is being determined *by* the person living with dementia and whatever 'nuggets of creativity' – to quote Jenny – that person offers. Both moments demonstrate the carer for people living with dementia – whether HCSW or artist facilitating a workshop – in a situation of pretend. One could see the particular choice of 'playing a friendly role' as serving a purpose (encouraging the person living with dementia to go to bed) and therefore being potentially coercive. Yet, by adding the angle of *artistry* and *craft* from the second case study, what is revealed is each care worker's 'magpie' ability to 'notice' a moment of significance for the other, and to then hold on to it as 'a way in ... [and] working with that'. In other words, the pretence is done within an ethos of respect, playfulness, and curiosity towards what the resident or person living with dementia finds important (the nightcap; the fingernails). The genuine willingness of the artists to connect can be seen in both instances: Bill described this act as just 'hanging out' and 'banter', insinuating a state of pleasure and without the external pressure of time. Jenny, in the other example, admits about not really knowing whether it works or not; and yet, the 'offer', to use her word, is there. When, then, does chumminess tip into disrespect? One could imagine Bill pretending to get drunk, for instance – or Jenny leaning a little too heavily into the fingernail colouring without being aware if Talia is even consenting to have her nails done, and, on top of this, making it her only point of attempted connection with Talia. These nuances are vital to acknowledge. What an arts-based lens provides is an articulation of the care worker's skills in honing (and refining) the subtle craft of 'disguise' so as to support and retain the person living with dementia's dignity.

It is important to note the difference between 'stepping into their own world' and 'clinical attitude disguised as chummy'. Improvising a 'way in' is at the centre of both practices; yet, the first has no significant purpose other than connecting with the individual, whereas the second is specifically aimed at 'getting something' from the person living with dementia. The decision to step into the resident's world, or that of the person living with dementia, does not necessarily mean the person has clinical intentions. For instance, neither the fishing line nor the sticker moments have ulterior motives (even if they, arguably, produce clinical benefits such as psychological safety and well-being). Here, we might say these are moments of care done mostly for their own, 'stand-alone', aesthetic purposes. In the whisky nightcap and fingernail moments however, staff chose to enter into aesthetic improvisations with people living with dementia in order to effect certain acts – getting the person (closer) to bed and getting the person to participate in the art project. Here, 'clinical attitude disguised as chummy' might be described as an aesthetic act for care's sake. In extrapolating the aesthetic elements in gestures of care, we can better trace the highly creative skills (improvisation, adaptability, and role-play) performed by carers regularly on the job. But, more importantly, we can also start noticing these abilities to creatively engage, connect, and gently form relationships, however fleeting, with people living with dementia.

## Conclusion

In this chapter, we have proposed elements of what might partially make up a practice of aesthetic care in dementia contexts. From observing two very different case studies under the umbrella of the CARE project, one in the context of 'health' in a NHS mental health ward for older people, and another in the context of 'arts' in a UK care home, we considered a total of four examples, or what we have at times dubbed 'moments' of aesthetic care, to represent two practices of care: 'stepping into their world' and 'clinical attitude disguised as chummy'.

In our discussion in each of the two case studies, we have sought to highlight the decisions made by care workers – be they the more task-oriented HCSWs or aesthetic-oriented artist Jenny Harris. It is in their decisions and subsequent care acts that we can identify the skills at play. These skills have been honed, refined, and crafted over time so that they, themselves, do not tend to notice them and rather 'take them for granted'. At times, when we asked these care professionals *why* they decided to perform a given action in a certain way, they would pause for thought or find it difficult to pinpoint a precise reason. Instead, they would respond, 'I just do it'. This idea of 'just doing' something without thought is also present in the examples provided in this chapter: the carers across both studies are employing embodied, sensory skills in their acts of care. If Daniel were to ignore the fishing line (Moment One in the first theme), he knows the person living with dementia might become agitated. And Jenny (Moment Two in the second theme) persists in painting her fingernails a different colour each week (indeed, saying 'yes, and' to Talia) in spite of shifts in Talia's sensorial participation in the activities, because she knows as a care worker that sensorial inclusion matters, especially for people living with dementia. For us both, such aesthetic ways of practising and *knowing* care are skills that do not fit neatly into either 'care' or 'aesthetic' skillsets.

While this chapter only goes so far in naming and valuing what indeed these professionals 'just do', there remains a dearth of research on the virtues of dementia aesthetic care in other parts of the world, especially non-English speaking and under presented cultural contexts. In ending this chapter, therefore, it is necessary to stress that further excavating of aesthetic care skills needs to be performed not only in global dementia academic studies and arts projects, but also in settings beyond dementia, social care, medicine, and health.

We end with our reflective response to the question posed at the beginning of this chapter: What might we learn from everyday practices of dementia care? We learn that aesthetics – the sensorial, embodied, and crafted – becomes increasingly pivotal in supporting people living with dementia not just in the doing of tasks, such as eating and getting dressed, but also in supporting their lived reality in a given moment. The context of dementia also teaches us that aesthetic care can be about legitimising seemingly silly, purposeless, or inappropriate acts such as sticking stickers on muffins. In offering alternatives to the currently dominant narrative of 'living well' with dementia (see, for example, Clare et al., 2025) and older ones about (only) loss, tragedy, and social death (Woods, 1989), aesthetic care might disrupt clinical intentions, strategies, and systems. Perhaps dementia's ability to disrupt the norm is the challenge to which any care act must respond.

## Acknowledgements

We would like to thank all participants in the study and the Arts and Humanities Research Council of the United Kingdom for their funding of these case studies under the 'Care Aesthetics: Research Exploration' project. Grant number: AH/W003104/1.

## Three Key Reading References

### *Reference 1*

Overboe, J. (2009). Affirming an impersonal life: A different register for disability studies. *Journal of Literary & Cultural Disability Studies*, 1 (3): 241–256. https://muse.jhu.edu/article/365199.

The late James Overboe contributed what he calls an 'impersonal register' to disability studies. In doing this, he considers two cases. Approaching a person living with dementia who apparently does not have the faculties needed to fulfil the normative notion of an autonomous, rational human and, reflecting on his own imminent death as a newborn baby who was indeed supposed to die (but did not), he compares and contrasts two disparate states of being as existing on an 'impersonal' plane. This existential life materialises when a person cannot necessarily access the means of codified communication, such as shared language nor even understand the intricacies of the world around them, or inside them.

### *Reference 2*

Gibson, J. (2020). *Dementia, Narrative and Performance: Staging Reality, Reimagining Identities*. London: Springer Nature.

Dementia performance scholar and practitioner Janet Gibson brings another refreshing perspective on dementia representation and aesthetics in her rigorously researched monograph. In it, she critically examines what she dubs as the 'right kind' of dementia story insofar as the West narrates them. Very much complementary to the work of Anna Basting's 'Timeslips' practice and the 'Shared Reading' method developed by Jane Davis (United States) and engaged with extensively by Aagje Swinnen (Netherlands), Gibson canvasses both challenges and opportunities for writers and artists working in dementia alike in a delicate balancing act of care.

### *Reference 3*

Bradwell, C. (2025). (not) lovely: Enacting solidarity in dementia care through participatory arts. *Journal of Aging Studies*, 75: Available: https://doi.org/10.1016/j.jaging.2025.101352; accessed 1 March 2026.

Chloé Bradwell's recent essay addresses a very interesting concern: When face-to-face with upset, sad, or angry residents, what can the artist do? The answer: validate these negative emotions in care residents through the skills artists already have, such as kinaesthetic attunement. Bradwell reconsiders the notion of 'well-being' in arts, health, and dementia contexts by concluding that the experience of grief is as integral to well-being as that of happiness. In the case of Entelechy Arts, a participatory arts company whose director is an author in the previous edited collection in the Care Aesthetics series (Maguire-Rosier et al., 2025), she describes the artist's kinaesthetically attuned validating role as a collective act of care.

## References

Barker, C. (1977). *Theatre Games: A New Approach to Drama Training*. London: Methuen Ltd.

Basting, A. (2020). *Creative Care: A Revolutionary Approach to Dementia and Elder Care*. London: HarperCollins.

Blum, N.S. (1994). Deceptive practices in managing a family member with Alzheimer's disease. *Symbolic Interaction*, 17 (1): 21–36. https://doi.org/10.1525/si.1994.17.1.21

Braun, V. and Clarke, V. (2022). *Thematic Analysis: A Practical Guide*. London: Sage.

Campbell, S., Dowlen, R., Keady, J. and Thompson, J. (2024). Care aesthetics and 'being in the moment' through improvised music-making and male grooming in dementia care. *International Journal of Education & the Arts*, 25 (si1.13). Available: https://journals.psu.edu.ijea/article/view/63522; accessed 1 March 2026.

Clare, L., Charlwood, C., Quinn, C. and Victor, C. (2025). *Living with Dementia Reconsidered*. Maidenhead: Open University Press.

Clarke, C.L., Wilcockson, J., Gibb, C.E., Keady, J., Wilkinson, H. and Luce, A. (2011). Reframing risk management in dementia care through collaborative learning. *Health & Social Care in the Community*, 19 (1): 23–32. https://doi.org/10.1111/j.1365-2524.2010.00944.x

Dowlen, R., McPherson, D.H.J., Swarbrick, C., Hoskin, L., Thompson, J. and Keady, J. (2024). Creating and reliving the moment: Using musical improvisation and care aesthetics as a lens of connection and self-expression for younger people living with dementia. *International Journal of Environmental Research and Public Health*, 21 (8): 972. Available: https://doi.org/10.3390/ijerph21080972; accessed 1 March 2026.

Fischer-Lichte, E. (2008). *The Transformative Power of Performance: A New Aesthetics*. London: Routledge.

Fleetwood-Smith, R., Tischler, V. and Robson, D. (2022). Aesthetics and dementia: Exploring the role of everyday aesthetics in dementia care settings. *Design for Health*, 6 (1): 91–113. https://doi.org/10.1080/24735132.2022.2074207

Fox, S., Thompson, J. and Keady, J. (2025). Meaningful moments of connection: How people affected by dementia and their carers living at home understand, interpret and experience everyday aesthetics. *International Journal of Geriatric Psychiatry*, 40 (8): e70136. Available: https://doi.org/10.1002/gps.70136; accessed 1 March 2026.

Gibson, J. (2020). *Dementia, Narrative and Performance: Staging Reality, Reimagining Identities*. London: Springer Nature.

Hendriks, R. (2017). Clown's view as respiciō: Looking respectfully to and after people with dementia. *Medicine Health Care Philosophy*, 20 (2): 207–217. https://doi.org/10.1007/s11019-016-9734-1

James, I.A., Wood-Mitchell, A.J., Waterworth, A.M., Mackenzie, L.E. and Cunningham, J. (2006). Lying to people with dementia: Developing ethical guidelines for care settings. *International Journal of Geriatric Psychiatry*, 21 (8): 800–801. https://doi.org/10.1002/gps.1551

Johnstone, K. (1981). *Impro: Improvisation and the Theatre*. London: Methuen Ltd.

Jones, L., Cullum, N., Watson, R., Thompson, J. and Keady, J. (2025). 'Only my family can help': The lived experience and care aesthetics of being resident on an NHS psychiatric/mental health inpatient dementia assessment ward – a single case study. *Ageing & Society*, 45 (6): 1143–1164. https://doi:10.1017/S0144686X24000096

Keady, J.D., Campbell, S., Clark, A., Dowlen, R., Elvish, R., Jones, L., Kindell, J., Swarbrick, C. and Williams, S. (2022). Re-thinking and re-positioning 'being in the moment' within a continuum of moments: Introducing a new conceptual framework for dementia studies. *Ageing & Society*, 42 (3): 681–702. https://doi.org/10.1017/S0144686X20001014

Kindell, J.A., Harman, K., Maguire-Rosier, K., Polonyi, R., Thompson, J. and Keady, J.D. (2025a). Exploring the everyday care practices of healthcare support workers when working with people with dementia admitted to National Health Service hospital wards in the United Kingdom: a qualitative systematic review of the literature. *Aging & Mental Health*, 29 (5): 915–927. https://doi.org/10.1080/13607863.2024.2447319

Kindell, J., Maguire-Rosier, K., Polonyi, R., Thompson, J., Cleasby, R., Watson, R. and Keady, J.D. (2025b). Healthcare support workers working with people with dementia on mental health wards: A practice model informed by care aesthetics. *Qualitative Health Research*, 1–14. Online First (December). Available: https://doi.org/10.1177/10497323251393890; accessed 1 March 2026.

Kitwood, T. (1997). *Dementia Reconsidered: The Person Comes First*. Buckingham: Open University Press.

Long, S., Irving, K. and Murphy, C. (2024). Is therapeutic lying contradictory to person-centred care? Toward understanding the connection. *Aging & Mental Health*, 28 (3): 520–530. https://doi.org/10.1080/13607863.2023.2202632

Maguire-Rosier, K. (2013). Mediating weeping woman: A live/screen performance study. *Macquarie Matrix*, 2 (2): 78–96.

Maguire-Rosier K. (2016). Moving 'Misfits'. *Australasian Drama Studies*, 69: 29–55.

Maguire-Rosier, K. (2018). *Politicising performances of 'care': Dance theatre by and with Australian artists with disability*. PhD thesis, Macquarie University. Available: https://figshare.mq.edu.au/articles/thesis/Politicising_performances_of_care_dance_theatre_by_and_with_Australian_artists_with_disability/19442402; accessed 1 March 2026.

Maguire-Rosier, K., Polonyi, R. and Thompson, J. (eds.) (2025). *Care Aesthetics and the Arts*. London: Routledge.

McPherson, D., Dowlen, R., Bithell, C., Gagatsis, A., Young, A., Hoskin, L., Thomas, M., Riley, C. and Keady, J. (2025). Music in mind training: Producing a theory of change model to evaluate the implementation of an improvisation-based music-making training programme for care home staff working with people with dementia. *Dementia: The International Journal of Social Research and Practice*, 24 (5): 866–883. https://doi.org/10.1177/14713012251319589/

Mental Health Act (1983). Available: https://www.legislation.gov.uk/ukpga/1983/20/contents; accessed 1 March 2026.

Murray, J., Thompson, J., Hill, M. and James, I. (2024). An ethnographic study to develop a taxonomy of lies for communicating with people with moderate to severe dementia. *Nursing Ethics*, 32 (1): 1–16. https://doi.org/10.1177/09697330241246087

Polonyi, R. (2023). *Threatening play: Radical spaces of ludic disruptions*. PhD thesis, The University of Manchester. Available: https://research.manchester.ac.uk/en/studentTheses/threatening-play-radical-spaces-of-ludic-disruptions/; accessed 1 March 2026.

Williamson, T. and Kirtley, A. (2016). What is truth? An inquiry about truth and lying in dementia care. *Mental Health Foundation*. Available: https://www.mentalhealth.org.uk/

explore-mental-health/publications/what-truth-inquiry-about-truth-and-lying-dementia-care; accessed 1 March 2026.

Woods, R.T. (1989). *Alzheimer's Disease: Coping with a Living Death.* London: Souvenir Press.

Zeilig, H., Killick, J. and Fox, C. (2014). The participative arts for people living with a dementia: A critical review. *International Journal of Ageing and Later Life*, 9 (1): 7–34. https://doi.org/10.3384/ijal.1652-8670.14238

# 7

# CREATIVE MOMENTS AND DEMENTIA

## Fostering relational, aesthetic approaches in care home settings

*Rebecka Fleetwood-Smith and Robyn Dowlen*

### Introduction

#### *Speculative route in*

> *You enter - a golden retriever from an animal rescue centre down the road, greets you. His breath hot, his fur silky and clean – smelling like lavender. The entrance is open and welcoming and leads you gently around to a café like space. There is a greeter rather than a receptionist. Well, a second (human) greeter if you count Noddy as the first. You hear laughter and music – somewhere in the home, housemates, house-friends, house-companions are making masks and playfully scaring one another. The walls are vibrant and full of life – they contain photographs and paintings, all beautifully framed yet mismatched. You're keen to know the stories behind the eclectic display. The smell of coffee wafts by and something has been freshly baked. Your body softens into the space; the trepidation felt on your journey here dissipates...*

When coming together to write this chapter, we spoke at length about our readings of current literature and what a care aesthetics lens may offer in developing understandings around creativity in the lives of people with dementia living in care homes. Through this chapter, we challenge dominant Western perspectives around creativity in the lives of people with dementia living in care homes – we draw on existing literature and our own research and practice as carried out in the United Kingdom (UK). We focus here on the lives of people living with dementia in care homes as over 70% of the UK care home population is estimated to live with a form of dementia (Alzheimer's Society, n.d.). During our discussions, we posed the prompt: '*Imagine if a care home was designed by artists, what would you*

DOI: 10.4324/9781003623441-10
This chapter has been made available under a (CC BY) 4.0 license.

*encounter and how would the space feel?'* We therefore begin this piece with this 'speculative route in' – an extract that combines freewriting that we undertook in response to this prompt. We share this writing as a tentative imagining. We write this as two white British cisgendered women who have had the privilege of engaging with the arts throughout our lives. In putting this chapter together, we acknowledge the privileges our backgrounds afford in shaping this imagining. We do not claim that this imagining is an ideal or perfect example (or that such a thing exists), but we used the activity to explore what a warm, lively, and curated space of care could look and feel like from our perspectives and what such imaginings offer our thinking about current practices. This was an experimental exercise which started from a position that centres rich aesthetic encounters. This endeavour reminds us of the work of Basting (2020), who wrote: 'One can spot a beautiful question because it gives the creative power to the listener, not the asker' (p. 79) whilst 'diagnostic questions, designed to seek out and identify losses revealed by brain changes, are not beautiful. They feel like sharp toothed traps' (p. 86). Through our 'speculative route in' we imagine otherwise to explore the antithesis to traditional institutions which typically centre efficiency and focus on risk management and containment all of which permeate the look and feel of these settings and the relations and interactions promoted within (see, for example, Buse and Twigg, 2016; Fleetwood-Smith et al., 2022).

This 'speculative route in' is a provocation to ask, 'What if?' So …

- **What if** the arts and creativity were not considered a 'nice to have' or an 'optional add on'?
- **What if** they were positioned as fundamental in the everyday lives of people with dementia living in (and beyond) care homes?
- **What if** they were not something to be measured, 'administered', or tested, but art for art's sake, with value held 'in the moment'?

Whilst this may be an idealised imagining, we suggest that such provocations are potentially valuable and revealing. We hope to use this chapter, and the lens of care aesthetics, to reimagine the role of creativity in the everyday lives of people with dementia in care home settings. In doing so, we build upon the work of Ruth Bartlett, Pia Kontos, and Anne Basting (see, for example, Bartlett and O'Connor, 2010; Kontos et al., 2017; Basting, 2020) to conceptualise the active roles that people living with dementia play in shaping creativity in the everyday, as well as the ways in which artists, professional care staff, family members and friends, and environments promote/facilitate these more spontaneous and improvised acts of creativity.

We first turn to current literature to examine the position and access to the arts and creativity as framed within the (bio)medical dementia context and how this context has been, and continues to be, detrimental in shaping understandings around creativity in the lives of people with dementia.

## Framing access to the arts

There has been a growing narrative of the positive value of the creative arts in the context of dementia over the past 20 years. There is a wide range of literature that showcases the broad nature of arts and cultural engagement in the context of dementia, including (but not limited to): visits to museums and galleries (Camic et al., 2019); music programmes led by professional orchestral musicians (Dowlen et al., 2022); devising theatrical performances centred on storytelling (Basting et al., 2016); as well as online music-making via Zoom during the COVID-19 crisis (Dowson et al., 2021). Alongside research in this area which has reported on the positive value of arts and cultural engagement for people living with dementia (see, for example, Zeilig et al., 2014; Dowson et al., 2021; Kinsey et al., 2021), there has also been growing advocacy for access to such experiences (see, for example, UK Music and Music for Dementia, 2022).

To critically explore the arts within the context of dementia, we must consider the (bio)medical model of dementia which sees the condition described as a 'disease' and perceived as a loss of 'normality' (such as described by Sabat, 2014). In practice, this has led to dementia being seen as something to be diagnosed and treated, involving, for instance, the management of 'difficult' behaviours resulting in people living with the condition becoming 'victims' and 'sufferers'. The impact that the medicalisation of the condition has on those living with dementia should not be underestimated, as Shakespeare et al. (2019) wrote:

> A person with dementia ends up being treated as dependent and denied a voice. Perhaps a better extrapolation of what happens when someone has dementia is that she is viewed in terms of her inabilities, whether these are cognitive, relational or functional, and in comparison to an expected norm of personhood. Her strength becomes invisible. Her emotional and social bonds stand for nothing. Her disease and difficulties become her defining features.
>
> *(p. 1082)*

This medicalisation of dementia has shaped the ways in which arts and creative experiences are framed, positioned, and often experienced by those with the condition. We see many narratives in this area that over-medicalise and 'interventionalise' creative practices, reducing the experiences of people living with dementia down to the 'problematic' symptoms they exhibit. For example, it is commonplace for creative experiences to be framed using medical language – something we see both in research and the media (Dowlen and Fleetwood-Smith, 2023). Within research literature to date, creative experiences have largely been framed as interventions aimed at reducing the so-called 'behavioural and psychological symptoms of dementia' or improving cognitive outcomes (James and Jackman, 2017; Kontos et al., 2017). Here, creative arts are considered as 'interventions' of which success, or failure, is measured against a reduction of these 'symptoms', or improvements in cognitive outcomes, such as a lessening of the signs of agitation or improving scores on areas of cognitive function following a time-limited arts-based intervention (de Medeiros and Basting, 2014). Studies that have used this approach to date have shown mixed findings, with a large number showing no significant reductions in 'symptoms' such as agitation or anxiety (Van der Steen et al., 2025). This has led to the dismissal of many of the positive findings associated with arts-based programmes in the context of dementia, with approaches that do not use standardised outcomes within randomised designs deemed to lack rigour or methodological quality (Gray et al., 2018).

Whilst such pre-post intervention approaches are reasonably typical within (bio)medical approaches to dementia research, they limit the inclusion of the voices of people living with dementia and rely heavily on the second-hand reporting of symptom severity by family members or formal carers. This has led to researchers questioning whether we are missing valuable parts of the lived experiences of people with dementia by only using pre-post intervention measures given the range of positive benefits that have been observed anecdotally and reported by people living with dementia themselves. For example, Gray et al. (2018) suggest a paucity in the field of arts and dementia of 'the assessment of artistic quality, aesthetic experience, cultural contributions, process, social impact and economic value' (p. 776). Thus, the (bio)medical model has infiltrated the ways in which the benefits of the arts are perceived in the context of dementia in terms of understanding or 'measuring' its impacts, yet the model permeates further into wider narratives of the arts in the lives of people with dementia.

In a recent publication by ourselves (Dowlen and Fleetwood-Smith, 2023), we examined the lack of criticality that has been applied to understanding of the arts and creativity in the context of dementia. Arguing that current positioning of the arts often sees the arts flattened, seen as something akin to a medicine that can be administered, and framed often from a purely positive stance. This traditional interventionist positioning of the arts in the context of dementia assumes both that people living with dementia are a homogenous group and that the arts simply provoke positive experiences. It also assumes that creative arts programmes and practices happen at a certain time on a certain day of the week, which neglects the wide and varied ways creative arts can be part of the everyday (Bellass et al., 2019). Creativity in the context of dementia, and the participation in creative practice, can also exacerbate feelings of loss and decline with Robertson and McCall (2020) finding that people required reassurance to minimise feelings of being tested, assessed, and measured. These assumptions, we argue, are limiting and perpetuate the stigmatisation of dementia whilst also neglecting the ways in which creativity and the arts present themselves in the everyday lives of people with dementia. By limiting our understandings of the creative arts to short-term, scheduled participation, we miss the rich and nuanced way that the creative arts can be spontaneously driven by people living with dementia (and noticed by others) in the everyday.

## Everyday creativity

Everyday creativity refers to the ways people engage in artistic or making practices as part of their daily lives. This includes not only participating in creative activities like drawing, singing, or crafting, but also how individuals respond to new or unfamiliar situations in imaginative or resourceful ways. Whilst these actions may vary widely between people and contexts, what distinguishes them as *creative* is the framing of such acts as personally meaningful or original. Richards (2018) argues that everyday creativity does not have to serve a practical purpose or be useful (although it can); its value lies in its significance to the individual or group involved. This framing becomes especially important in dementia contexts, where subtle, embodied, and momentary acts may hold deep creative and relational meaning, even if they are not recognised or noticed as such in conventional terms.

Creativity is seen to be a central tenet of the everyday experience of dementia, showcasing how people living with dementia can exert agency and capacity through their everyday actions. Bellass et al. (2019), for example, discuss the importance of recognising everyday forms of creativity in the context of dementia, advocating for a broader understanding of creativity beyond traditional arts-based interventions. They do not dismiss the value of more structured arts programmes but emphasise that the use of the arts in the context of dementia cannot be an all-or-nothing approach (it does not have to be stimulation or nothing at all). Everyday creativity in dementia is much less explored and understood than the more traditional programme-based or intervention-based arts activities. Attending to everyday creativity necessitates shifting attention from the 'uncovering exceptional' encounters to understanding creativity as central to everyday lives. This shift is more in line with approaches to understanding 'everyday' or 'relational' citizenship in the context of dementia, including the mundane, unremarkable, and routine parts of life (Kontos et al., 2017; Nedlund et al., 2019).

Whilst there has been less exploration of the role and value of everyday creativity in a dementia context, several researchers are beginning to shift understanding of creativity to the everyday in response to the overmedicalisation of the arts within this context. It reflects shifts within wider discourses in the arts and cultural sector, which highlight the value of everyday engagement with the arts in fostering social inclusion, community connection, and well-being beyond the confines of formal practices, state-funded institutions, and conventional cultural venues. Traditional arts institutions, for example, often operate within cognitive-normative and physically inaccessible frameworks that unintentionally exclude people living with dementia (Zeilig et al., 2014). As Basting (2009) and others argue, this exclusion is reinforced by dominant biomedical narratives and an over-reliance on memory and verbal fluency as prerequisites for participation. Even initiatives aiming for inclusion frequently fall short in addressing the specific needs and capacities of people living with dementia. Attending to everyday creativity thus invites a more nuanced understanding of agency and citizenship in dementia, grounded not in 'exceptional' creative acts, but in the ordinary rhythms, gestures, and improvisations of daily life. Foregrounding everyday creativity in the context of dementia necessitates a reorientation of how agency and expression are understood, meaning the embodied, affective, and relational ways of being can be privileged.

This orientation towards everyday creativity resonates strongly with moment-based approaches to dementia, which similarly emphasise the value of attending to the here-and-now of lived experience rather than measuring participation against external benchmarks of ability or productivity (Keady et al., 2022; Campbell et al., 2024; Dowlen et al., 2024). A moment-based lens encourages sensitivity to the fleeting, embodied, and relational expressions through which people living with dementia assert presence and agency. It is in that sense, when we refer to *creative moments* in this chapter, we are drawing together the framing of creativity and the principles of a moment-based approach and care aesthetics, to draw attention to the ordinary, improvised, and affective dimensions of expression that might otherwise be overlooked.

## Relational citizenship and creativity

Increased attention to the everyday experience of dementia and a person's everyday actions involves attending not only to what a person says but also how a person uses their body. The 'bodily turn' in the social sciences and humanities (Martin, 1992) has been instrumental in expanding understandings of dementia and researchers suggest it may have vast implications in developing care practices that are flexible, responsive, and malleable (see, for example, Downs, 2013; Ward et al., 2014). An embodied understanding of selfhood places the body at the centre of a reconceptualisation of dementia and requires disregarding the body as secondary, to embrace the notion that a person *is* their body, *its* movements, *its* habits, *its* gestures, and so forth (Kontos, 2004, 2005). Building upon the notion of embodied selfhood, Kontos and colleagues (2017, 2020) claim that dementia care paradigms traditionally neglected the body, and that this has resulted in the silencing of bodily expressions. Indeed, Kontos et al. (2017) proposed a new model of care to embrace the role of the body and foreground and attend to such expressions. Relational citizenship centres on the importance of interdependence and relational practices between people. The model of care is underpinned by: (i) the concept of citizenship (i.e., interdependence, reciprocity); (ii) treating the person living with dementia as active partners in their own care; and (iii) the theory of embodied selfhood (i.e., that the body is expressive and communicative of the self). Kontos et al. (2017) argue that 'relational citizenship more inclusively and unconditionally provides for the recognition and support of membership in, and contributions to, social collectivity' (p. 194). The repositioning of the body, as Kontos et al. (2020) argue, is critical as embodied expression is a fundamental way in which people living with dementia engage in the world. Thus, Kontos et al. (2020) suggest that relational citizenship 'more comprehensively recognises the human rights of persons living with dementia' (p. 5).

Creativity is considered a central tenet of relational citizenship due to the ways in which creative practices involve responsive, expressive, and lively forms of engagement which centre multisensory ways of being-in-the-world. This, Kontos et al. (2021) argue, involves considering creativity beyond structured activities, to understand the opportunities that open-ended creative practices have in enabling people living with dementia to express themselves and develop their skills. When speaking to the role of creativity in the lives of people with dementia, Kontos et al. (2021) not only talk to engagement with specific creative practices but also suggest an expanded understanding to embrace the multiplicity of ways in which people are creative in their daily lives (i.e., everyday creativity). Within this understanding of everyday creativity, they suggest that imaginative, humorous, and playful engagement, as enacted through the body, should be embraced.

To date, relational citizenship has been explored through and in relation to dance, drama, and elder-clowning (Kontos et al., 2017, 2021) whilst materiality is implicitly explored; we suggest that a more explicit approach to illuminating relations between people and 'things' within dementia care environments would allow us to explore the micro-practices that make up creative moments within these environments. This may allow us to expand understanding of relational citizenship and everyday creativity. For example, Bradwell (2025) presents the power of the arts in fostering solidarity through enabling people living with dementia to express feelings of sadness and anger. In her analysis, she presents the importance of attending to micro-practices to reveal the enmeshed ways in which creativity and care are practised and the space for expression that this creates. Attunement to such micro-practices, we posit, illuminates the nuanced, intricate, and fine-grained practices (between and beyond people) that shape and make creative moments within dementia care settings. Cultivating attunement involves relational, multisensory, and embodied practices in which attentiveness is given to the interdependent things at play (Hatton, 2021). We have argued elsewhere (Dowlen and Fleetwood-Smith, 2023) that the tendency to equate the elusiveness of creative moments in the lives of people with dementia as something other-worldly negates the care and skills of all those involved in such encounters. We suggest here that this also negates the many things that make up such creative moments; for instance, the architecture, the materials within the setting, and how the space feels.

## Applying a relational, aesthetic lens

Attention to aesthetics within dementia studies has gained traction in recent years (see, for example, Halpern et al., 2008; Buse and Twigg, 2018; Fleetwood-Smith et al., 2022; Thompson, 2023; Campbell et al., 2024; Fox et al., 2025). Here, we draw on the notion of everyday aesthetics (Saito, 2007, 2017, 2023) and care aesthetics (Thompson, 2020, 2023) to examine the ways in which aesthetics and relational citizenship connect and how the bringing together of these may be of great interest in considering moments of everyday creativity within the lives of people living with dementia.

Everyday aesthetics involves considering the ways in which our daily lives are shaped by our aesthetic encounters. This shifts traditional Western understandings of aesthetics beyond our engagement with, and appreciation of, art, to understand that aesthetics surrounds us. Saito (2017) writes, for instance, 'if the humdrum nature of daily life is a dreary drudgery, it does not render it anesthetic; rather, it is still an aesthetic texture of everyday life, though negatively experienced' (p. 28). This understanding of aesthetics has been applied in thinking through experiences of people with dementia living in a care home (Fleetwood-Smith et al., 2022), demonstrating how people perform and express aesthetic preferences through their bodies, whilst also indicating the ways in which stigmatising notions of dementia shape the aesthetics of care environments. This attention speaks to importance of 'things' and 'materials'. In a recent study, Fox et al. (2025) explored the notion of everyday aesthetics within people living with dementia's homes and found that objects, tastes, and smells were meaningful and supported moments of connection to a person's identity and culture and fostered social connections.

As also shared in the Introduction to this book, James Thompson's (2023) recent extensive work on care aesthetics draws upon feminist ethics of care to consider connections between arts and care practices to ultimately examine how care encounters are enmeshed with aesthetic sensibilities. Care aesthetics can be considered from a macro level e.g., the political, societal, and environmental, to a micro level e.g., fine-grained, everyday practices of care. At a micro-level care, aesthetics involves attending to the embodied and sensory to identify the intricate practices involved in moments of care. This attention, Thompson (2023) suggests, involves noticing and spotlighting processes and practices that are typically deemed 'elusive'. This fine-grained approach can allow us to examine what makes up potentially 'good' moments of care.

Whilst there may be a tendency to focus on 'positive' examples, Thompson (2023) indicates that the care aesthetics lens can also reveal 'careless' practices. Careless practices here could be read in a multitude of ways, at a micro level; for example, assumptions made about a person living with dementia's quiet participation in an activity and curtailing their involvement due to this. As West et al. (2024) note, holding space for 'lulls' and 'quiet moments', and embracing the uncertain ways in which practices unfold, is paramount in supporting creative moments with people living with dementia. Considering careless practices at a macro level could involve, for example, the ways in which creative programmes are funded and the frequent subjective well-being metrics used. For instance, as Hatton (2021) writes, arts organisations may unintentionally collude with the wider neoliberal agenda that places the responsibility with an individual to maintain their own well-being, negating the responsibility of health and social care services. Here, Hatton (2021) details a shift in focus – one that places people living with dementia within an interconnected caring network and de-emphasises the individual. Foregrounding the web of interdependencies at play within dementia care speaks to burgeoning approaches that advocate de-centring the person living with dementia (see, for example, Katz and Leibing, 2023) thus challenging dominant Western perspectives around selfhood. Recent critical dementia scholarship de-centres the person living with dementia to emphasise relational, connective, and collective approaches. For instance, Hulko (2023) de-centres dementia as an 'individual experience' and focuses instead on how people living with dementia are shaped 'by socio-cultural practices and discourses' (p. 228), thereby identifying how the individualism inherent in dominant Western discourse negates the complex intersections that impact the lives of people living with dementia.

When we bring this thinking to our focus on everyday creativity in the lives of people with dementia in care home settings, we can consider the ways in which it is impossible to disentangle the creative moment from the specific time, place, and context in which it unfolds. This involves noticing and elucidating the ways in which people, environments, and materials are contingent, unfixed, and ever-changing. This counters pervasive narratives that see people living with dementia as a homogenous group and focuses on 'recall', 'maintenance', and 'preservation' – all of which suggest a sense of fixedness and containment, implying that people living with dementia and their wants, needs, preferences, and so forth, can be pinned down and readily 'accessed'. We instead consider everyday creativity and citizenship as being in a constant state of becoming. Cultivating awareness of the material, sensory, and embodied (Hatton, 2021) within everyday creative moments in dementia care environments can offer vast opportunities to reimagine dementia care settings and practices (and conceptualisations of dementia more broadly). As Basting (2020) posits, 'the arts offer a chance for people with dementia to connect with the people who have forgotten them – their communities at large' (p. 16).

## Creative moments in practice – illustrative examples

We centre this section around the presentation of a selection of creative moments from our work with people living with dementia. We draw on the work of Keady et al. (2022) to consider these creative moments from our respective work. The moments presented here are considered through two concepts that act in dialogue with each other: *spontaneous creative moments* and *enabled creative moments*. We consider spontaneous creative moments as those that unfold in the everyday either outside a specific creative activity or within a facilitated session, but beyond its expected remit, initiated by a person living with dementia. They carry a sense of open-endedness, often being unexpected, improvised, and unprompted, gaining significance through the attentiveness and responsiveness of the people or things that are present. Enabled creative moments occur within the structure of a planned creative activity or session. These often involve engagement with more formal or recognised creative practices, supported through interactions with artists, care staff, family members, or friends. Both forms of creativity are relational: they arise within shared spaces of attention and care, and both invite us to consider how attunement to the embodied, sensory, and affective aspects of interaction shapes opportunities for creative expression.

These two forms of creativity are not discrete or hierarchical, but part of a dialogic process. For example, attending to spontaneous, everyday expressions can heighten awareness of a person's creative agency, prompting the development of more structured opportunities for engagement. In turn, participation in such enabled creative moments can deepen relationships, build mutual attunement, and sensitise those around the person to their embodied and relational modes of expression, making it more likely that spontaneous moments will be recognised and valued in everyday life. This cyclical interplay resonates with both relational citizenship (Kontos et al., 2017), a moment-focused approach to dementia (Keady et al., 2022), and care aesthetics (Thompson, 2023) in its focus on sustained attentiveness.

We now turn to illustrative examples, drawing on multiple studies in which we have had the privilege of working creatively with people living with dementia, both in the flow of their everyday lives and within the context of more structured creative activities. Whilst it is not possible to disentangle these forms of creativity, we hope to show how such moments can develop and evolve over time, shaping and being shaped by their relationships and environments in which they occur. All studies have ethical permissions via the institutions in which they were granted: Patient and Public Involvement and Engagement (PPIE) project led by Manchester Metropolitan University Health and approved by the Education Ethics Committee (reference number: 63966), and Rebecka's doctoral research approved by the NHS Research Ethics Committee (reference number: 18/LO/1707). Pseudonyms/codes have been used to protect the confidentiality of those who have been involved in research or PPIE work.

### *Going with the flow of the moment – Robyn Dowlen*

It is an unusually warm day in March when I arrive at the care home. It is a space that I have visited a couple of times before in setting up for a PPIE project led by Sarah Campbell and supported by myself and Rebecka. We have been trying since November to get a date in the diary to visit to run a workshop around everyday moments with the residents, but there have been staff changeovers and bouts of illness in the care home, which have led to many cancellations. We arrive with many sensory objects that are themed around the everyday: soaps, perfumes, jewellery, gardening gloves, photographs of green spaces, combs etc. We are waiting for a while in the reception area. We are nervous about the workshop because it feels as though the care home is not ready for our arrival and staff are, perhaps, not completely sure what it is we have come there to do.

Greta Santagata, the filmmaker, has accidentally gone to the wrong care home and so we wait for a while in the long corridor off reception. We are offered a cup of tea while we wait. When Greta arrives, we help bring her camera equipment through to the area in the care home where people with dementia live. We enter that space through a key code protected door. The space is bright and warm, many of the residents are sat outside with some members of the care staff. Others are having their lunch at the tables within the communal room that have yellow tablecloths. We all feel a bit flustered, it is hot, and we were expecting the room to be ready for us to run the workshop in the short amount of time we had. But the space is not ready, and it feels like we are hovering over people while they eat, which is an uncomfortable feeling.

Suddenly, a resident who is being pushed in a wheelchair whizzes past me and says, 'I'm sorry my dear but I'm just popping off to the shops, I've got your number though, so I'll give you a call on the way back'. 'Of course!' I respond, 'It's always so wonderful to see you, you've got my number. I look forward to hearing from you!' She wasn't off to the shops, she was going to be taking part in the workshop, but I went along with it, breaking the tension in the room of these new people who were unknown within their space. This interaction happens at such speed that I'm only thinking about it after it happened.

We set up the workshop ready for filming. The residents sit around the table and are a little uncertain of what it is they are meant to be doing. But that is the point of this exercise, it is to use everyday objects to elicit conversations, sensory experiences, changes in atmosphere. But it takes a bit of warming up. The presence of a filmmaker and camera equipment is also a little disorientating, so we make sure to restate what's happening. The workshop is full of energy and full of people living with dementia showcasing the different ways in which they use objects and the memories associated with different things that we have brought along with us. One of the smells leads to a resident beginning to sing (although I can't remember the song) and I join in with her. Music was not an element of the workshop that was planned, but we sing a couple of songs together. The rest of the group don't join in, but I turn to face her, and we try to awkwardly remember the lyrics to what very well-known songs should be.

There are many moments like this throughout the workshop. Even though there was a chaotic beginning to our presence in the space, the residents have eased into us being there. So much so that after we have cleared away and are having a debrief two of the residents decide to join us and engage in what feels like a stand-up comedy routine. Telling stories of their husbands, laughing and joking, bringing a warm presence to the beige room that we are in. We laugh, and we joke along with them. It brings a sense of ease to everyone in the room. When they leave, we note that this is why we love doing this type of work. It's for these moments. We get tied up in the bureaucracy of *doing* research when we really want to be *doing* care aesthetics in these moments. The spontaneous creativity of the residents in these moments allowed us to focus in on the ways that we could enable creativity in the short time we were present with them.

These moments (the imagined shopping trip, the unplanned songs, and the impromptu comedy routine) illustrate the dynamic interplay between spontaneous and creative moments. They emerged from the residents' own initiatives but were sustained through mutual recognition, responsiveness, and an openness to improvise. With regard to relational citizenship, these were acts through which residents expressed agency, humour, and identity, and through which we could recognise and affirm their place in the shared social world of the care home. From a care aesthetics perspective, the atmosphere, sensory prompts, and quality of our presence together created conditions for these moments to flourish. This interplay reminds us that whilst structured activities can enable creativity, attentiveness to the everyday and the unexpected is what allows these moments to surface. Taking this more porous approach allows us to gain a nuanced understanding of the value of creative arts in upholding meaningful moments for a person living with dementia in their everyday lives. It invites us to see creativity not only as an event to be delivered, but also as a way of being with each other 'in the moment', woven into thresholds, pauses, and transitions as much as into planned activities. In this sense, the arts become less a separate intervention and more of a mode of care, a texture of daily life that honours presence, fosters connection, and sustains a sense of belonging.

### *Creative material moments – Rebecka Fleetwood-Smith*

Here, I present two short extracts. The first moment reflects on a moment within a PPIE workshop (situated within the same session presented above) and the second presents a moment that unfolded during my PhD research (Fleetwood-Smith, 2020).

The first extract shares a reflection on engaging with a specific moment during the PPIE project led by Sarah Campbell (please see Chapter 5 for a further example of Sarah's work) and supported by Robyn and myself and speaks to the fragility of a creative moment as held within the care home setting:

> I am removed watching this – it is not how I usually work, and I am disappointed that I could not attend the session in person. As I sit watching, listening, and re-watching (without audio) the recording of the session, I am acutely aware that there is a sense of familiarity within the session – I have known similar encounters within care home settings. I am familiar with the overlapping discussions and questions. The concurrent moments that unfold come into being and slip away as different people engage with materials and with each other. I am helping to edit the films, watching with 'fresh' eyes. I am innately drawn to the 'quiet' moments, the passing and sorting of items, the flicker of an expression, the way the rhythm of a song is felt through the movement of someone's hands. As I make notes and suggestions, there is one moment that feels striking as it speaks to the complexity of this work. I pause and skip backwards to revisit the moment. Sarah is working with someone and offers her a satsuma to smell – she holds it close, just beneath the person's nose. At the same time, you can hear someone off camera say, 'she'll try and eat it'. The person Sarah is working with pretends to take a big bite of it (it's unpeeled), she laughs (as does Sarah) her

> shoulders move as she does so, and she smiles. The moment feels humorous, playful, and natural. As Sarah peels the satsuma the person is offered a satsuma segment by someone unseen by the camera. The moment is fleeting – if watched without sound, you would not know the concern raised by the person off camera.
>
> Context: Rebecka, a reading of a creative material moment from PPIE work led by Sarah Campbell in collaboration with Robyn Dowlen.

My reading of this is limited to my role as a collaborator and as someone who watched the footage and was not there. I do not know the care home site, or the people involved. However, the moment felt akin to many that I have noticed and felt during my time working in health and social care settings. A sense of cautiousness and risk aversion can hang heavy in these complex sites – this is typically at odds with the sense of permissiveness and openness inherent in creativity. Disentangling the practices which understandably necessitate caution and risk aversion (e.g., administering of medicine, supporting people during personal care) with creative ways of being that allow space for things to unfold is complex and subjective. Yet, as Thompson (2023) presents, all require an embodied and multisensory attentiveness. This extract speaks to the ways in which creative moments may be enabled, or curtailed, depending on the interdependent things at play.

The second extract, taken from my PhD research (Fleetwood-Smith, 2020), was part of a research encounter in which I explored everyday clothing practices in a care home setting. During the research, I worked with people living with dementia, care home staff, and creative practitioners. The research involved using creative, multisensory ways of working to explore practices. The following brings together research fieldnotes and reflexive notes:

> I had been working with this participant over a series of multisensory encounters, when this moment unfolded. We had built rapport and had a sort of rhythm to the way in which we worked together. During the encounters, I would invite her to reflect on her clothing. We would work together in a quiet space and encounters ranged anywhere from thirty minutes to an hour or so. The sessions would often involve travelling down unanticipated routes – gently guided by the prompts and questions that I used. I lightly scaffolded sessions to ensure that the time together was guided by the research. This was often difficult and sensitive, the encounters often felt like an opportunity for participants to take up space, to be heard, listened to, and engaged with beyond task-orientated care practices. Some participants brought specific objects or things with them into the sessions, other participants would explore what they were carrying on their person – it was very much dependent on the individual and how we worked together. I vividly remember this moment. When working with this participant, she commented on the large resin ring that I was wearing on my right index finger. The ring is quite distinctive, it was inexpensive, and I wear it most days. Without it my hand feels bare – the habitual weight and feel of it is important to me. Yet,

when the participant asked if it was heavy, I instinctively took it off, balanced it in my palm, and then handed it across. She examined it – turning it over in her hands. Then she balanced it in the centre of her palm, seemingly weighing it. She proceeded to try it on – moving it from thumb to index finger and so on. As she did so, she recited a rhyme from her childhood. The improvised moment was playful and joyful and unexpected for both of us. As she continued moving the ring and splaying her fingers, she translated the rhyme for me saying that it was both wonderful and difficult (I assumed it was the translation that may have been difficult to recollect). The moment came to a close as she handed the ring back and I put it back on.

Context: Rebecka, a reading of a creative material moment from her PhD research

This moment was held within a research encounter, centred around clothing practices, yet it was improvised, relational, and unfolded due to a sense of openness and togetherness. It was meaningful and prompted the embodied sharing of a memory through engagement with an unexpected object. Opportunities to engage with things, to handle, look through, explore, move, manipulate, and arrange are often limited within care home settings. Yet, there are vast opportunities for material things to support and enable everyday creative moments, whether that be someone rearranging a series of objects on a shelf or using something to express themselves.

## Conclusion and our speculative route out

The examples in this chapter show that creativity in the context of dementia is rarely confined to the walls of planned arts activities. It emerges in everyday exchanges, in improvised humour, in sensory responses, and in the gentle negotiation of shared spaces. These moments matter. They are where relational citizenship and care aesthetics meet, where we see agency enacted, identity affirmed, and connections forged in ways that may be fleeting but are no less significant.

Recognising these moments is not something that is accidental. It requires a model of care and practices that values attentiveness, makes space for the unplanned, and treats everyday interactions as creative opportunities. If we know what to look (and sense) for, we may begin to see and feel it more. And the more we notice and feel, the more we may create conditions where such moments arise. This noticing is both a skill and an ethic (Thompson, 2023): it demands time (something that is often stretched to its limit in care environments), curiosity, and a willingness to go with the flow of the creative moment. We recognise the unique position we held within these contexts, where we had the luxury to attend to, and enter into, moments that were initiated by people living with dementia. This is a luxury that many people who support the care of people living with dementia do not necessarily have. In this chapter, we have referred specifically to the possibilities of creative moments – this is not to simplify the complex, difficult, and challenging moments that occur within these settings all of which similarly necessitate careful, attentive practices to shift, limit, and (where possible) end such moments. We also raise here the trappings of this work, as we discuss the importance of noticing (and feeling) attentive practices that make room for such creative moments, we realise that there is a risk that creative moments are positioned, or considered only possible, through activation and thus suggesting that a person living with dementia lacks agency. This is not what we are suggesting. We do, however, argue that care models and care environments could better foster creative moments through attention to relational, everyday, embodied, and multisensory aesthetic encounters.

### *Speculative route out*

We want to end this chapter in a similar way to how we began it, by stepping out of the care home and into the wider context that surrounds (and facilitates) a careful approach to valuing the arts and creativity in the lives of people with dementia. As chapter authors, we came together again through a freewriting exercise, based on the question for our speculative route in, but this time asking, 'What would need to change in the structures and systems that uphold care in order for this to be a reality?' This may seem fruitless and simply an exercise in utopian speculative thinking given the challenging times we currently live in, but we hope it emphasises the macro-level changes required for the arts and creativity to be meaningfully valued in the lives of people living with dementia:

> *Creativity would not be 'a nice to have' but something that was embedded throughout the life course. We would not need to argue for the value of the arts, its presence would be seen, felt, and recognised. Artists would be valued for the ways in which they bring energy into care spaces and people living with dementia would engage in the arts in endless ways – the good, the bad, the ugly, and everything in between. Rather than being done 'against the odds', creativity would be woven throughout health and social care settings. People living with dementia would be held within their communities. Care homes would be important, multi-use spaces in our communities that invite people in rather than being 'unseen' locked spaces. The arts and social care would be well resourced promoting networks that foster creativity and connection. Productivity and efficiency would be de-emphasised to focus on meaningful and effective practices. Practitioners in health and social care would be valued and their skills upheld, recognised, and foregrounded as care-full, aesthetic, and relational.*

Finally, we close this chapter with a series of provocations for research and practice to deepen our understanding of creativity in the everyday lives of people with dementia. These prompts are intended to spark discussion, challenge assumptions, and invite new ways of thinking. We offer them with an awareness of the systemic challenges that shape the care of people living with dementia, and the opportunities that arise when those challenges are met with creativity and attentiveness:

- **What if** care environments were designed not just for safety and efficiency, but to prompt and respond to spontaneous creative acts? What would this look and feel like?
- **What if** training for care staff included skills in noticing, amplifying, and responding to embodied and relational forms of expression? What would this training look and feel like in practice?
- **What if** arts and dementia policy shifted from measuring programme outputs to valuing micro-interactions as markers of creative and cultural participation? Who do we need to convince that this shows value?
- **Who notices** these moments now, and who is missing from that conversation?
- **How might** we make the tools, language, and confidence to recognise everyday creativity to everyone in a care home, from cleaners to managers to visiting family?

The challenge now is not simply to notice these moments, but to embed the skills, sensibilities, relationships, and spaces that allow them to flourish. This will take us some way to making creativity an everyday right of citizenship for people living with dementia, one that is realised through aesthetic practices that value atmosphere, sensory richness, and relational presence as much as planned activities.

## Dedication

During the final stages of writing this chapter, Robyn and her family lost a close family friend. Ronni was a wonderfully creative person and a full-time carer for her mum, Sheila, who lived with dementia. She cared for Sheila with extraordinary love and creativity, and sadly, they died within two weeks of each other. They could often be found at dementia-friendly productions of musicals at the Chichester Festival Theatre where the staff ensured both Sheila and Ronni could continue to share their love of theatre and the arts. Ronni was an incredible advocate for her mum and truly embodied what it means to care creatively. These acts of care often go unseen, taking place behind closed doors, carried out with careful skill and humour. We hope that ongoing work within care aesthetics and dementia continues to shine light on such practices.

## Three Key Reading References

### *Reference 1*

Basting, A. (2020). *Creative Care: A Revolutionary Approach to Dementia and Elder Care*. New York: HarperCollins.

Basting's *Creative Care* offers a powerful reimagining of dementia care, centred on creativity as a transformative force. Drawing on decades of practice, she demonstrates how storytelling, improvisation, and imagination can generate connection and dignity beyond biomedical models. Her vision extends beyond activities to organisational culture, asking: 'what if we could pour [creativity] into the water of an organization so it spread through its systems to all its staff, the elders, and their families?' (p. 234). This question challenges us to think of creativity not as an optional enrichment but as a structural principle shaping relationships, atmospheres, spaces, and routines.

### *Reference 2*

Bellass, S., Balmer, A., May, V., Keady, J., Buse, C., Capstick, A., Burke, L., Bartlett, R. and Hodgson, J. (2019). Broadening the debate on creativity and dementia: A critical approach. *Dementia: The International Journal of Social Research and Practice*, 18 (7–8): 2799–2820. https://doi.org/10.1177/1471301218760906

Bellass et al. (2019) highlight the value of everyday creativity in this paper. Their work critiques the narrow views of creativity as the production of artistic outputs or participation in formal arts programmes. Instead, they foreground small, often overlooked acts (such as humour, play, improvisation, or inventiveness in daily routines) as important forms of creative expression. By recognising these moments, they demonstrate how creativity is woven through ordinary encounters and relationships, offering continuity of identity and fostering connection. Importantly, they situate creativity within a social and political context, attending to power dynamics, access, and the conditions that enable or constrain participation. Their framing supports a care aesthetics perspective that values the subtle, relational, and often fleeting creative acts through which people living with dementia assert agency and belonging.

### *Reference 3*

Kontos, P., Miller, K.L. and Kontos, A.P. (2017). Relational citizenship: Supporting embodied selfhood and relationality in dementia care. *Sociology of Health & Illness*, 39 (2): 182–198. https://doi.org/10.1111/1467-9566.12453

This paper is central to reframing dementia care through the lens of relational citizenship. Building on the concept of embodied selfhood, the authors argue that citizenship cannot be reduced to cognitive capacity or verbal expression but is continually enacted through embodied, relational practices. Drawing on ethnographic insights, they show how gestures, rhythms, touch, and aesthetic encounters allow people living with dementia to assert identity, agency, and belonging within shared social worlds. Relational citizenship thus recognises the mutual, co-constructed nature of care, in which creativity and responsiveness are foundational for sustaining personhood.

## References


Alzheimer's Society. (n.d.). *Facts for the media about dementia.* Available: https://www.alzheimers.org.uk/what-we-do/news-and-media/facts-media; accessed 1 March 2026.

Bartlett, R. and O'Connor, D. (2010). *Broadening the Dementia Debate: Towards Social Citizenship*. Bristol: Policy Press.

Basting, A. (2020). *Creative Care: A Revolutionary Approach to Dementia and Elder Care.* New York: HarperCollins.

Basting, A., Towey, M. and Rose, E. (2016). *The Penelope Project: An Arts-Based Odyssey to Change Elder Care*. Iowa: University of Iowa Press.

Basting, A.D. (2009). *Forget Memory: Creating Better Lives for People with Dementia.* Baltimore: John Hopkins University Press.

Bellass, S., Balmer, A., May, V., Keady, J., Buse, C., Capstick, A., Burke, L., Bartlett, R. and Hodgson, J. (2019). Broadening the debate on creativity and dementia: A critical approach. *Dementia: The International Journal of Social Research and Practice*, 18 (7–8): 2799–2820. https://doi.org/10.1177/1471301218760906

Bradwell, C. (2025). (not) lovely: Enacting solidarity in dementia care through participatory Arts. *Journal of Aging Studies*, *75*, 101352. Available: https://doi.org/10.1016/j.jaging.2025.101352; accessed 1 March 2026.

Buse, C. and Twigg, J. (2016). Materialising memories: Exploring the stories of people with dementia through dress. *Ageing & Society*, 36 (6): 1115–1135. https://doi.org/10.1017/S0144686X15000185

Buse, C. and Twigg, J. (2018). Dressing disrupted: Negotiating care through the materiality of dress in the context of dementia. *Sociology of Health & Illness*, 40 (2): 340–352. https://doi.org/10.1111/1467-9566.12575

Camic, P.M., Hulbert, S. and Kimmel, J. (2019). Museum object handling: A health-promoting community-based activity for dementia care. *Journal of Health Psychology*, 24 (6): 787–798. https://doi.org/10.1177/1359105316685899

Campbell, S., Dowlen, R., Keady, J., and Thompson, J. (2024). Care aesthetics and 'being in the moment' through improvised music-making and male grooming in dementia care. *International Journal of Education & the Arts*, 25 (si1.13). Available: https://journals.psu.edu/ijea/article/view/63522; accessed 1 March 2026.

De Medeiros, K. and Basting, A. (2014). "Shall I compare thee to a dose of donepezil?": Cultural arts interventions in dementia care research. *The Gerontologist*, 54 (3): 344–353. https://doi.org/10.1093/geront/gnt055

Dowlen, R. and Fleetwood-Smith, R. (2023). From symptoms to citizenship: A critical reading of the perceived value of arts and culture in a dementia context. In J. Fletcher and A. Capstick (eds.) *A Critical History of Dementia Studies*. London: Routledge, pp. 138–154.

Dowlen, R., Keady, J., Milligan, C., Swarbrick, C., Ponsillo, N., Geddes, L. and Riley, B. (2022). In the moment with music: An exploration of the embodied and sensory experiences of people living with dementia during improvised music-making. *Ageing & Society*, 42 (11): 2642–2664. https://doi.org/10.1017/S0144686X21000210

Dowlen, R., McPherson, D.H.J., Swarbrick, C., Hoskin, L., Thompson, J. and Keady, J. (2024). Creating and reliving the moment: Using musical improvisation and care aesthetics as a lens of connection and self-expression for younger people living with dementia. *International Journal of Environmental Research and Public Health*, 21 (8): 972. Available: https://doi.org/10.3390/ijerph21080972; accessed 1 March 2026.

Downs, M. (2013). Embodiment: The implications for living well with dementia. *Dementia: The International Journal of Social Research and Practice*, 12 (3): 368–374. https://doi.org/10.1177/1471301213487465

Dowson, B., Atkinson, R., Barnes, J., Barone, C., Cutts, N., Donnebaum, E., Hung Hsu, M., Lo Coco, I., John, G., Meadows, G., O'Neill, A., Noble, D., Norman, G., Pfende, F., Quinn, P., Warren, A., Watkins, C. and Schneider, J. (2021). Digital approaches to music-making for people with dementia in response to the COVID-19 pandemic: Current practice and recommendations. *Frontiers in Psychology*, *12*. Available: https://doi.org/10.3389/fpsyg.2021.625258; accessed 1 March 2026.

Fleetwood-Smith, R. (2020). *Exploring the significance of clothing to people living with dementia using Sensory Ethnography.* PhD thesis, The University of West London. Available: https://repository.uwl.ac.uk/id/eprint/7758/1/Rebecka%20Fleetwood-Smith_Thesis_2020.pdf; accessed 1 March 2026.

Fleetwood-Smith, R., Tischler, V. and Robson, D. (2022). Aesthetics and dementia: Exploring the role of everyday aesthetics in dementia care settings. *Design for Health*, 6 (1): 91–113. https://doi.org/10.1080/24735132.2022.2074207

Fox, S., Thompson, J. and Keady, J. (2025). Meaningful moments of connection: How people affected by dementia and their carers living at home understand, interpret and experience everyday aesthetics. *International Journal of Geriatric Psychiatry*, 40 (8): e70136. Available: https://doi.org/10.1002/gps.70136; accessed 1 March 2026.

Gray, K., Evans, S.C., Griffiths, A. and Schneider, J. (2018). Critical reflections on methodological challenge in arts and dementia evaluation and research. *Dementia: The International Journal of Social Research and Practice*, 17 (6): 775–784. https://doi.org/10.1177/1471301217734478

Halpern, A.R., Ly, J., Elkin-Frankston, S. and O'Connor, M.G. (2008). "I know what I like": Stability of aesthetic preference in Alzheimer's patients. *Brain and Cognition*, 66 (1): 65–72. https://doi.org/10.1016/j.bandc.2007.05.008

Hatton, N. (2021). *Performance and Dementia: A Cultural Response to Care*. Springer International Publishing. Available: https://link.springer.com/book/10.1007/978-3-030-51077-0; accessed 1 March 2026.

Hulko, W. (2023). Revolutionising dementia policy and practice: Guidance from 'the memory girl', an accomplice. In R. Ward and L. J. Sandberg (eds.) *Critical Dementia Studies: An Introduction.* London: Routledge, chapter 16. Available: https://www.taylorfrancis.com/chapters/oa-edit/10.4324/9781003221982-21/revolutionising-dementia-policy-practice-wendy-hulko?context=ubx&refId=9a5c7e53-ae8b-4411-807c-457da8753800; accessed 1 March 2026.

James, I.A. and Jackman, L. (2017). *Understanding Behaviour in Dementia that Challenges: A Guide to asAessment and Treatment*. London: Jessica Kingsley.

Katz, S. and Leibing, A. (2023). 'Lost in time like tears in rain': Critical perspectives on personhood and dementia. In R. Ward and L. J. Sandberg (eds.) *Critical Dementia Studies: An Introduction.* London: Routledge, chapter 6. Available at: https://www.taylorfrancis.com/books/oa-edit/10.4324/9781003221982/critical-dementia-studies-richard-ward-linn-sandberg?refId=11c60a23-97d4-4a27-b200-1ff68986d09d&context=ubx; accessed 1 March 2026.

Keady, J.D., Campbell, S., Clark, A., Dowlen, R., Elvish, R., Jones, L., Kindell, J., Swarbrick, C. and Williams, S. (2022). Re-thinking and re-positioning 'being in the moment' within a continuum of moments: Introducing a new conceptual framework for dementia studies. *Ageing & Society*, 42 (3): 681–702. https://doi.org/10.1017/S0144686X20001014

Kinsey, D., Lang, I., Orr, N., Anderson, R. and Parker, D. (2021). The impact of including carers in museum programmes for people with dementia: A realist review. *Arts & Health*, 13 (1): 1–19. https://doi.org/10.1080/17533015.2019.1700536

Kontos, P. (2004). Ethnographic reflections on selfhood, embodiment and Alzheimer's disease. *Ageing & Society*, 24 (6): 829–849. https://doi.org/10.1017/S0144686X04002375

Kontos, P. (2005). Embodied selfhood in Alzheimer's disease: Rethinking person-centred care. *Dementia: The International Journal of Social Research and Practice*, 4 (4): 553–570. https://doi.org/10.1177/1471301205058311

Kontos, P., Miller, K.L. and Kontos, A.P. (2017). Relational citizenship: Supporting embodied selfhood and relationality in dementia care. *Sociology of Health & Illness*, 39 (2): 182–198. https://doi.org/10.1111/1467-9566.12453

Kontos, P., Grigorovich, A. and Colobong, R. (2020). Towards a critical understanding of creativity and dementia: New directions for practice change. *International Practice Development Journal*, 10 (3) [online]. Available: https://doi.org/10.19043/ipdj.10Suppl.003; accessed 1 March 2026.

Kontos, P., Grigorovich, A., Kosurko, A., Bar, R.J., Herron, R.V., Menec, V.H. and Skinner, M.W. (2021). Dancing with dementia: Exploring the embodied dimensions of creativity and social engagement. *The Gerontologist*, 61 (5): 714–723. https://doi.org/10.1093/geront/gnaa129

Martin, E. (1992). Body narratives, body boundaries. In L. Grossberg, C. Nelson and P. Treichler (eds.) *Cultural Studies*. New York: Routledge, pp. 409–423.

Nedlund, A.C., Bartlett, R. and Clarke, C.L. (2019). *Everyday Citizenship and People with Dementia*. Edinburgh: Dunedin Academic Press.

Richards, R. (2018). *Everyday Creativity and the Healthy Mind: Dynamic New Paths for Self and Society*. London: Palgrave Macmillan.

Robertson, J.M. and McCall, V. (2020). Facilitating creativity in dementia care: The co-construction of arts-based engagement. *Ageing & Society*, 40 (6): 2155–1174. https://doi.org/10.1017/S0144686X18001575

Sabat, S. (2014). A bio-psycho-social approach to dementia. In M. Downs and B. Bowers (eds.) *Excellence in Dementia Care: Research into Practice*. Maidenhead: Open University Press, pp. 107–121.

Saito, Y. (2007). *Everyday Aesthetics*. Oxford: Oxford University Press.

Saito, Y. (2017). *Aesthetics of the Familiar: Everyday Life and World-Making*. Oxford: Oxford University Press.

Saito, Y. (2023). Living with everyday objects: Aesthetic and ethical practice. In E. K. Man and J. Petts (eds.) *Comparative Everyday Aesthetics: East-West Studies in Contemporary Living*. Amsterdam: Amsterdam University Press, pp. 9–20.

Shakespeare, T., Zeilig, H. and Mittler, P. (2019). Rights in mind: Thinking differently about dementia and disability. *Dementia: The International Journal of Social Research and Practice*, 18 (3): 1075–1088. https://doi.org/10.1177/1471301217701506

Thompson, J. (2020). Towards an aesthetics of care. In A. Stuart Fisher and J. Thompson (eds.) *Performing Care: New Perspectives on Socially Engaged Performance*. Manchester: Manchester University Press, pp. 36–38

Thompson, J. (2023). *Care Aesthetics: For Artful Care and Careful Art*. London: Routledge.

UK Music and Music for Dementia. (2022). *Power of Music: A plan for harnessing music to improve our health, wellbeing and communities*. Available: https://musicfordementia.org.uk/wp-content/uploads/2022/04/Power-of-Music-Report.pdf; accessed 1 March 2026.

van der Steen, J.T., van der Wouden, J.C., Methley, A.M., Smaling, H.J., Vink, A.C. and Bruinsma, M.S. (2025). Music-based therapeutic interventions for people with dementia. *Cochrane Database of Systematic Reviews*, (3). Available: https://doi.org/10.1002/14651858.CD003477.pub5; accessed 1 March 2026.

Ward, R., Campbell, S. and Keady, J. (2014). 'Once I had money in my pocket, I was every colour under the sun': Using appearance biographies to explore the meanings of appearance for people with dementia. *Journal of Aging Studies*, 30: 64–72. Available: https://doi.org/10.1016/j.jaging.2014.03.006; accessed 1 March 2026.

West, J., Zeilig, H., Cape, T., Payne, L. and Whistler, C. (2024). Making a living moment more resonant: An exploration of the role of the artist in co-creative work with people living with dementia. *Wellcome Open Research*, 8, 580. Available: https://doi.org/10.12688/wellcomeopenres.19357.3; accessed 1 March 2026.

Zeilig, H., Killick, J. and Fox, C. (2014). The participative arts for people living with a dementia: A critical review. *International Journal of Ageing and Later Life*, 9 (1): 7–34. https://doi.org/10.3384/ijal.1652-8670.14238

# 8

# INTEGRATING AESTHETICS, NEUROAESTHETICS, AND POLYVAGAL THEORY TO DEVELOP A NOVEL CONCEPTUAL FRAMEWORK FOR PERSON-CENTRED DEMENTIA CARE

*Sarah Fox*

## Author note

I have included a 'Glossary of Key Terms' in Box 8.1 (situated at the end of this chapter) to provide further information on terms that may be unfamiliar to the reader and require additional explanation. At first use only, the terms included in Box 8.1 are marked with a * in this chapter.

## Introduction

I spent most of my early career meandering between disciplines, searching for a path which reflected the duality of my interests and identity. As a teenager, I dreamed of becoming an illustrator. I drew immense joy from copying the elegant curves and fluid physiques of the Lion King's characters (Minkoff and Allers, 1994) and was amazed to learn how the animators travelled to Africa to observe lions in the wild so they could reliably translate their movements onto the screen. However, this early dream, as is often the case for childhood dreams, did not come to pass and instead I chose to follow a science, technology, and engineering career path at university.

Driven by curiosity about how the brain works, and what happens when things go wrong, my PhD studies at The University of Manchester focused on how communication between different parts of the brain involved in forming, consolidating, and storing memories changed as the pathology of Alzheimer's disease spread (Fox, 2014). In many ways, the elegance and creativity of the scientific method mirrored the attributes I once found in art. However, as I reached the conclusion of my first postdoctoral position in 2016, I found myself reflecting on the animators I used to admire, remembering how they did not just draw lions from static images

DOI: 10.4324/9781003623441-11
This chapter has been made available under a (CC BY) 4.0 license.

or memory, but they travelled to observe them in their natural environments. Having no personal experience of dementia at this time, my knowledge about the topic was drawn from academic papers, mouse models, and the gentle fireworks of chattering neurons. I knew there was something missing. Soon after concluding my first postdoctoral position, I sidestepped the lab bench and moved into the field of Patient and Public Involvement and Engagement (PPIE), discovering the ideology 'nothing about us without us' which helped to meet this 'missing' need. This was met through my work with Greater Manchester Mental Health's Dementia Research Centre (https://gmmh.nhs.uk/greater-manchester-dementia-research-centre/; accessed 1 March 2026) and Dementia United (https://dementia-united.org.uk/; accessed 1 March 2026), Greater Manchester's Integrated Care Partnership's programme for dementia, both of which facilitate the involvement of people living with dementia in a range of local, regional, and national strategic and research initiatives.

After several years working closely with people living with dementia and their carers in Greater Manchester, seeing first-hand the impact our health and social care system had on their lives, in 2022, I applied for, and took the opportunity to become, a DEM-COMM postdoctoral Fellow, a scheme funded by the National Institute for Health and Care Research (NIHR) and the Alzheimer's Society and based at The University of Manchester at the NIHR Applied Research Collaboration-Greater Manchester (https://healthinnovationmanchester.com/our-work/arc-gm/Applied; accessed 1 March 2026). My introduction to this DEM-COMM position was serendipitous insofar as due to my previous research experience, Dementia United had asked me to join a call with The University of Manchester to discuss four proposed postdoctoral Fellowship projects funded as part of the DEM-COMM scheme. As I was taking notes about how Dementia United might support these Fellowships, I became increasingly distracted by discussion of one project; this was proposed by James Thompson and John Keady (and editors of this volume) and involved researching everyday aesthetics* in dementia care. Following on from a positive experience in 2021, as an Atlantic Fellow for Equity in Brain Health (see: https://www.gbhi.org/; accessed 1 March 2026) where I worked closely with creative professionals, and alongside my experiences in PPIE, I could not help but see myself in this work. After some soul-searching about leaving my colleagues and projects at Dementia United, I applied for the 'everyday aesthetics and dementia' Fellowship and was thrilled to be offered the position, setting me on a path to integrate my practical experience and creative interests in dementia research.

As of October 2025 (when this chapter is being written), I am researching at the intersection of social science, art, and healthcare, and I can see how my academic and professional background offer a unique perspective for understanding dementia from a lived, aesthetic, and neurobiological perspective. The challenges faced by people living with dementia are neither uniquely psychosocial nor uniquely biological. It is the interplay of these factors combined with an individual's everyday environment, resources, values, and preferences which drives their experience of dementia, suggesting the importance of a bio–psycho–social–physical model of dementia care (Keady et al., 2013).

## The landscape

Throughout my employment in integrated care, I spent a lot of time listening to the voices of those affected by dementia and one resounding message rose to the surface which has recently been articulated in a Care England (2025) report, namely: 'Despite its scale, the current dementia care system remains fragmented, underfunded, and difficult to navigate, leaving many individuals and families unsupported' (p. 8). This concerning situation sometimes circulates around the fragmentation of access to medical care, but it may also be focused on the distinct lack of 'something' just as intrinsic to everyday life, namely, access to environments and experiences that enable people living with dementia and their carers to live well with the condition. Indeed, the Mayor of Greater Manchester, Andy Burnham, made a similar observation when he stated:

> You have got to start with the person not the patient, prioritise social, cultural and creative interventions to prevent the risk of cognitive decline. In a 21st century NHS we need to turn things around.
>
> *(Franklin Gould, 2021)*

It is only relatively recently that health and social care policy and practice have begun to catch up with these lived narratives and concerns. For instance, in the early 20th century, dementia was considered predominantly through a biomedical lens with a focus on medical management of symptoms rather than on improving quality of life and well-being. However, mainly stemming from the seminal work of Professor Tom Kitwood in the late 1980s and into the 1990s (see, for example, Kitwood, 1997), narratives shifted to include reference to person-centred care, acknowledging the effect the interplay of biological, social, and environmental factors has on the ability of a person living with dementia to live well and retain their personhood.

The ideas behind person-centred care have spawned a wealth of research and policy which focus on the everyday experiences of people living with dementia. Policy frameworks such as the UK Prime Minister's challenge on dementia 2020 (Department of Health, 2015), and research from national initiatives like the IDEAL study (Clare et al., 2025) and the Neighbourhoods study (Keady, 2024), increasingly recognised that this form of well-being is not achieved through clinical care alone, but through a multidisciplinary approach that brings together biomedical, neurological, psychosocial, and aesthetic understandings of dementia as it is lived every day.

In this chapter, I will discuss how current research concerning the aesthetic, physiological, social, and psychological aspects of dementia may be drawn together to develop a novel integrative framework for aesthetic dementia care. I focus on the three fields independently these being aesthetics*, neuroaesthetics*, and Polyvagal Theory*, before moving to discuss their conceptual overlaps and divergences, ultimately suggesting where the fields interweave and where they can inform one another.

## An introduction to the core lenses

Drawing on my cross-disciplinary background and work to date alongside people with lived experience of dementia, I have identified three intersecting conceptual lenses which, I believe, when combined, offer the foundations for a novel framework for person-centred dementia care. These are:

1. Aesthetics, which highlight the sensory and embodied experiences that impact an individual's emotional connection to their lived environments and relationships with those around them.
2. Neuroaesthetics, which considers how the brain processes and responds to aesthetic experiences, offering a neurological basis for understanding the potential impact of aesthetic experiences in both health and disease.
3. Polyvagal Theory, which examines how social, relational, and environmental experiences impact the autonomic nervous system (ANS)* and how these can be harnessed therapeutically to foster experiences of safety and connection.

In the sections that follow, I explore each of these lenses independently, starting with aesthetics, and then move to integrate these into a coherent framework with implications for dementia care, policy, and practice.

### *Aesthetics*

When Alexander Gottlieb Baumgarten (1750) first coined the term aesthetics in the 18th century, he positioned it as a distinct form of knowing, separate from logical and conceptual knowledge and instead derived from the senses, intuition, and perception. Whilst the term has traditionally been associated with artistic beauty, modern thinkers such as Thomas Leddy (2015) and Yuriko Saito (2010) have stressed a continuity between the aesthetics of art and everyday life. They suggest that our sensuous engagement with the physical and social world represents an aesthetic experience which is separable from our logical and conceptual interactions.

Drawing from both my personal and academic experiences, I suggest that aesthetic experiences provide a layer of experiential, sensory safety, and connection for (all) people living with dementia, which is accessible despite cognitive decline.

This next section therefore explores how aesthetics may help to sustain a sense of identity and support well-being for those living with dementia whilst cognitive capacities change.

*Everyday aesthetics, identity, and dementia*

Several months ago, I was walking through a street in Greater Manchester with my husband and his family. This street was part of a bustling Jewish community, the air was filled with the smell of traditional foods, whilst distinctive kippahs and the occasional shtreimel hurried by. My husband's mother, who is a practising progressive Jew, turned to us with a smile and commented on how safe and homely the street felt, reflecting on how nice it was to be enwrapped in the culture she identified with: 'Doesn't it just feel so comfortable?' she observed, questioningly. My response was stilted, since my experience of this environment seemed at odds with hers. As a non-religious woman, dressed in bright summer clothes, which were by no means immodest but also not modest enough by orthodox religious standards, I actively felt out of place.

Yuriko Saito, in Media and IAFOR (2015), defines everyday aesthetics as 'the aesthetics of objects, environments and situations from our everyday life', also suggesting that the aesthetic tone of everyday experiences is self-defined by the individual. At the time, my own experience struck me as being an interesting example of everyday aesthetics and how this concept interacts with an individual's sense of felt and known identity. The aesthetic environment of that street, built from the sights, sounds, smells, and social atmosphere, triggered in both my mother-in-law and me a unique experience, one which we translated into an affective experience as it filtered through the lens of our own histories, cultures, and identities.

My personal example illustrates how an aesthetic experience can emotionally affect an individual and how the valence of this effect may be guided by the individual's unique social, cultural, and personal identity. This relationship between aesthetic experience, identity, and well-being has important implications for people living with dementia.

Today, many academics and clinicians favour an approach which assumes selfhood to be underpinned by a mixture of cognition, social interactions, and bodily sources of agency (Sabat, 2005; Keady et al., 2013; Kontos and Martin, 2013; Hughes, 2014; Jones et al., 2025; Kindell et al., 2025). Therefore, even when cognition falters, an individual's identity and personhood can be maintained through aesthetic experiences and connections, including social interactions, preconscious bodily behaviours, and experiences. Indeed, growing evidence also suggests that despite cognitive decline, people living with dementia maintain the ability to recognise, appreciate, and engage in aesthetic experiences (Halpern et al., 2008).

Returning to my personal illustration, for my mother-in-law, the smells and sounds of a traditional Jewish neighbourhood evoked feelings of comfort and belonging based on her autobiographical history and experiences. For people living with dementia, similarly meaningful aesthetic cues may provide a bridge to identity, offering continuity, reassurance, and a sense of safety and well-being. Indeed, access to the benefits of such experiences may not require bespoke interventions since these experiences are embedded in everyday 'ordinary' environments and interactions, thus offering an accessible everyday approach to person-centred dementia care.

### *Care aesthetics**

This field focuses on the felt, embodied, and relational dimensions that shape how care is given and received. To illustrate the meaning of care aesthetics, Thompson (2023) uses a particularly poignant example in his book *Care Aesthetics: For Artful Care and Careful Art* where he observes the work of a physiotherapist providing rehabilitation to one of his colleagues who was significantly injured in a war zone. He describes how the practitioners' attentive, gentle touch transformed the rehabilitation process, going beyond the purely mechanical or functional elements of physiotherapeutic practice, and infusing the care with an artistry based on trust, attention, and sensory awareness. This forms a counterpoint to the visceral observation of care used by Kitwood (1997) when he outlined the debilitating elements of 'malignant social psychology' where residents in a care home were left sitting on commodes in a semi-public space whilst staff carried on with other tasks or conversations nearby. Both examples illustrate an aesthetic of care, whereas one is artful and beautiful, the other may be seen as dehumanising and disconnected. Whilst care aesthetics is often discussed as a relational practice, it can also be observed in the environments, atmospheres, and policies of care settings.

As there is conceptual divergence between 'everyday' and 'care aesthetics', both draw from Baumgarten's (1750) concept of an aesthetic form of knowing and therefore, from this point on in this chapter, I will use the term 'aesthetics' when referring broadly to aesthetic experiences which may encompass concepts from both 'care' and 'everyday' conceptual positioning. That said, I will also use the terms 'care aesthetics' or 'everyday aesthetics' specifically if I need to reference these concepts independently.

### *Aesthetics: an expansive definition for a unique experience*

As discussed by Leddy (2015) and Saito (2010), the definition of everyday aesthetics is expansive and subjective. Leddy (2015) explores this span when he discusses 'garbage moments' in his essay *Experience of Awe: An Expansive Approach to Everyday Aesthetics*. Here, Leddy (2015) reflects on whether an act as mundane as taking out the garbage could ever be considered aesthetic, referencing a cartoon called 'Rose is Rose' where a character experiences moments of awe whilst taking out the family's garbage. This reflection aligns with my belief that we cannot be prescriptive regarding what we define as an aesthetic experience, and that we must appreciate the aesthetic value of a given moment as defined subjectively by the person experiencing it. Indeed, in a recent publication (Fox et al., 2025), I probed how people living with dementia and their carers experience and identify aesthetic moments in their own daily lives. Whilst the language of aesthetics was unfamiliar to this demographic, the underlying theoretical concept of everyday aesthetics was easily grasped. Using the alternative term 'meaningful moments of connection' (put forward by people living with dementia during a consultation meeting early on in my study) as a proxy for everyday aesthetics, participants identified a range of aesthetic moments in their everyday lives spanning sensory, physical, relational, and cognitive experiences which were based on their biographical histories and preferences. These meaningful moments of connection were then linked with subjective identity and well-being.

Whilst my research findings provided interesting insights, it has been the resulting conversations and public support which have impacted me the most. Almost without fail, public and professional presentations of this work drew out vivid reflections from audience members with their own lived experience. However, this also leads to a concern about how aesthetic experiences are defined, and whether the expansive subjectivity of my findings (Fox et al., 2025), alongside Leddy's (2015), Saito's (2001, 2010) and Thompson's (2023) definitions of aesthetics, may hinder their adaptation into the kind of structured framework that clinical professionals might apply to their practice. Yet, whilst the interpretation of an aesthetic experience is inevitably subjective and shaped by personal biography, the underlying biological responses it elicits may be consistent across individuals. Hence, I believe that understanding of the neurocognitive and psychological mechanisms which underpin aesthetic experiences may offer an objective cornerstone for a future aesthetic-based care framework, a concept I will return to later in this chapter.

### *In summary*

Aesthetic experiences, shaped by sensory input, culture, and personal history, can support identity, well-being, and a sense of continuity for people living with dementia, even amidst cognitive decline. Everyday objects, environments, and artful, caring relationships all have the potential to create meaningful and emotionally resonant moments. By recognising the subjective, yet biologically grounded nature of these experiences, we can identify a promising pathway for person-centred dementia care.

## *Neuroaesthetics*

The field of neuroaesthetics explores how the brain and nervous system process and respond to aesthetic experiences. This field draws on a variety of methods, such as functional magnetic resonance imaging, electroencephalogram, and physiological measurements (including heart rate and skin conductance) to trace responses to aesthetic stimuli, ranging from music, visual art, dance, and natural environments (Chatterjee, 2011). Whilst the history and scope of neuroaesthetic research is broad, here I will focus on theories and studies which I believe hold particular relevance for the discussion of aesthetics in dementia care. For those interested in learning more about neuroaesthetics, I recommend reviews conducted by Cinza and Vittorio (2009), Chatterjee (2011), Chatterjee and Vartanian (2014) and Ligaya et al. (2020).

### *Beauty and the brain*

In a recent *Perspectives* paper by Nadal and Skov (2024), the authors proposed a sensory valuation account of aesthetic experiences. They suggested that, from a neurological perspective, aesthetic experiences are not unique and may not be linked solely to stimuli traditionally regarded as artful or beautiful, i.e., there is no unique brain region which solely processes artful stimuli. Rather, they suggested that neural responses, traditionally observed in neuroaesthetic studies, activated a network of brain regions known as the mesocorticolimbic reward system* and that activation of this system is the same for art and non-art stimuli (Grewe et al., 2010). Interestingly, Nadal and Skov (2024) also found that responses to pleasurable stimuli are not unique to humans, with many mammals showing activation of equivalent neural systems to those activated by pleasurable experiences in human subjects. This suggests that the brain networks which process aesthetic stimuli may have evolved from more primitive systems whose role it was to assess the hedonic and survival value of everyday experiences, such as food or survival threats. Over time, these systems may have evolved to include assessment of more abstract, artistic, and cultural objects and experiences. To the best of my knowledge, a direct comparison has yet to be made between everyday aesthetics and Nadal and Skov's (2024) account. Nonetheless, a conceptual overlap is apparent in the suggestion that the same brain regions which respond to art and beauty may also process everyday pleasurable experiences with less 'traditional' artistic or cultural value, such as enjoyable food and good company, arguably aesthetic experiences in themselves.

When considering aesthetic care, this neurological framework may help us to understand how people experience everyday aesthetics and why this experience might be functionally different to those living with dementia. For example, Nadal and Skov's (2024) hypothesis regarding the mesocorticolimbic reward system might provide a roadmap for how aesthetic experiences are processed by the brain. Their theory highlights several distinct brain regions which work together to evaluate an aesthetic experience. This means we can break down an aesthetic experience into a computation which combines sensory input (visual imagery, smells, touch, etc.), executive and semantic processing (existing knowledge, situational expectations, etc.), and physiological state (homeostatic, autonomic and endocrine information representative of physiological states, hunger, pain, etc.). This enables a better understanding of the range of factors that directly impact the computation of an emotional outcome based on an aesthetic experience.

During my time as a PPIE officer at Dementia United, I worked with someone who had a phobia of barking dogs and this individual also struggled with sensory difficulties as part of their dementia. They once described a panic attack in a public bathroom because the sound of the hand dryer reminded them of barking. This case illustrates how altered sensory processing can profoundly shape the hedonic and emotional quality of an everyday experience. Thus, when developing aesthetic-based care frameworks, it will be essential to recognise how sensory differences, physical factors such as infection or hunger, memories, and aesthetic preferences all impact an individual's experience of an environment or interaction.

Another brain network thought to be involved in aesthetic processing is known as the default mode network (DMN)*. In their unifying model, Menon (2023) suggested that the DMN brings together regions of the brain which combine language, autobiographical memory*, and knowledge about the world (semantic memory*) with the overall purpose of creating an internal narrative and subjective continuity of internal mental thoughts; a sense of self and place within the wider world. This model suggests that the DMN network informs a unique multifaceted narrative linked to our sense of self, based on our histories, experiences, likes, and dislikes.

Interestingly, alongside its proposed role in maintaining a sense of self, the DMN is also activated by aesthetic experiences. A study by Vessel et al. (2012) found that images rated by study participants as 'highly aesthetic' activated the DMN, whilst those rated as 'less aesthetic' did not. Since DMN activity is predominantly linked to periods of self-reflection and is traditionally suppressed by physical tasks, activity of the DMN during presentation of external stimuli is rare. This may reflect a unique property of intensely aesthetic stimuli in increasing internalised self-reflection.

Whilst the stimuli used in Vessel et al.'s (2012) study (images of artwork) aligns better with a traditional view of art-focussed aesthetics, rather than everyday aesthetics, the broader methodology was reflective of Saito's (2001) suggestion that 'it is generally agreed that aesthetic objects do not constitute a set of special objects but rather are determined by our [in this case the study participant's] attitudes and experiences' (p. 1). Specifically, participants in Vessel et al.'s (2012) study rated the images they viewed based on their own aesthetic preferences on a scale of 1–4. This methodology encouraged participants to make their own judgement regarding the aesthetic quality of the study images.

This work suggests that the mesocorticolimbic reward system and the DMN may work together to evaluate aesthetic experiences with the mesocorticolimbic reward system evaluating the reward value of an aesthetic experience, whilst the DMN weaves these experiences into an individual's personal narrative, linking momentary aesthetic pleasure with a sense of self and personal narrative. These theories also speak to my recent study (Fox et al., 2025) which indicated that self-reported aesthetic stimuli are linked with a sense of self for people living with dementia. Therefore, further research is warranted to explore how aesthetic-induced mesocorticolimbic and DMN activity might impact personal narratives and self-identity for people living with dementia.

In the preceding sections, I have considered how everyday and care aesthetics might form the basis of a new framework of aesthetic care for people living with dementia. I have also highlighted how insights into the brain regions involved in processing aesthetic stimuli can inform this work. So far, these approaches have emphasised the aesthetic world and the brain but have paid less attention to the body, the medium through which the two are integrated. To address this, I will now turn to Polyvagal Theory, which examines how social, relational, and environmental cues shape the nervous system's responses. Polyvagal Theory offers therapeutic perspectives on how aesthetic elements of care and environments foster safety, connection, and autonomic regulation.

### *In summary*

Neuroaesthetics demonstrates that aesthetic experiences, whether derived from traditional art or everyday encounters, can engage both the brain's reward systems and the DMN. These networks integrate sensory input with memory, emotion, and self-identity, whilst individual preferences, personal histories, and bodily states further shape each experience, making it deeply personal. Such insights illuminate how the aesthetic and relational elements of care influence brain function, and how a person living with dementia may interpret their environment differently depending on their history, preferences, physiological state, and cognitive abilities.

## *Polyvagal Theory*

Neuroaesthetics helps us understand how the brain responds to aesthetic experiences, but it does not fully explain how these experiences are felt in the body. Polyvagal Theory fills this gap by showing how the nervous system translates sensory and social cues into feelings of safety, connection, or stress. I believe that insights from this field will act as a conduit, explaining how the physical and relational aesthetic environment communicates with the brain and ultimately impacts our emotional reactions and experiences.

In 2023, soon after my return to academia and whilst I was just beginning to research everyday aesthetics and dementia, a colleague of mine shared with me Gulino's (2023) contemporaneous article on glimmers*. This article referred to the work of psychotherapist Deb Dana (2024a) who, in a web-based overview, described glimmers as 'micro-moments of regulation that foster feelings of well-being'. I read this piece at around the same time I was discovering Thomas Leddy's (2015) work on awe, everyday aesthetics, and well-being and, in my mind, the two begin to converge conceptually. Dana's (2024a) definition of a glimmer, and the examples she also used in her web-based overview, i.e., 'A glimmer could be as simple as seeing a friendly face, hearing a soothing sound, or noticing something in the environment that brings a smile' seemed to overlap with Leddy's (2015) and Saito's (2001, 2010) descriptions of everyday aesthetics. This raised a question for me: Was this an example of the same, or similar, concept being viewed and described through different lenses, one artistic and one psychological?

Dana's (2023) therapeutic practice is based on a theory developed by neuroscientist Stephen Porges. Porges (2007, 2022, 2025) believes that contemporary strategies for health and well-being fail to acknowledge how feelings of safety are essential for well-being and how they emerge from inside the body, specifically via the ANS. Interestingly, Porges (2022) links his idea of 'feeling safe' with the 'felt sense' described by Gendlin (1997) and referenced by Rogers (1951) in his book *Client-Centred Therapy*. The way Rogers (1951) describes the idea of a 'felt sense' as a 'sensuous form of knowledge', echoes Baumgarten's (1750) description of aesthetics, thus further linking aesthetics with Polyvagal Theory.

According to Porges (2022), the ANS is organised along an evolutionary hierarchy. The most primitive system being the unmyelinated branch of the vagus nerve (the dorsal vagal complex) which supports immobilisation responses, such as freeze or shutdown; the sympathetic adrenal system which leads to mobilisation (fight-or-flight); and the most evolutionarily recent addition, the myelinated vagus (the ventral vagal complex) which facilitates social communication, homeostasis, self-soothing, and calm. These three circuits are dynamic, adaptive, and can function together to form hybrid states in response to varying levels of safety, threat, and danger.

Both Porges (2007, 2022) and Dana (2023) observed that a process termed 'neuroception'* functions below the level of conscious awareness to determine how specific features of the environment are translated into changes in autonomic state. Neuroceptive processes integrate information from internal cues, such as visceral sensations like hunger or nausea, with external environmental signals. Consequently, autonomic responses are complex, influenced by both internal and external factors. Feedback loops also exist between these inputs; for instance, during a state of defence (fight-or-flight), relaxation of inner ear muscles enhances sensitivity to low-frequency sounds, such as those made by predators. This illustrates how autonomic states can bias sensory processing, promoting hypervigilance and threat detection whilst potentially obscuring cues of safety. Such mechanisms may explain why individuals in agitated states may misinterpret stimuli and react more strongly to physical or environmental stressors. Thus, Porges (2007, 2022, 2025) describes autonomic state as an intervening variable both modulating response to stimuli and being modulated by it.

Whilst, to the best of my knowledge, there has not been any research investigating the connection between neuroaesthetics and Polyvagal Theory, it is worth noting that the mesocorticolimbic reward system shares bidirectional connections with the ANS. This raises the possibility that polyvagal glimmers may impact neuroaesthetic processing systems (such as the mesolimbic reward system) via their effect on the ANS (Barbieri et al., 2023). Therefore, the ability to understand the experiences which cause glimmer/trigger-induced autonomic shifts may be particularly relevant in dementia care, especially in circumstances where autonomic triggers are associated with complex behaviours and where use of aesthetic glimmers could act as safety cues, accessible even in the later stages of the disease (Fox et al., 2026).

Porges (2007, 2022) and Dana (2023) through their discussion of glimmers and co-regulation* also form a bridge between the concepts underpinning care aesthetics and Polyvagal Theory. Geller and Porges (2014) discuss co-regulation and how therapeutic presence can facilitate a sense of safety. They suggest that co-regulation may be achieved through social safety cues, for example, facial expression, touch, gestures, or prosodic vocalisations. This description largely mirrors the way Jones et al. (2025) described aesthetic care practice on a mental health ward for people living with dementia, specifically in an example where the importance of sensory experiences such as 'hugs', 'holding hands', 'rubbing cheeks', 'tone of voice', 'gaze', and 'eye contact' was described. Co-regulation may also occur through aesthetic moments of shared awe or pleasure, for example, listening to music, watching birds from a window, or discussing memories (Mol et al., 2010; Fox et al., 2025). Thus, by viewing aesthetic experiences like a gentle touch from a loved one, or listening to music, through a polyvagal lens, they might be re-framed as therapeutic regulatory experiences. These experiences bring with them a sense of safety, connectivity, and identity which remain accessible for people living with dementia, including those living through the later stages of the condition.

### *In summary*

Polyvagal Theory provides a framework for understanding how the nervous system translates sensory and social cues into feelings of safety, connection, or stress. Even small aesthetic 'glimmers', brief, meaningful sensory experiences, can help regulate autonomic states, supporting both well-being and the preservation of identity. When combined with insights from aesthetic and neuroaesthetic research, polyvagal-informed approaches offer a novel avenue for dementia care, leveraging sensory and relational experiences to foster emotional regulation, engagement, and a strengthened sense of self.

## Developing a conceptual framework

In this section, I explore where I believe there to be meaningful conceptual crossover between aesthetic theory, neuroaesthetics, and Polyvagal Theory, with a focus on how these lenses may combine to inform a practice-focused framework for aesthetic dementia care. At this stage, I have organised this framework into two interrelated layers. The first, I refer to as the 'psychotherapeutic layer', which considers how the therapeutic implications of Polyvagal Theory and practice might be linked with current understandings of aesthetic care for people living with dementia. The second, I term the 'neurophysiological layer' which seeks to bring Polyvagal Theory into conversation with neuroaesthetics to explore how the brain and ANS respond to aesthetic stimuli. These two layers are not intended as fixed or discrete categories, but as points of entry into the same set of processes each informing and reinforcing the other.

### *Psychotherapeutic layer*

Current research suggests that practices which place focus on the aesthetic elements of care and the lived environment may be uniquely beneficial for people living with dementia (Kontos and Martin, 2013; Buse and Twigg, 2018; Fleetwood-Smith et al., 2022; Treadaway et al., 2023; Fox et al., 2025; Jones et al., 2025). To highlight a recent example, Fleetwood-Smith et al. (2022) explored the effect of everyday aesthetics for people living with dementia in care homes. She found that participants responded to, and engaged with, aesthetic elements of their environments and that positive connections were formed when care home staff engaged in discussions about aesthetics with residents. Her work calls for a rebalancing of design priorities from an almost exclusive focus on physical safety towards a greater emphasis on comfort, beauty, and connection. In contrast, my own research (Fox et al., 2025) highlighted how people living with dementia and their care partners used everyday aesthetic experiences as an anchor that connects them with place, with others, and with their own sense of identity and personhood. In my study, aesthetic moments were identified by both the person living with dementia and, where present, one or more care partners. Some moments occurred organically as part of everyday activities (for example, stopping to look at flowers in a garden), whilst others were curated by either the person living with dementia or by their carer (for example, the presence of mementos around the home to spark positive autobiographical memories or planned trips to meaningful locations). The findings from both these studies (Fleetwood-Smith et al., 2022 and Fox et al., 2025) suggest that greater attention needs to be paid to the aesthetic environments and experiences accessible to people living with dementia, since access to these spaces, places, objects, and meaningful moments of connection supports well-being and a sense of identity.

The aesthetics of care also extends beyond environmental design into the sensory, embodied, and relational dimensions of practice. As shared earlier, Jones et al. (2025) wrote vividly about sensory, embodied, and relational care practices alongside the contribution of atmospheres to the aesthetic register of the care environment. Kindell et al. (2025) expanded on this work by developing a practice model for healthcare support workers (HCSWs) observing how they drew on a spectrum of senses and embodied practices to become 'co-present' with the people living with dementia they cared for on mental health wards for older people. Both studies highlighted the importance of sensory and embodied care practices, including: bodily forms of connection, for example, in the HCSW practice of kneeling, holding hands, and linking arms; vocal forms, for example, in HCSWs adjusting the tone and volume of their voice, humming, singing, and whispering; and sensory awareness, for example, in the way HCSWs spent time listening and watching.

Although these observations focus on dementia care practice through the lens of care aesthetics, they closely parallel principles within polyvagal-informed practice. In her book *Polyvagal Practices*, Dana (2023) describes how we move in and out of different autonomic states many times each day, and that the goal of polyvagal therapy is not to prevent these shifts but to find our way back to a ventral state of safety. Dana (2023) suggests several methods to encourage a shift towards safety, many of which overlap with the meaningful moments of connection highlighted in my own work on everyday aesthetics (Fox et al., 2025), and with those discussed by Fleetwood-Smith et al. (2022). For example, Dana (2023) suggests that it is important to find experiences which can bring a person back to a state of safety and provides examples of how this could be achieved, including:

- Noticing places which bring you a sense of regulation and connection.
- Finding objects that bring 'ventral energy', including things you wear.
- Observing soundscapes and music that engenders a feeling of safety and 'remembering safety', including mentally revisiting moments of previous ventral connection.

Dana (2024a) names these moments 'glimmers', a term that captures their fleeting, yet potent capacity, to evoke connection and calm. As seen in my own work, and shared in this chapter, these 'glimmers' seemingly dovetail well with the everyday aesthetic moments highlighted by people living with dementia, including connections with objects, clothing, activities, reminiscence, and lived environments (Fox et al., 2025).

An interesting alignment is also seen in the language between the two lenses. Dana (2024b) commonly uses the term 'anchor' in her writing. In my study (Fox et al., 2025), one of my participants, 'Sky', used the same terminology as Dana to describe how their family 'anchored' them, as follows (slightly abridged):

> The thing I crave the most […] is my parents because they're my anchor […]. I feel like I'm fighting in a jungle, and you lose yourself. Sometimes there's no one to ground you, remind you of who you are and where you come from and yeah, they don't tell you they… just, just being around them makes you know, you know. (p. 5)

Whilst connection with others can be a form of everyday aesthetics, care aesthetics explicitly focuses on relational and sensory aspects of care (Thompson, 2023). Kindell et al. (2025) refer to these relational acts as co-presence, a concept which mirrors Porges' (2022) notion of co-regulation in which individuals reciprocally calm one another through cues such as facial expression, eye contact, posture, and tone of voice. Porges (2022) situates this as a neurophysiological process, first shaped in infancy that remains fundamental to human safety and connection throughout life. In his recent publication, Porges (2025) suggests that: '…rather than asking whether a policy 'works', polyvagal-informed design asks whether it stabilizes autonomic regulation and supports access to the social engagement system' (p. 181). This analysis may also speak to the work of Baart and Timmerman (2024) in suggesting the need for an institutional realignment away from bureaucracy, metrics, and protocols and towards relational care practices namely, recognition, connection, dignity, and responsiveness – practices which encourage aesthetic connection and autonomic safety.

When considering care for people living with dementia, Polyvagal Theory provides a psychotherapeutic and neurological framework for how co-regulation and glimmers (aesthetic and caring moments) might be harnessed therapeutically to improve well-being and engender a sense of safety. This may be particularly important for people living with dementia who can struggle with autonomic dysregulation and whose cognitive symptoms lead them to feel unsafe in everyday situations. Whilst polyvagal therapy provides a tested therapeutic practice, care and everyday aesthetics offer greater insight into what constitutes a 'glimmer' and co-regulation for people living with dementia, and how these may be optimised in a care setting to restore a sense of safety and connection (see, also, Fox et al., 2026).

### *Neurophysiological layer*

If the psychotherapeutic layer brings focus to lived experience and practice, the neurophysiological layer considers how these moments of safety and connection might be understood in terms of brain–body processes. Furthermore, there are undoubtedly interesting conceptual links to be explored regarding how the brain responds to aesthetic stimuli and how this leads to feelings of well-being, connection, identity, and safety, especially for individuals living with dementia whose cognitive abilities will change over time as neural pathology spreads.

Polyvagal Theory focuses on the central role the ANS plays in shaping our responses to the environment, both modulating response to external and internal stimuli and being modulated by them. Whilst elements of Porges' (2022) theory, including his focus on the ANS, have been critiqued (Grossman, 2023), conceptual crossover within the field of neuroaesthetics may expand on these ideas, specifically by exploring how higher cortical networks might also be involved (via the ANS) in processing polyvagal triggers and glimmers.

From a dementia care perspective, understanding the biological correlates of aesthetic processing may provide a deeper understanding of how aesthetic experiences are perceived by people living with dementia. Specifically, there is scope to further explore how pathology-induced changes in memory (autobiographic and semantic), sensory processing, and autonomic activity (Femminella et al., 2014) impact the way people living with dementia experience and respond to aesthetic stimuli in their day-to-day lives. Considering the work of Menon (2023), we may also further explore the potential link between aesthetic experiences, self-reflection, and identity through activation of the DMN.

Finally, research from Blain-Moraes's lab in Montreal, Canada (Lai Kwan et al., 2019; Fu et al., 2021) illustrates how physiological changes linked with aesthetic experiences might be observed in real time. In these studies, meaningful (or significant) moments were detected using wearable, intelligent assistive technology measuring electrodermal activity, skin temperature, and heart rate or blood volume pulse; these being measures of autonomic activity. These measurements not only facilitated detection of significant and meaningful moments (Lai Kwan et al., 2019) but also enabled researchers to calculate moments of interpersonal connection between individuals (Fu et al., 2021). Whilst further study is necessary, this may be reflective of everyday aesthetic experiences and co-presence/co-regulation in these moments. Arguably, such methods open up possibilities for identifying the moments that matter most in care, offering both a means to evaluate aesthetic interventions, and a way to better understand the biological pathways through which they take effect.

### *Bringing it together*

Bringing these layers into conversation creates space for a richer account of how aesthetic experience contributes to safety, connection, and identity in dementia care. Polyvagal Theory and therapy speak to the importance of autonomic regulation in these processes, whilst neuroaesthetics offers both mechanistic insight and the possibility of real-time measurement. Together, they suggest a way of mapping aesthetic moments to shifts in physiological state, optimising care practices for co-regulation, and designing person-centred environments which are respectful of sensory and cognitive differences and invite glimmers of safety and belonging. This process is summarised in Figure 8.1.

## Next steps

Based on the observation of conceptual overlap between these three disciplinary fields, I believe that the first step towards developing an integrative framework for aesthetic care practice in dementia will be to build a concept synthesis framework (Jabareen, 2009) which systematically combines aesthetics, neuroaesthetics, and Polyvagal Theory. This form of analysis will draw on grounded theory methods to ensure synthesis is systematic, grounded in evidence, and structured. A concept synthesis would facilitate a deep dive into these fields, probing for related concepts; for example, polyvagal glimmers, aesthetics, and aesthetic stimuli in the field of neuroaesthetics, and concept deviations where knowledge from one field may build upon the others. This framework should also be grounded in lived experience and academic understanding of dementia care, ensuring the resulting framework is directly relevant to dementia care practice, but with acknowledgement that the underlying concepts will stretch beyond this specific clinical focus. Such an analysis will highlight areas where further research is required to fill gaps

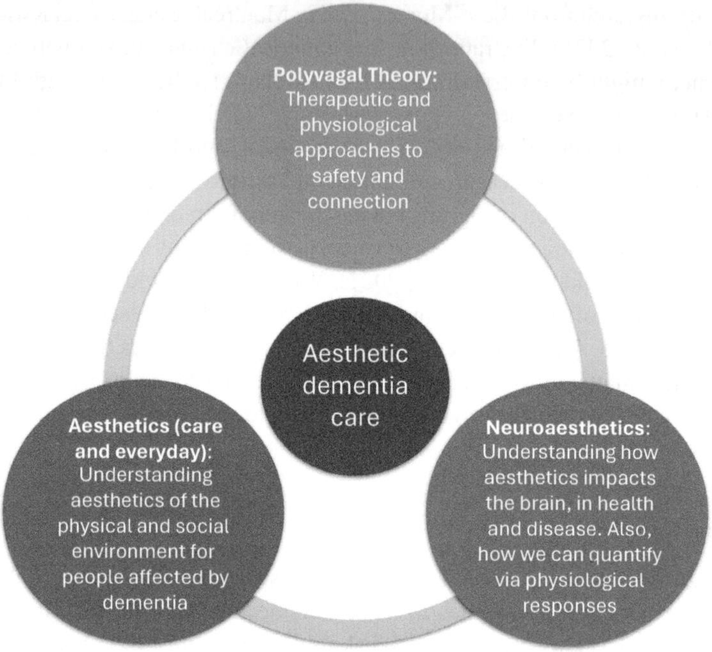


FIGURE 8.1 Mapping aesthetic moments.

in our current understanding, and where knowledge from one field may be combined with learning from another to develop a more holistic approach to aesthetic dementia care.

In parallel to developing a concept synthesis framework, it is also important to ensure this work is grounded in an understanding of how it will impact people affected by dementia. To achieve this, it is important not only to continue work to identify meaningful, aesthetic experiences for people living with dementia but also to further probe how those with lived experience engage with, and understand, these experiences. This may be achieved through a mixture of concept mapping (Burke et al., 2005), a participatory research method to embed the voice of lived experience in theory development, and further research into how the concept of meaningful moments and co-regulation may be embedded into current dementia care policy, research, education, and practice.

## Conclusion

To the best of my knowledge, this is the first time that the three areas of aesthetics, neuroaesthetics, and Polyvagal Theory have been brought into the same conversation. Whilst our understanding of the pathological underpinnings of Alzheimer's disease and other dementias has advanced, their impact on the person's psychosocial selves and lived experience remains beyond the reach of medicine alone. Indeed, Saito's (2010), Leddy's (2015), and Thompson's (2023) theories – which embody Baumgarten's (1750) sensory and perceptual understanding of knowledge – suggest how the sensory and aesthetic layer of everyday life can shape well-being. These ideas, when placed alongside an understanding of the neural correlates of aesthetic perception and psychological approaches to safety and autonomic regulation, suggest therapeutic possibilities for enhancing safety, connection, and identity through aesthetic practices. In my opinion, only by bringing together multiple perspectives might a fuller understanding of the whole be approached.

## BOX 8.1 GLOSSARY OF KEY TERMS

**Aesthetics:** Traditionally, referring to art and beauty, but here it refers to how people experience the world through the senses, sights, sounds, smells, touch, and atmosphere and how these shape feelings of comfort, safety, and connection.

**Autobiographical memory:** Recollection of personally experienced events and life episodes, integrating both the factual and emotional details of one's past.

**Autonomic Nervous System:** The body's automatic 'control system' that regulates heartbeat, breathing, and stress responses. According to Polyvagal Theory, it has three main branches:

- **Ventral vagal system** (calm, social engagement, and connection)
- **Sympathetic system** (fight-or-flight response)
- **Dorsal vagal system** (shutdown, freeze, or withdrawal)

**Care aesthetics:** The 'look and feel' of care itself. The sensory, embodied, and relational qualities of how care is given and received. For example, a gentle tone of voice, attentive touch, or a calm atmosphere.

**Co-regulation:** The process by which two people help regulate each other's nervous systems through presence, tone, touch, or shared experiences.

**Default Mode Network:** A brain system active when we reflect on ourselves, our memories, and our place in the world. Research shows it also activates during meaningful aesthetic experiences, linking them to self-reflection and identity.

**Everyday aesthetics:** Ordinary sensory and emotional experiences in daily life (e.g., the smell of baking bread, the feel of holding hands) that can bring comfort and reinforce identity.

**Glimmers:** A term from therapy for micro-moments of safety and connection (e.g., a smile, birdsong, and a hug). These can regulate the nervous system and restore calm.

**Mesocorticolimbic reward system:** A brain network that processes pleasure and reward. It responds not only to art and beauty, but also to everyday experiences like food, music, or companionship.
**Neuroaesthetics**: The study of how the brain and nervous system respond to aesthetic experiences. It helps explain why everyday moments can trigger feelings of pleasure, safety, or connection.
**Neuroception:** The body's unconscious way of scanning the internal and external environment for safety or threat, shaping how people feel and react.
**Polyvagal Theory:** A model of how the nervous system detects safety or threat in everyday situations. It explains why people feel calm and connected in some environments and anxious or withdrawn in others.
**Semantic memory:** The store of general world knowledge, facts, concepts, and meanings. This may be derived from, but no longer tied to a specific autobiographical experience which formed a more generalised belief. For example, being bitten by a dog may lead to the generalisation that dogs are dangerous.

## Three Key Reading References

### *Reference 1*

Nadal, M. and Skov, M. (2024). The sensory valuation account of aesthetic experience. *Nature Reviews Psychology*, 4 (1): 49–63. Article e21852. https://doi.org/10.1038/s44159-024-00385-y

The paper proposes that aesthetic experience is not uniquely human but arises from neurobiological sensory valuation processes shared across species, where hedonic responses are shaped by both stimulus properties and the individual's learned experiences, physiological state, and behavioural context.

### *Reference 2*

Fox, S., Thompson, J. and Keady, J. (2025). Meaningful moments of connection: How people affected by dementia and their carers living at home understand, interpret and experience everyday aesthetics. *International Journal of Geriatric Psychiatry*, 40 (8): e70136. Available: https://doi.org/10.1002/gps.70136; accessed 1 March 2026.

This study explores how people living with dementia and their carers perceive and experience everyday aesthetics, highlighting how these meaningful moments of connection shape their understanding, interpretation, and quality of daily life at home.

### *Reference 3*

Porges, S.W. (2025). Polyvagal theory: Current status, clinical applications, and future directions. *Clinical Neuropsychiatry,* 22 (3): 169–184. https://doi.org/10.36131/cnfioritieditore20250301

This article reviews the current status of Polyvagal Theory, outlining its clinical applications in understanding autonomic regulation and social engagement, and discusses directions for future research and therapeutic practice.

## References

Baart, A. and Timmerman, G. (2024). *Relational Caring and Presence Theory in Health Care and Social Work, A Care-Ethical Perspective*, Bristol: Bristol University Press.

Barbieri, P., Sarasso, P., Lodico, F., Aliverti, A., Murayama, K., Socco, K. and Ronga, I. (2023). The aesthetic valve: How aesthetic appreciation may switch emotional states from anxiety to curiosity. *Philosophical Transactions of the Royal Society London, Series B, Biological Sciences*, 379 (1895): 20220413. Available: https://doi.org/10.1098/rstb.2022.0413; accessed 1 March 2026.

Baumgarten, A.G. (1750). *Aesthetica*, Impens: Ioannis Christiani Kleyb 1.

Burke, J.G., O'Campo, P., Peak, G.L., Gielen, A.C., McDonnell, K.A. and Trochim, W.M.K. (2005). An introduction to concept mapping as a participatory public health research method. *Qualitative Health Research*, 15 (10): 1392–1410. https://doi.org/10.1177/1049732305278876

Buse, C. and Twigg, J. (2018). Dressing disrupted: Negotiating care through the materiality of dress in the context of dementia. *Sociology of Health & Illness*, 40 (2): 340–352. https://doi.org/10.1111/1467-9566.12575

Care England (2025). *The current state of dementia diagnosis and care in England.* Available: https://www.careengland.org.uk/wp-content/uploads/2025/07/The-Current-State-of-Dementia-Diagnosis-Care-in-England-3.pdf; accessed 1 March 2026.

Chatterjee, A. (2011). Neuroaesthetics: A coming of age story. *Journal of Cognitive Neuroscience*, 23 (1): 53–62. https://doi.org/10.1162/jocn.2010.21457.

Chatterjee, A. and Vartanian, O. (2014). Neuroaesthetics. *Trends in Cognitive Sciences*, 18 (7): 370–375. https://doi.org/10.1016/j.tics.2014.03.003

Cinza, D. and Vittorio, G. (2009). Neuroaesthetics: A review. *Current Opinion in Neurobiology*, 19 (6): 682–687. https://doi.org/10.1016/j.conb.2009.09.001

Clare, L., Charlwood, C., Quinn, C. and Victor, C. (2025). *Living with Dementia Reconsidered,* Maidenhead: Open University Press.

Dana, D. (2023). *Polyvagal Practices, Anchoring the Self in Safety*, New York: W.W Norton & Company Inc.

Dana, D. (2024a). *What is a Glimmer?* Available: https://www.rhythmofregulation.com/glimmers; accessed 1 March 2026.

Dana, D. (2024b). *Anchored: How to Befriend Your Nervous System Using Polyvagal Theory*, London: Vermilion

Department of Health (2015). *Prime Minister's challenge on dementia 2020.* Available: https://www.gov.uk/government/publications/prime-ministers-challenge-on-dementia-2020/prime-ministers-challenge-on-dementia-2020; accessed 1 March 2026.

Femminella, G. D., Rengo, G., Komici, K., Iacotucci, P., Petraglia, L., Pagano, G., de Lucia, C., Canonico, V., Bonaduce, D., Leosco, D. and Ferrara, N. (2014). Autonomic dysfunction in Alzheimer's disease: Tools for assessment and review of the literature. *Journal of Alzheimer's Disease*, 42 (2): 369–377. https://doi.org/10.3233/JAD-140513

Fleetwood-Smith, R., Tischler, V. and Robson, D. (2022). Aesthetics and dementia: Exploring the role of everyday aesthetics in dementia care settings. *Design for Health*, 6 (1): 91–113. https://doi.org/10.1080/24735132.2022.2074207

Fox, S. (2014). *Oscillations memory and Alzheimer's disease*. PhD thesis, The University of Manchester. Available: https://www.librarysearch.manchester.ac.uk/permalink/44MAN_INST/1r887gn/alma992983202547201631; accessed 1 March 2026.

Fox, S., Davies, J., Dowlen, R., Keady, J., Thompson, J. and Watson, R. (2026). Feeling safe, feeling connected: Aesthetic and polyvagal approaches to dementia care. *Frontiers in Dementia (Perspective article)*, 12 January 2026: 1–7. Available: https://doi.org/10.3389/frdem.2025.1735205; accessed 1 March 2026.

Fox, S., Thompson, J. and Keady, J. (2025). Meaningful moments of connection: How people affected by dementia and their carers living at home understand, interpret and experience everyday aesthetics. *International Journal of Geriatric Psychiatry*, 40 (8): e70136. Available: https://doi.org/10.1002/gps.70136; accessed 1 March 2026.

Franklin Gould, V. (2021). *A.R.T.S. for Brain Health Social Prescribing: transforming the diagnostic narrative for dementia from despair to desire*. Available: https://artsfordementia.org/wp-content/uploads/2024/01/Arts-for-Brain-Health-Final-Report.pdf; accessed 1 March 2026.

Fu, D., Incio-Serra, N., Motta-Ochoa, R. and Blain-Moraes, S. (2021). Interpersonal physiological synchrony for detecting moments of connection in persons with dementia: A pilot study. *Frontiers in Psychology*, 12: 749710. Available: https://doi.org/10.3389/fpsyg.2021.749710; accessed 1 March 2026.

Geller, S.M. and Porges, S.W. (2014). Therapeutic presence: Neurophysiological mechanisms mediating feeling safe in therapeutic relationships. *Journal of Psychotherapy Integration*, 24 (3): 178–192. https://doi.org/10.1037/a0037511

Gendlin, E. (1997). *Experiencing and the Creation of Meaning: A Philosophical and Psychological Approach to the Subjective*. Studies in Phenomenology and Existential Philosophy, Illinois: Northwestern University Press.

Grewe, O., Kopiez, R., Altenmuller, E. and Katzur, B. (2010). Chills in different sensory domains: Frisson elicited by acoustical, visual, tactile and gustatory stimuli. *Psychology of Music*, 39 (2): 220–239. https://doi.org/10.1177/0305735610362950

Grossman, P. (2023). Fundamental challenges and likely refutations of the five basic premises of the polyvagal theory. *Biological Psychology*, 180: 108589. Available: https://doi.org/10.1016/j.biopsycho.2023.108589; accessed 1 March 2026.

Gulino, E. (2023). 'Glimmers' can make us happier - & they're all around us. *Refinery*, 29. Available: https://www.refinery29.com/en-us/how-glimmers-work-polyvagal-theory?utm_campaign=later-linkinbio-refinery29&utm_content=later-35578031&utm_medium=social&utm_source=linkin.bio; accessed 1 March 2026.

Halpern, A.R, Ly, J., Elkin-Frankson, S. and O'Connor, M.G. (2008). "I know what I like": stability of aesthetic preference in Alzheimer's patients. *Brain and Cognition*, 66 (1): 65–72. https://doi.org/10.1016/j.bandc.2007.05.008

Hughes, J.C. (2014). The aesthetic approach to people with dementia. *International Psychogeriatrics*, 26 (9): 1407–1413. https://doi.org/10.1017/S1041610214001100.

Jabareen, Y. (2009). Building a conceptual framework: Philosophy, definitions, and procedure. *International Journal of Qualitative Methods*, 8 (4): 49–62. https://doi.org/10.1177/160940690900800406

Jones, L., Cullum, N., Watson, R., Thompson, J. and Keady, J. (2025). 'Only my family can help': The lived experience and care aesthetics of being resident on an NHS psychiatric/mental health inpatient dementia assessment ward – a single case study. *Ageing & Society*, 45 (6): 1143–1164. https://doi:10.1017/S0144686X24000096

Keady, J. (ed.) (2024). *Reconsidering Neighbourhoods and Living with Dementia: Spaces, Places and People*, Maidenhead: Open University Press/McGraw-Hill.

Keady, J., Jones, L., Ward, R., Koch, S., Swarbrick, S., Hellstrom, I., Davies-Quarrell, V. and Williams, S. (2013). Introducing the bio-psycho-social-physical model of dementia through a collective case study design. *Journal of Clinical Nursing*, 22 (19–20): 2768–2777. https://doi.org/10.1111/j.1365-2702.2012.04292.x

Kindell, J., Maguire-Rosier, K., Polonyi, R., Thompson, J., Cleasby, R., Watson, R. and Keady, J.D. (2025). Healthcare support workers working with people with dementia on mental health wards: A practice model informed by care aesthetics. *Qualitative Health Research*, 1–14. Online First (December). Available: https://doi.org/10.1177/10497323251393890; accessed 1 March 2026.

Kitwood, T. (1997). *Dementia Reconsidered: The Person Comes First*, Buckingham: Open University Press.

Kontos, P. and Martin, W. (2013). Embodiment and dementia: Exploring critical narratives of selfhood, surveillance, and dementia care. *Dementia: the International Journal of Social Research and Practice*, 12 (3): 288–302. https://doi.org/10.1177/1471301213479787

Lai Kwan, C., Mahdid, Y., Motta Ochoa, R., Lee, K., Park, M. and Blain-Moraes, S. (2019). Wearable technology for detecting significant moments in individuals with dementia. *Biomedical Research International*, 6515813. Available: https://doi.org/10.1155/2019/6515813; accessed 1 March 2026.

Leddy, T. (2015). Experience of awe: An expansive approach to everyday aesthetics. *Contemporary Aesthetics (Journal Archive)*, 13 (8). Available: https://digitalcommons.risd.edu/liberalarts_contempaesthetics/vol13/iss1/8; accessed 1 March 2026.

Ligaya, K., O'Doherty, J.P. and Starr, G.G. (2020). Progress and promise in neuroaesthetics. *Neuron*, 108 (4): 594–596. https://doi.org/10.1016/j.neuron.2020.10.022

Media and IAFOR (2015). Everyday aesthetics and world-making. Available: https://www.youtube.com/watch?v=ktwTiUl_fEQ; accessed 1 March 2026.

Menon, V. (2023). 20 years of the default mode network: A review and synthesis. *Neuron*, 111 (16): 2469–2487. https://doi.org/10.1016/j.neuron.2023.04.023

Minkoff, R. and Allers, R. (1994). *The Lion King*, Burbank, CA: Walt Disney Pictures.

Mol, A., Moser, I. and Pols, J. (2010). *Care in Practice: On Tinkering in Clinics, Homes and Farms*, London: Transaction Publishers.

Nadal, M. and Skov, M. (2024). The sensory valuation account of aesthetic experience. *Nature Reviews Psychology*, 4 (1): 49–63. Article e21852. https://doi.org/10.1038/s44159-024-00385-y

Porges, S.W. (2007). The polyvagal perspective. *Biological Psychology*, 74 (2): 116–143. 4(2):116–43. https://doi.org/10.1016/j.biopsycho.2006.06.009

Porges, S.W. (2022). Polyvagal theory: A science of safety. *Frontiers in Integrated Neuroscience*, 16: 871227. Available: https://doi.org/10.3389/fnint.2022.871227; accessed 1 March 2026.

Porges, S.W. (2025). Polyvagal theory: Current status, clinical applications, and future directions. *Clinical Neuropsychiatry*, 22 (3): 169–184. https://doi.org/10.36131/cnfioritieditore20250301

Rogers, C.R. (1951). *Client-Centred Therapy*, Boston: Houghton-Mifflin.

Sabat, S. (2005). Capacity for decision-making in Alzheimer's disease: Selfhood, positioning and semiotic people. *Australian & New Zealand Journal of Psychiatry*, 39 (11–12): 1030–1035. https://doi.org/10.1080/j.1440-1614.2005.01722.x

Saito, Y. (2001). Everyday aesthetics. *Philosophy and Literature*, 25 (1): 87–93. https://doi.org/10.1353/phl.2001.0018

Saito, Y. (2010). *Everyday Aesthetics*, Oxford: Oxford University Press.

Thompson, J. (2023). *Care Aesthetics: For Artful Care and Careful Art*, London: Routledge.

Treadaway, C., Seckam, A., Fennell, J. and Taylor, A. (2023). HUG: A compassionate approach to designing for wellbeing in dementia care. *International Journal of Environmental Research and Public Health*, 20 (5): 4410. Available: https://doi.org/10.3390/ijerph20054410; accessed 1 March 2026.

Vessel, E.A., Starr, G.G. and Rubin, N. (2012). The brain on art: Intense aesthetic experience activates the default mode network. *Frontiers in Human Neuroscience*, 6. Available: https://doi.org/10.3389/fnhum.2012.00066; accessed 1 March 2026.

# PART 3

# Care aesthetics, outside spaces, and everyday design

# 9

# GARDENING AS AN AESTHETIC PRACTICE FOR PEOPLE LIVING WITH DEMENTIA

*Rita Newton, Daniel Atherton, Ozichi Brewster, Emmanuel Tsekleves and John Keady*

## Introduction

In the UK, as in other parts of Western Europe and the world, the domestic homes in which we live come in many different shapes, sizes, designs, locations, year of build, structure, and levels of affordability and accessibility. Whether we live in a brand new top floor flat with a view over an evolving city landscape, or a terraced house on a suburban street, or a smallholding in a remote and rural community, what unites each of our living spaces is that the windows in our home will connect us to a view of the outside and, if we are fortunate, to a door that will enable us to access a private outside space. That private outside space could be a balcony attached to a flat, a backyard in a terraced home, or a front and back garden in a detached or semi-detached house. The spaces inside and outside our homes also act as a keeper of our memories, relationships (both human and inter-species), and material possessions, whilst also making constant demands on our time and personal finances for upkeep. Moreover, these stories of home also connect to the neighbourhood in which our home is located and the social, spatial, and relational networks that constitute the fabric of our everyday lives, both in the present and across time.

Within this positionality, our life-long exposure and attachment to our domestic home(s) help us to frame our experience, interaction, and expectations about its outside and green spaces and our embodied practices and memories about the domestic (home) garden. For instance, we can usually reminisce with some fondness about our experiences of playing as children outside our childhood home and remember with pride the successful growing of fruit, vegetables, and/or herbs in the domestic garden that could then be used for home cooking and food preparation. This association between personal memories, biographical identity, and the

DOI: 10.4324/9781003623441-13
This chapter has been made available under a (CC BY) 4.0 license.

role played by the domestic garden in our everyday lives was addressed in a recent study by Lauwerijssen et al. (2025) who conducted 20 oral history interviews with older people in the Netherlands about their domestic gardens. Lauwerijssen et al. (2025) found that the environment where a person grew up was 'a foundational space for participants to develop a connection to gardens' (p. 6) and the authors went on to argue that spending time in the domestic garden influenced the meaning and attachment that older people placed in their gardens and that domestic garden use changed across the lifespan.

These are important points as it reminds us that we all have an identity that is aligned to the outside spaces of our homes (even if we did not, or currently do not, have such access) and that such an exposure helps to frame our own interaction, and expectation, of a domestic garden. At one level, this connection is only natural as it has been documented for some time that being outdoors and engaging in the natural world has a restorative, relaxing, and connecting impact on what it is to be human and to 'Be-in-the-world' (Kaplan, 1995; and see Julian C. Hughes' chapter at the start of this book). This need for engagement in the garden and green spaces of our domestic homes was also seen in a large-scale UK-based questionnaire study by Chalmin-Pui et al. (2021) who found that gardening at home on a frequent basis (i.e., at least two to three times a week) corresponded with the greatest perceived health benefits for those doing the gardening. However, paradoxically, the authors reported that this was not the main motivation shared by participants about why they gardened; instead, that was related to the simple pleasure that gardening brought to their lives and to the aesthetic value in seeing plants and flowers grow, bloom, and change over the seasons. There was also a reported sense of achievement in planting and making a domestic garden look neat and tidy, especially at the front of the house.

To loosely apply these findings to ourselves as a UK-based authorship situated in different rural/urban locations and living in different types of housing, we spent a little time together jotting down how gardens and gardening at home was represented in our everyday lives:

i When we go to our bookcase at home and can select a book about gardening, gardens, plants, planting, and 'how to garden'. The selection of books we own, and use, are mainly written by 'celebrity' names in gardening, such as Alan Titchmarsh, Monty Don, Bob Flowerdew, and Charlie Dimmock.
ii When we are exposed to gardening products at our local supermarket, including the opportunity to buy a variety of low-cost plants, ornaments, compost, birdboxes, pots, and gardening equipment, such as a rake, hoe, spade, secateurs, and garden shears.
iii When we visit national superstores focused on products for the home/home improvements (e.g., B&Q, HOMEBASE, B&M, and The Range), where we can not only buy a number of the garden products that are available in the supermarkets but also purchase 'bigger ticket' items such as sheds, trellising, fencing,

a wheelbarrow, lawnmowers, hosepipes, planters, pots, troughs, rotating washing lines, outdoor barbeques, paving stones, patio sets, garden benches, leaf-blowers, and so on. We can also do this viewing and ordering online.

iv When we purposively decide to visit a local garden centre to access specialist advice about our gardens/gardening requirements and have an opportunity to buy 'quality' plants, compost, seeds, and gardening materials.

v When we are exposed to the plethora of programmes about gardening, garden makeovers, and 'how to garden' which are broadcast on the television, radio, and other media, including podcasts such as 'Gardener's Question Time' through BBC Radio 4.

The list could go on. Where we had more difficulty was in focusing down on thinking about the availability of gardening books, products, and specialist services/advice on domestic gardens/gardening aimed specifically at the experience of people living with dementia and/or caring for a person with dementia living at home. Similarly, until recently, most housing adaptation literature/advice for people living with dementia has failed to include the domestic garden/outside spaces of the home within its remit with the weight of attention placed on the inside spaces of the house, particularly the kitchen, bathroom, and bedroom (Newton et al., 2023). Indeed, when gardens have been mentioned in the housing adaptation literature, it is couched in the language of its therapeutic impact (Whear et al., 2014) and its dementia-friendly design (Motealleh et al., 2019) rather than on the act of enabling people living with dementia to simply carry on with accessing and using their garden at home and continuing their identity of 'being a gardener'.

This was a surprise as for people with dementia living at home, access to the outside spaces of the house, and the local neighbourhood, does not stop once a diagnosis of dementia is made (Campbell et al., 2023; Keady, 2024). Indeed, it was over a decade ago that Mapes (2012) suggested that being outdoors can help a person living with dementia to orientate themselves to the changing seasons and engender a sense of place/belonging (see also Tsai et al., 2020). In addition, other authors have highlighted that being outdoors is important for people living with dementia as it can, for example, give an opportunity for social encounters to take place (Duggan et al., 2008; Phinney et al., 2016) and lead to a general lowering of stress levels through an appreciation of the natural world (Edwards et al., 2013). At present, the literature on outdoor spaces accessed by people living with dementia is heavily weighted towards this 'away-from-home' activity and includes studies on tending to community gardening and allotments (Noone et al., 2017; Noone and Jenkins, 2018), spending time in day farms (Ibsen and Eriksen, 2021), and visiting green spaces such as parks and woodlands (Mmako et al., 2020).

In contrast, and as a context for her Economic and Social Research Council (ESRC) Collaborative Studentship Competition (CASE)-funded PhD study, Rita, as the lead author of this chapter, conducted the first systematic narrative review of the literature to explore the everyday experiences of people living with dementia in using and accessing their garden in the domestic home (Newton et al., 2021; John and Emmanuel were included as co-authors in this published review paper in their role as Rita's ESRC CASE PhD supervisors). This review explored the experiences of people living with dementia, including family/carers as appropriate, in accessing and using their garden in both the domestic home and care home settings. Initially, Rita wanted to simply review the literature on the access and use of the domestic (home) gardens of people living with dementia, but the review parameters had to be extended to include care home gardens as there was simply not enough studies published anywhere in the world to undertake a review on this topic alone. At the time of searching for review papers between October 2019 and September 2020, Rita could only find five articles (out of 23 eventually included in the review) that mentioned this specific access and use (Newton et al., 2021). Once retrieved, findings from the 23 included studies were then thematically analysed and three independent but, at times, intersecting themes emerged from this process, namely (1) enabling a sense of life continuity and identity; (2) connecting to nature and to the moment; and (3) managing everyday risks. As Newton et al. (2021) concluded, the narrative review confirmed that relatively little was known about the domestic garden and the everyday experience of living with dementia and the significant value people gain from 'simply being in a garden and its capacity to substantially improve quality of life' (p. 10).

Developing the above point, the following two data extracts focused on the access and use of the domestic garden, are taken from Rita's published literature review as examples underpinning the theme 1 heading and help to provide a flavour of some of the situations faced by people living with dementia and family carers in their everyday lives:

> My father is a gardener and I have a patio with pots so…I let him do whatever he likes and then I go round afterwards and sort it out again because he does some weird things now. He's still got the mind that he had before – it just doesn't always show.
>
> *(Chung et al., 2017, p. 7)*

> I want to go to the shed [in the garden] to get a chisel or something, and by the time I unlock the door I've forgotten what I was looking for and this sort of thing. So, to make life a little easier I have…different coloured buckets so I put my spanners in one and other things in that, so I sort of set things out.
>
> *(Allen et al., 2019, p. 1207)*

Since Rita's review, Christina Buse and her colleague (2023) – and see Christina's Chapter (2) in Part 1 of this book that details her own autobiographical narrative of caring at home for her mum which includes mention of the domestic garden – conducted a pilot study with six households in the UK during March to July 2020 (data collection occurred during the onset of the COVID-19 pandemic) that explored the participants' experiences of domestic gardens for people living with dementia. Using creative social research methods, including the use of video and the work of an illustrator, Buse et al. (2023) highlighted the significance of domestic gardens for the person living with dementia's sense of identity, everyday practices, and social connections. However, Buse et al. (2023) stated that a limitation of their work was that it failed to capture a 'year-long' and seasonal representation of garden access and use by people living with dementia, and that this overall perspective was missing from the literature. Interestingly, Rushton et al. (2025) have recently extended the critical discourse on identity and suggested that the domestic garden for people living with dementia can also act as a site for the nuanced and embodied expression of agency.

This chapter will now develop the domestic garden as an everyday creative and aesthetic space for people living with dementia by focussing on two case studies. The first will draw on the findings of Rita's part-time ESRC-funded PhD study that explored how people living with dementia used and accessed their domestic garden over a year, albeit from a cross-sectional perspective. In this case study, we will tell the story of how a set of season-specific posters was developed and exhibited in partnership with Daniel (co-author) and Ozichi (co-author) at the Royal Horticultural Society (RHS) Garden Bridgewater in Salford, Greater Manchester, as part of the ESRC Festival of Social Science (FOSS) during 2024. The second case study will share an extract from a conversation conducted between Rita and Ozichi (who is the therapeutic gardener at RHS Garden Bridgewater) which took place at the time of Rita's ESRC FOSS exhibition and in the Community Wellbeing Garden at RHS Garden Bridgewater. The conversation communicates Ozichi's skills, passion, and knowledge about gardening practices and its relationship to vulnerable groups. Images of each of the exhibited posters will be shared in case study 1 and photographs taken by either Rita or John at the time of the study will be shared in both case studies; the selected photographs have been chosen to support the narrative storyline in each case study.

## Case study 1

As the posters and their contents used in the RHS FOSS exhibition were drawn directly from Rita's PhD study, we will start this first case study by providing a brief overview of the study design and methods that informed this work. We will then share the story of our partnership together and the contents of the posters used in the exhibition, before concluding with attendance and some anonymous evaluation data from the 2024 ESRC FOSS event.

### *An overview of Rita's PhD study design and methods*

The primary aims of Rita's PhD study were twofold, namely (i) to explore how people living with dementia and their household access and use their garden at home on an everyday basis; and (ii) to use creative social research methods to capture domestic garden biographies over all four seasons of the year. Data collection to meet these study aims took place in the Northwest of England in 2023 and participants were recruited through visiting community support groups for people living with dementia in the Northwest of England and undertaking an in-person presentation about the study aims and its ambition. This process eventually resulted in seven households coming forward to volunteer to take part in the study. In the study design, a household comprises a person with dementia living at home and in a supportive relationship with a person sharing the same domestic space. An overview of the participants who took part in the study, their household demographics and property type, is shown in Table 9.1.

As seen in Table 9.1, the type of neighbourhood varied across the households from residential suburbs typically on the edge of town, to mixed-use urban areas close to a city centre. There were no households in what we would intuitively understand as rural areas. Households 1, 2, 5, and 7 were located on quiet roads, including cul-de-sacs, whilst households 3, 4, and 6 were located on more busy roads. Additionally, households 1 and 5 were located close to a very busy motorway. The number of visits Rita undertook to each household, and the visiting time frame aligned to the season of the year, is shown in Table 9.2.

To comply with our ethics approval permissions, each household contact lasted a maximum of six weeks and data collection was purposively sampled over a one-year time frame so that all seasons of the year could be represented in the study findings. Weather permitting, most visits conducted by Rita to the participant's household were undertaken outside in the domestic garden or backyard, with participants preferring the conversations and observations to take place in the more private garden/space at the rear of the home. With the informed consent of all household participants, including the person living with dementia, Rita used a range of creative social research methods in her household contacts, including participant observation, impromptu conversations, photographs, fieldwork notes, and a reflexive journal.

To ensure that the person living with dementia continued to have capacity to consent to take part in the study and understood its purpose, Rita used the process consent method (Dewing, 2002, 2007) at the start of each household contact. No visits needed to be rearranged due to capacity issues and there was no sign of distress shown by the participants during any of Rita's visits. All data was transcribed and data analysis, including visual data, was coded and followed Braun and Clarke's (2019) approach to reflexive thematic analysis. Ethnographic typologies were collated for each participating household and Rita was the main researcher who analysed and collected the data in all seven households.

In this chapter, all participant names are pseudonyms in line with Health Research Authority Social Care Research Ethics Committee permissions and the approved study protocol (study reference: 22/IEC08/0013).

**TABLE 9.1** Participating household demographics and property type

| *Household* | *Participant* | *Gender* | *Age* | *Relationship* | *Diagnosis of dementia and date* | *Gardener* | *Property type* | *Tenure* | *Front garden (size is approximate)* | *Back garden (size is approximate)* |
|---|---|---|---|---|---|---|---|---|---|---|
| 1 | Linda | Female | 70 | Mother | Yes 2014 | Yes | Terraced house | Owner occupier | Car parking, hard landscaping; 31m² | Lawn, raised beds, and sunroom; 82m² |
| | Janet | Female | 46 | Daughter | No | Yes | | | | |
| 2 | Jack | Male | 82 | Husband | Yes 2021 | No | Detached house | Owner occupier | Open-plan garden and driveway; 115m² | Lawn, borders, seating, shed, and small pond; 100m² |
| | Ann | Female | 71 | Wife | No | Yes | | | | |
| 3 | Ron | Male | 84 | Husband | Yes 2020 | Yes | Detached house | Owner occupier | Landscaped garden and driveway; 200m² | Landscaped garden, seating, pergola, shed, and outbuildings; 347m² |
| | Ruby | Female | 77 | Wife | No | Yes | | | | |
| 4 | Simon | Male | 68 | Husband | Yes 2022 | No | Terraced house | Owner occupier | Hard-surfaced garden with wall and planting; 12m² | Hard-surfaced garden with seating and shed; 18m² |
| | Zoe | Female | 69 | Wife | No | Yes | | | | |
| 5 | Phillip | Male | 78 | Husband | Yes 2019 | Yes | Semi-detached bungalow | Social housing tenant | Communal lawn and footpath; 35m² | Hard-surfaced garden with raised beds, seating, summerhouse, and greenhouse; 60m² |
| | Elizabeth | Female | 77 | Wife | No | Yes | | | | |
| 6 | Margaret | Female | 77 | Wife | Yes 2017 | No | Terraced house | Owner occupier | Hard-surfaced garden with wall and planting; 7m² | Hard-surfaced back yard with seating, and shed; 26m² |
| | Michael | Male | 79 | Husband | No | Yes | | | | |
| 7 | Catherine | Female | 79 | Wife | Yes 2022 | Yes | Detached house | Owner occupier | Open-plan garden and driveway; 82m² | Lawn, borders, seating, shed, and greenhouse; 142m² |
| | David | Male | 82 | Husband | No | No | | | | |

**TABLE 9.2** The number of Rita's visits to each household

| *Household* | *Visits* | | |
|---|---|---|---|
| | *Garden Ethnography* | *Feedback (garden biography)* | *Validating the typologies* |
| 1 | 5 | 1 | 1 |
| 2 | 4 | 0 | 0 |
| 3 | 6 | 1 | 1 |
| 4 | 6 | 1 | 1 |
| 5 | 5 | 1 | 1 |
| 6 | 3 | 0 | 0 |
| 7 | 3 | 0 | 0 |

### *Curating a partnership with RHS Garden Bridgewater*

As so little was known about gardening at home and the experience of living with dementia, we wanted to share the findings of Rita's mixed-methods qualitative study with the public to raise awareness about this everyday practice and challenge the stigma that is all too often associated with a life with dementia (Kim et al., 2023). An opportunity arose in the spring of 2024 to apply for a small amount of funding held at The University of Manchester to be part of the annual ESRC FOSS Manchester event which takes place across Greater Manchester. For information, Greater Manchester, which hosts the cities of Manchester and Salford and is situated in the Northwest of England, has a population of 2.868 million people and the region includes areas of high deprivation as well as affluence and significant cultural diversity (see Greater Manchester Population Statistics, n.d.).

The ESCR FOSS is a national event which takes place annually for three consecutive weeks between the middle of October and the beginning of November and it is an opportunity for social science researchers across the UK to share the findings of their work with the public. Importantly, one of the underpinning values of any national ESRC FOSS event is that access should be free of charge to the public and enable visitors to share feedback on its impact, creativity, and personal meaningfulness. As The University of Manchester held the ESRC budget to hold an ESRC FOSS event in Greater Manchester, and supported partnership working with community, charitable, and creative organisations, in May 2024 it was a relatively straightforward decision for Rita to reach out to Daniel, in his role as RHS Interpretation Manager North with responsibility for public engagement, to explore the possibility of hosting a poster exhibition of her PhD work at the RHS Garden Bridgewater in Salford. The poster exhibition was to cover all four seasons of the year.

In no small measure, this decision to reach out to Daniel was influenced by the local, national, and worldwide reputation of the RHS, its charitable status, and mission to 2030 which is spelt out as follows:

> Our vision is a world where gardening is embraced as a way of life – a source of joy and fulfilment, building healthier lives, stronger communities, and thriving environments. To achieve this, our mission is to be there for everyone on their lifelong adventure with gardening.
>
> *(RHS, 2023, p. 4)*

To underpin this mission statement, the RHS listed six priorities in their strategy report 'A lifelong adventure with gardening' (RHS, 2023) to drive forward these organisational values: (i) open up gardening for anyone, anywhere; (ii) grow our story to share the joy of gardening; (iii) build horticulture for the future; (iv) deliver science solutions for people, gardens, and nature; (v) champion the essential role of gardening; and (vi) unlock our potential. As it impacts and intersects with the work shared in this chapter, the RHS mission statement wording 'to be there for everyone on their lifelong adventure with gardening' and their six underpinning priorities was made real in the RHS Garden Bridgewater through the establishment of a Community Wellbeing Garden. This Community Wellbeing Garden was the first permanent garden to be created within an RHS garden anywhere in the UK with health and well-being at its core. A photograph of the Community Wellbeing Garden is shown in Image 9.1.

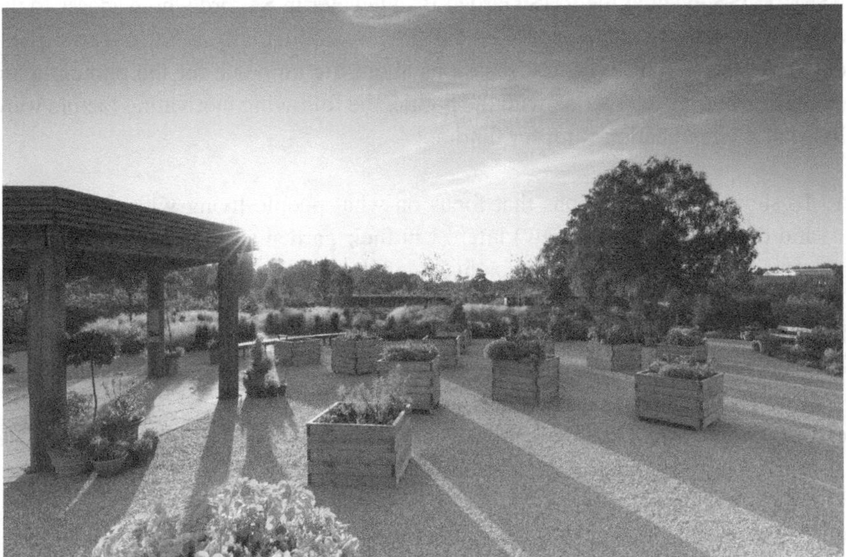

**IMAGE 9.1** A view of the Community Wellbeing Garden at RHS Garden Bridgewater

*Source:* © RHS/Josh Kemp-Smith.

According to RHS Garden Bridgewater, three values underpin the Community Wellbeing Garden. The first is an idea of a garden as a place of sanctuary; the second is a garden as a space which offers the community an opportunity to grow, reflect, meet others, and 'get moving'; and third, a garden that is purpose-built to be a constantly evolving space which responds to the needs and wishes of its users and visitors. An activity area is located at the centre of the Community Wellbeing Garden which is connected to the rest of the garden through its circular paths, raised beds, and raised planters. Dedicated seating areas are purposively situated in the garden to encourage rest, relaxation, and reflection and it is split into three zones: woodland, activity, and memory. The memory garden is described as having a more traditional cottage-style planting that is intended to evoke feelings of nostalgia and familiarity and be a safe and connecting space for people living with dementia and/or other neurodegenerative conditions. We will return to the Community Wellbeing Garden when we describe the location and contents of the exhibition boards and during case study 2 when sharing the conversation between Rita and Ozichi.

### *Applying to hold the ESRC FOSS Manchester exhibition*

As an authorship, and led by Rita who completed the ESRC FOSS compulsory training in May 2024 to enable her to lead an application, we therefore joined forces and submitted a bid for funding to The University of Manchester to host an ESRC FOSS event at the RHS Garden Bridgewater in Salford where access to the residents of Salford is free each Tuesday (known colloquially as Salford-free Tuesdays). As we started to have discussions about the rationale for the photographic exhibition and its interaction with the public, the following motivating factors were listed in the application form for funding:

a To showcase photographs that focus on what people living with dementia do and their continued (or new) interest in their garden at home, this will help to combat stigma and the social exclusion of people with dementia in everyday life and activities.
b To communicate the powerful effects that being outdoors has for people living with dementia and the continuity of everyday roles and interests, and how gardening changes over the seasons.
c For the display to enable visitors to reflect on their own lives and experiences where the lived experience of dementia may be present either in the past or in the present day.
d To enhance my (Rita's) skills in communicating social science and creative/participatory social research methods to a non-academic audience and visitors to the exhibition.

After some discussion, the title of the photographic exhibition was subsequently agreed as 'Gardening with Dementia: the power of nature and the outdoors' as this seemed to capture the vision and values of our intentions and work together. Daniel was keen for the exhibition to be available to all visitors to RHS Garden Bridgewater for the full three-week duration of the ESRC FOSS event, although evaluation and attendance by Rita would only take place on the Salford-free Tuesdays. Moreover, as the poster boards and photographic exhibition were to be situated outdoors for the duration of the ESRC FOSS, it was therefore logical to plan for the photographic exhibition to be positioned adjacent to the Community Wellbeing Garden so that the values of both could be aligned.

After a peer review and competitive selection process, our application for funding (which totalled £500) was successful and our subsequent publicity information to advertise the event on the ESRC FOSS (Manchester) website was written as follows:

> A photographic exhibition that celebrates the powerful connection between home and garden for people living with dementia in Northwest England. The exhibition is a partnership between the Royal Horticultural Society, The University of Manchester and Lancaster University and shows how people living with dementia access and use their garden over each season of the year. The exhibition also includes quotes by people living with dementia about their garden and the importance of being outdoors.

Moreover, in addition to other approaches to raising awareness about the exhibition, including through social media and the networks of the RHS and Creative Manchester at The University of Manchester, we also had a series of postcards printed for distribution to local organisations just in case access to digital media might be an issue for anyone interested in knowing about and attending the event. This postcard is shown in Image 9.2.

It is important for us to share that the photograph in Image 9.2 was taken by Rita in line with her research permissions and showed a participant with dementia's (Linda – household 1; and see Table 9.1) gardening clothes and material objects that were purposively assembled and displayed by Linda to show her readiness to garden at home. The items were placed by her back patio door which led directly out to the garden. As can also be seen in Image 9.2, it was the Salford-free Tuesdays that were advertised on the postcard, in keeping with the accessibility ethos and values of the ESRC FOSS and us as an authorship. Just for clarity, the shared October and November dates on Image 9.2 relate to 2024.

### *Designing and showing the exhibition posters*

During August and September 2024, Daniel worked closely with Rita in planning and setting out the contents and images of each of the exhibition posters. A decision was taken early on by the team to have an Introductory poster that would spell out what the exhibition was about and include a photograph of Rita, and then four

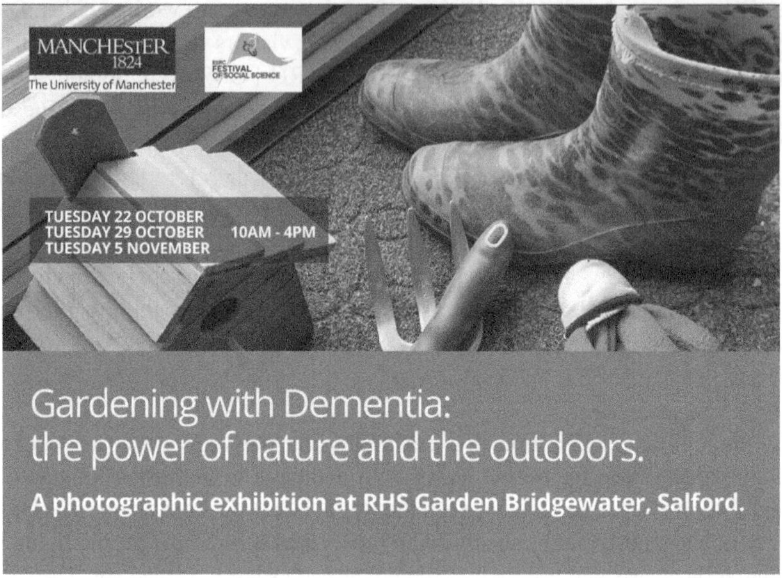
MANCHESTER
1824
The University of Manchester
FESTIVAL OF SOCIAL SCIENCE
TUESDAY 22 OCTOBER
TUESDAY 29 OCTOBER
TUESDAY 5 NOVEMBER
10AM - 4PM
Gardening with Dementia:
the power of nature and the outdoors.
A photographic exhibition at RHS Garden Bridgewater, Salford.

**IMAGE 9.2** Advertising postcard for the ESRC FOSS event at RHS Garden Bridgewater.

separate posters each of which would focus on data from each season so that a journey through a year could be taken by those visiting and viewing the exhibition posters. The contents of each poster were to include photographs taken by Rita during her time visiting the different gardens and symbolise each of the seasons that the posters intended to represent. The quotations included on each of the four posters that represented each season of the year were also to be written so that they only shared the experiences of people living with dementia and were shared without reference to their household number or name (see Table 9.1). This decision was taken intentionally to avoid complicated name-alignment text on the Introductory poster. The images were selected to showcase the person living with dementia's continued involvement in everyday gardening and connection with the spaces outside the home and that this act remained an integral part of the person's sense of self and identity. It was also decided to keep the text minimal on the four 'seasonal' poster boards and to also let the images convey a meaning and interpretation in the mind of the viewer.

Once the text and images relating to each poster were supplied by Rita, through his considerable design skills, Daniel took charge of setting out each of the five posters for printing in time for the start of the exhibition at RHS Garden Bridgewater. Furthermore, as the posters were to be located outside and face the vagrancies of the weather in Greater Manchester during mid-October to early November, Daniel and Ozichi sourced five oak poster boards from their supply stock at RHS Garden Bridgewater for their display. It was important to the RHS, as it was for us all, that a focus on the use of sustainable and recyclable materials was a core value of the exhibition before, during, and after it had concluded.

Therefore, under the guidance of Daniel, each of the five posters to be attached to the oak poster boards was printed on Foamalux®, a material that is 100% recycled and recyclable.

With all the pieces of the exhibition just about in place, under the supervision of Daniel and Ozichi, the gardening team at RHS Garden Bridgewater then fixed the five oak poster boards in place and *en route* to the Community Wellbeing Garden so that it would be seen by all visitors to the garden, not just those who might have a special interest in viewing the exhibition. Once the poster boards were firmly secured in the earth, Rita then attended RHS Garden Bridgewater before its opening hours to work with Daniel in attaching the five posters to the poster boards using Velcro®. With this final act, the 'Gardening with Dementia: the power of nature and the outdoors' poster exhibition, as part of the ESRC FOSS Manchester, was ready for public display starting on 19 October 2024. Image 9.3 shows where and how the poster boards were positioned at RHS Garden Bridgewater.

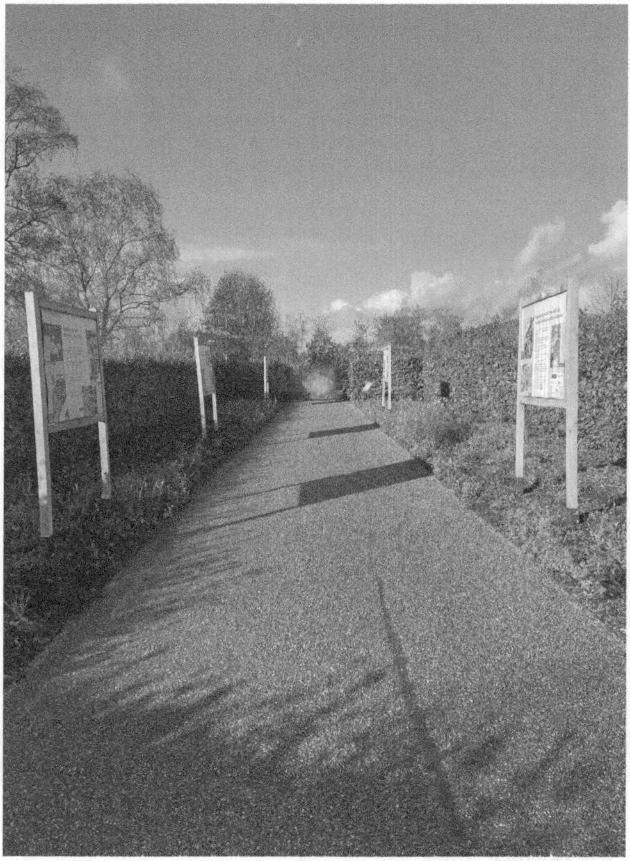

**IMAGE 9.3** The position of the oak poster boards and exhibition posters adjacent to the Community Wellbeing Garden.

As you look at Image 9.3, the poster board displaying the Introductory poster is the first one on the right-hand side of the photograph and directly opposite it is the poster board and poster for spring. The next poster board down the path after spring display is the poster for summer, then autumn (situated on the opposite side of the path). The exhibition concludes with winter, the third and furthest away poster on the left-hand side of Image 9.3. This ordering of the posters was intentional as we

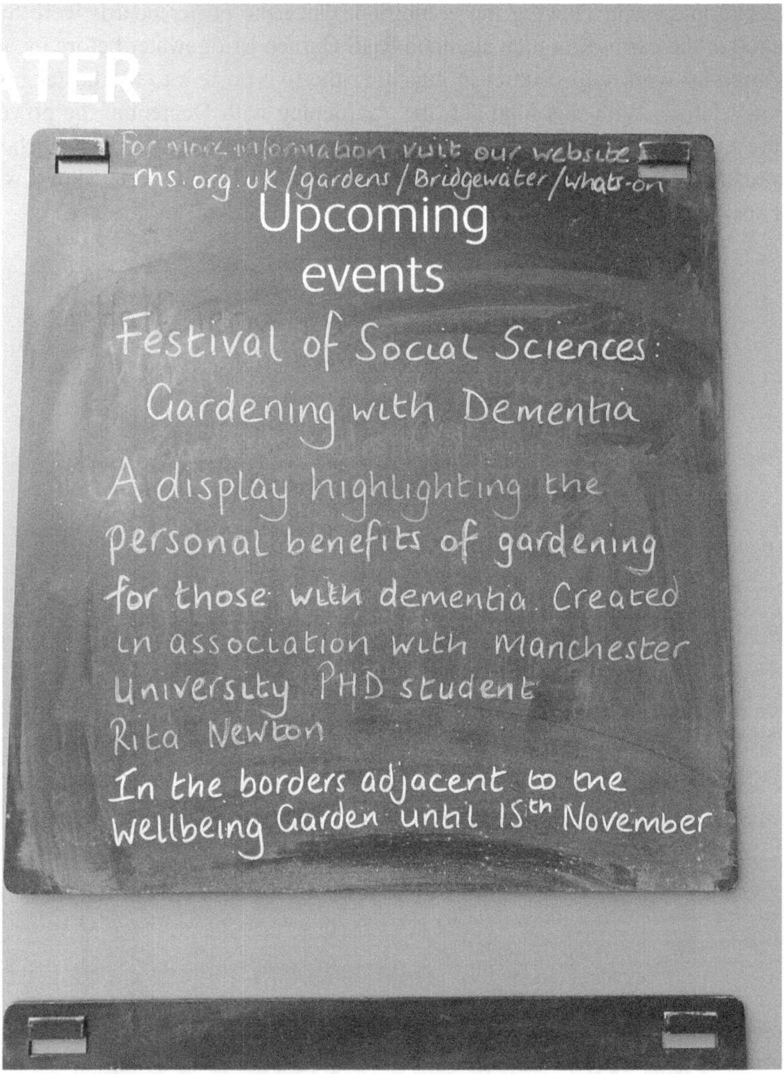


IMAGE 9.4 The 'blackboard and chalk' advertising for the ESRC FOSS exhibition at RHS Garden Bridgewater.

wanted the exhibition to start with spring with its seasonal focus and imagery on growth and new beginnings; a symbolism we wanted to align to the experience of living well with dementia. In the middle of Image 9.3, at the end of the path beyond the gate (which is opened during RHS opening hours) is the entrance to the Community Wellbeing Garden.

Once the exhibition was ready to be viewed and open to the public, and as seen in Image 9.4, the RHS's focus on sustainability was carried through to the 'blackboard and chalk' advertising of the ESRC FOSS event which was positioned at the main entrance to the RHS Garden Bridgewater in Salford for the duration of the exhibition.

We will now share and briefly summarise the contents on each of the five posters used in the exhibition, starting with the Introductory poster.

## The five exhibition posters

### *Introductory poster*

The Introductory poster shown in Image 9.5 starts by repeating the title of the ESRC FOSS exhibition and, whilst the reproduction of the poster in this chapter is in black and white, the actual colours used were different shades of green to subliminally associate the display with the greenspaces of the domestic (home) and/

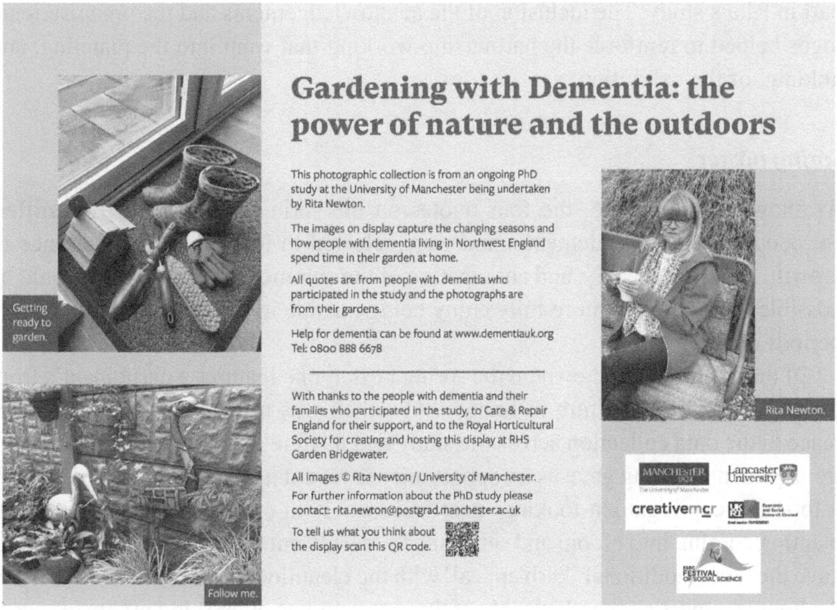


**IMAGE 9.5** Exhibition introductory poster.

or its outside spaces. The title of the exhibition is written in dark green. On the top left-hand side of the poster, the included photograph of 'Getting ready to garden' was the same picture as used in the postcard advertising (see Image 9.2). This tied the two accounts together and made sure that anyone attending the event informed by the postcard advertising knew that they were in the right place.

The included photograph of Rita was taken in the back garden of one of the participant's homes and the picture was edited to remove the image of a person living with dementia who, at the time, was seated on the garden bench next to Rita. This was to comply with our research ethics permission not to reveal faces or other identifying features of people living with dementia in the research work. Including the picture of Rita also helped viewers and visitors to the exhibition to identify Rita when she attended the display in-person each Salford-free Tuesday to talk about the posters with anyone who might be interested in hearing more about them and to collect evaluation data about the exhibition from any willing visitor. The Introductory poster also included a QR code that could be scanned on a mobile telephone by anyone who was able to do this and wanted to give feedback on the exhibition. Some of the anonymous evaluation data is shared at the end of this case study.

The Introductory poster was also designed to include (i) a national contact number to inform any visitors of help and advice that is available for those living with, or caring for, a person living with dementia; and (ii) a reminder that all quotes in the four-seasons display posters were by people living with dementia who took part in Rita's study. The inclusion of the acknowledgements and the organisational logos helped to reinforce the partnership working that went into the planning, and holding, of the exhibition.

### *Spring poster*

As shown in Image 9.6, the four quotes on the spring poster were from different people living with dementia and were selected to focus on the importance of growth, activities, beauty, and anticipation of the summer months when it would be possible to once again more fully enjoy being outside in the garden and for longer periods of time.

Of the five pictures shown on the spring poster, one features a participant's front garden (lower right picture in Image 9.6) which was a relatively unusual occurrence in the data collection across the study and its timeline. However, showing the front garden in spring gave us an opportunity to reveal just how much display work it took to keep a garden looking 'neat and tidy' with current and previous years' planting coming into bloom and set against a freshly cut lawn. Such an aesthetic act gave the home additional 'kerb appeal' with the cleanliness and order in the front of the house suggesting that the inside of the house and its other (hidden) green spaces would be as equally 'neat and tidy' and cared about.

The photographs on the spring poster also represented work that was conducted in the garden, such as washing down patio furniture and tidying up the garden

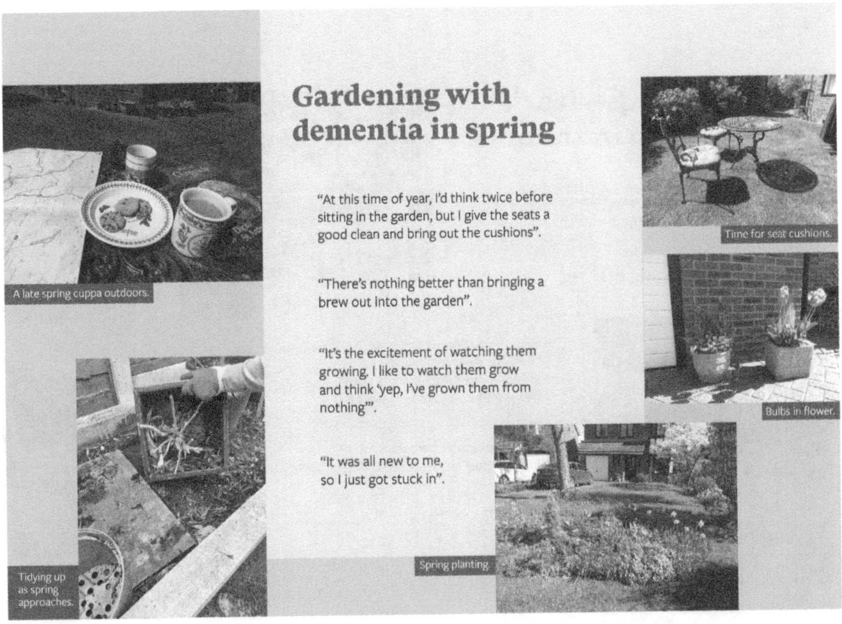
Gardening with dementia in spring
"At this time of year, I'd think twice before sitting in the garden, but I give the seats a good clean and bring out the cushions".
"There's nothing better than bringing a brew out into the garden".
"It's the excitement of watching them growing. I like to watch them grow and think 'yep, I've grown them from nothing'".
"It was all new to me, so I just got stuck in".
A late spring cuppa outdoors.
Time for seat cushions.
Bulbs in flower.
Tidying up as spring approaches.
Spring planting

**IMAGE 9.6** Spring poster.

after the ending of winter and the difficulty in those months of getting out into the garden. Domestic gardens therefore encouraged people living with dementia to socialise, engage with the outside spaces of their home, and to literally have their hands in the earth clearing, digging, sorting, and planting. Such focused work helped all those viewing the garden to appreciate its beauty, such as that contained in the stone pots and flowers in Image 9.6.

### *Summer poster*

The photographs and the text in Image 9.7 were primarily selected to represent the peacefulness and warmth of the summer months, the greenery and colours of nature, and the fact that people living with dementia wanted their identity as a gardener to be acknowledged and seen.

The photographs and selected quotes in Image 9.7 also highlighted that, at times, the domestic garden contained material structures, such as a shed, that were used by people living with dementia as part of their everyday lives and interaction with the greenspaces of their home. As seen in the quote in the poster that begins 'Even if I can't remember what I've done during the day …', the garden, and the act of gardening, enabled people with dementia to live 'in the moment' and be immersed in the task in hand.

Like a photograph in Image 9.6, one of the photographs in Image 9.7 shows a person living with dementia wearing gardening gloves and dressing for the garden which was perhaps symbolic of the transformation of the person living with

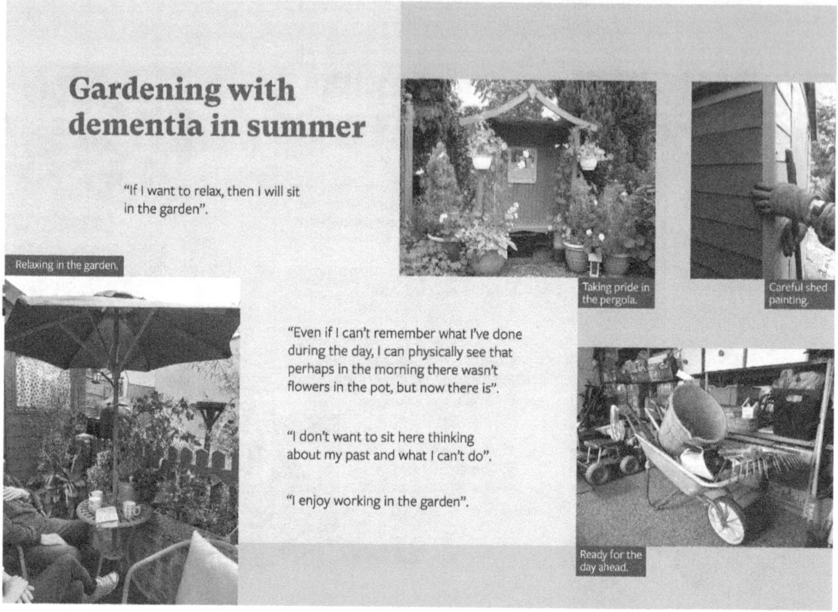


IMAGE 9.7 Summer poster.

dementia's identity into a gardener and that being in the garden was also 'work'. This material transformation is also perhaps one way to delineate the act of gardening and being a gardener from a state of relaxing and sitting quietly under a garden umbrella, as also seen in one of the photographs in Image 9.7.

### *Autumn poster*

The photographs and four quotes by people living with dementia in Image 9.8 reveal a change in use and activity in the garden and introduces a 'planning ahead' narrative that is focused on planting for the garden for next year.

The photograph which is positioned top right in Image 9.8 includes two recycling bins situated in the far corner of the patio, and they perhaps represent the necessary, but unavoidable, clutter of everyday domestic life. Next to the recycling bins is a large water butt for catching and recycling rainwater. The same photograph also contains a bird table and an attached fat ball feeder for the birds that ostensibly reveals that garden use, planning, and care extends to wildlife and to their welfare both in autumn and in the winter months to come.

Some of the photographs in Image 9.8 also capture the growing of fruit in the garden and reveal that the summer plants are starting to lose their bloom and need to be carefully pruned to enable regrowth the following spring/summer. It is a seasonal change that aligns itself to the rhythmic cycle of nature and to our

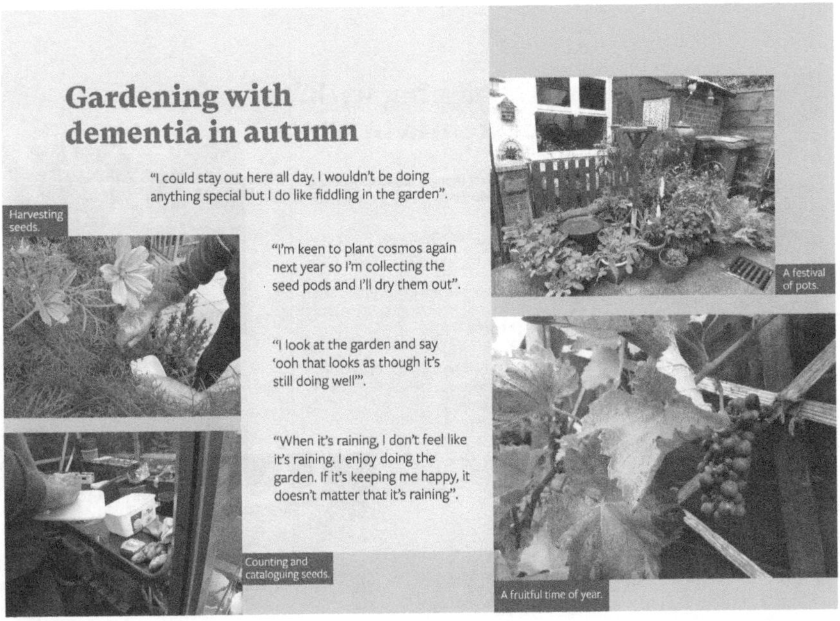


IMAGE 9.8 Autumn poster.

own transitional life experiences. As shown in the photograph situated bottom left in Image 9.8, planting and cataloguing seedlings in the greenhouse also instils a future narrative for the person living with dementia and continues their identity as a gardener.

### *Winter poster*

As can be seen in Image 9.9, the five photographs and four quotations by people living with dementia reveal an engagement with the garden in the winter months, even though the greenery and growth shown in the other three seasonal posters have largely disappeared.

The photographs and supporting text in Image 9.9 indicate that everyday work in the garden still goes on, albeit at a slower pace and in a more subdued way. The photograph located top right in Image 9.9 is the only one of the four seasons in the ESRC FOSS exhibition that shows an inside view of a person living with dementia's home. It reveals how a connection to the outside continues, as can be seen in preparing to feed the visiting squirrel(s) to the back garden and in the view of the patio door leading out to the garden with the wellington boots strategically placed on the doormat. These liminal and threshold spaces would therefore appear to be important connections in the everyday life of people with dementia using and accessing their garden in winter.

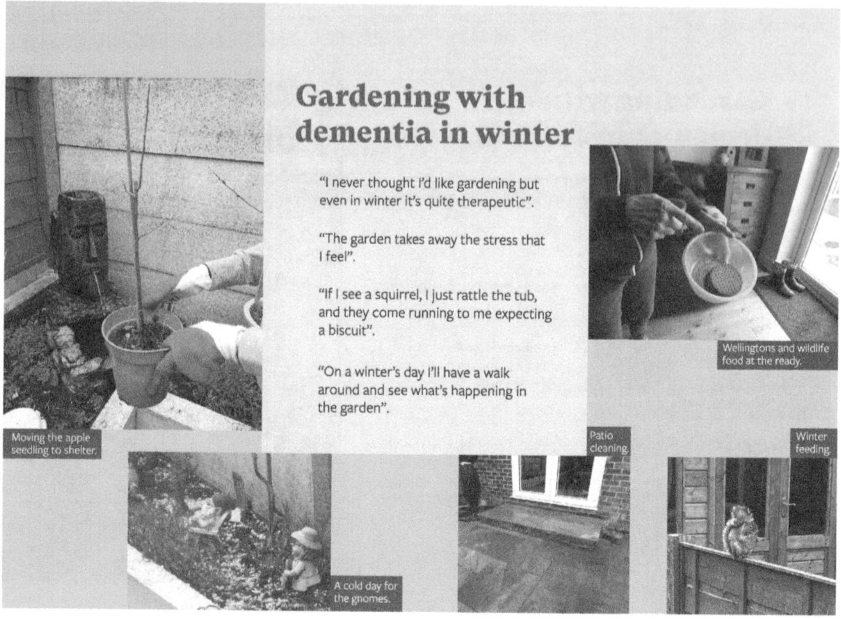


IMAGE 9.9 Winter poster.

As also seen in the photograph on the lower left of Image 9.9, the garden is a place for fun and remembrance as seen in the picture of the garden gnomes covered in frost. Whilst it was not made clear in the supporting text, the placement and positioning of the garden gnomes was deliberate and an act of associated remembrance as the gnomes represented the person living with dementia and her husband, who had died several years earlier. This placement in the garden could be seen as a continued display of the home and an act imbued with personal and relational significance.

### *ESRC FOSS visitor numbers and evaluation outcome*

The number of Salford residents attending RHS Garden Bridgewater on Salford-free Tuesdays was recorded as being 2,014 on the 22 October 2024 (Rita conducted 47 face-to-face discussions with visitors that day about the exhibition); 1,440 on the 29 October 2024 (Rita conducted 31 face-to-face discussions with visitors that day about the exhibition); and 665 on the 5 November 2024 (Rita conducted 17 face-to-face discussions with visitors that day about the exhibition). The variance in visitor attendance between the numbers attending on 22 and 29 October as compared to the November date was that the October visiting times coincided with the school holidays and around 25% of the total visitor numbers on those days were children.

The evaluation of the ESRC FOSS exhibition was overwhelmingly positive with the following three (anonymous) examples helping to illustrate this:

> This morning, I had the opportunity to take a closer look at the posters on dementia and gardening. I wanted to take a moment to express my sincere appreciation for the thoughtful and sensitive way this topic was presented. The posters are beautifully crafted, both informative and compassionate, shedding light on the importance of horticulture for those affected by dementia.
>
> The message resonated deeply with me on a personal level. My friend's father is currently navigating the difficult journey of dementia and seeing how the garden can serve as a source of comfort, engagement, and connection is truly meaningful. Your work in making this connection visible and accessible to visitors is inspiring.
>
> Thank you for your dedication to raising awareness of the healing power of nature, especially for those facing such challenging circumstances. It is initiatives like these that remind us of the incredible impact gardens can have on wellbeing and community.

The conclusion of the ESRC FOSS exhibition brought with it an opportunity to think about developing more information and help for those people living with dementia who wanted to continue to access and use their garden at home and to continue their identity as a gardener. It is this emphasis that broadly sits at the heart of case study 2, as we will now share.

## Case study 2

This second case study showcases a conversation between Rita and Ozichi: just as a reminder, Ozichi is a therapeutic gardener at RHS Garden Bridgewater and helped to set up and facilitate the ESRC FOSS exhibition. Ozichi has long-standing experience of being alongside people living with dementia in the outdoors and has a responsibility for the Community Wellbeing Garden. The conversation took place between Rita and Ozichi (see Image 9.10) during the time of the ESRC FOSS exhibition and is about the Community Wellbeing Garden, as well as being conducted in that space.

### Rita in conversation with Ozichi

*Rita:* So, what is the Community Wellbeing Garden at RHS Garden Bridgewater and how did it come about?

*Ozichi:* In 2018 or thereabouts there was a big community consultation to ask people in Salford what they would want in a wellbeing garden and some of those ideas from the consultation were incorporated into the design. There is a grass mound and that was influenced by a particular organisation where their wheelchair users were saying *'You don't really*

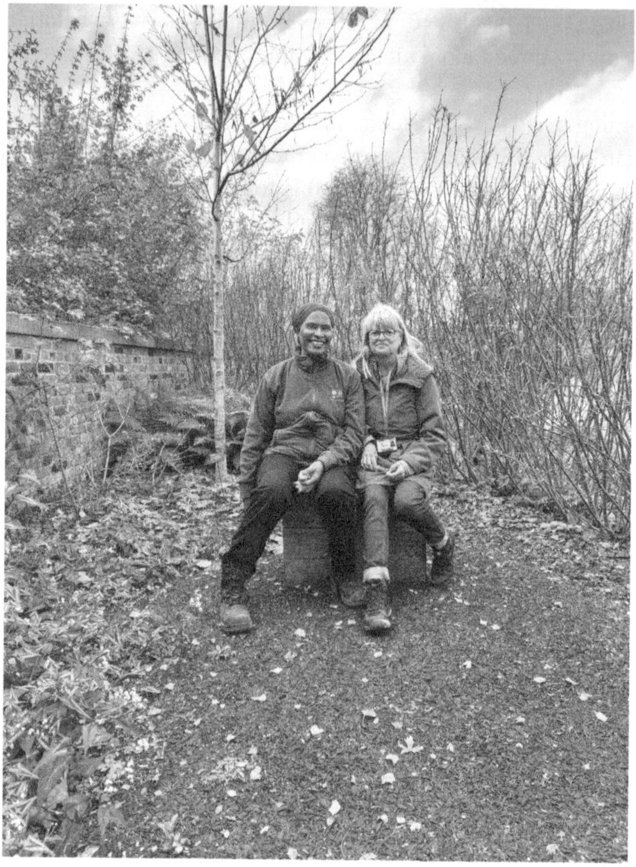

IMAGE 9.10 Rita and Ozichi seated in the Community Wellbeing Garden.

*Source:* Photograph taken by John Keady and shared with the permission of Rita and Ozichi

*access grass anymore as somebody in a wheelchair'* and so the grass lawn is a bit higher so people in a wheelchair can touch the grass, or sit on it, or place their feet on it from their wheelchair. However, regardless of whether you are in a wheelchair or not, you can interact with the grass mound, and we often see people walking on it or touching it with bare feet. It is a design that works for everyone. Personally, I like to lie on it and close my eyes for a few minutes. It is like a grass sofa. The action of lying on the earth automatically does something that engages your body into relaxation, it just happens. The grass mound does get roped off over winter so that it can recover and dry out.

It is why I enjoy being a community gardener, because a garden is more than just something to look at and look at all the beauty in it, but as something that you interact with. You begin to engage with plants in a way that you get to know them like knowing a person – it becomes something in which you acquire knowledge and begin to discover. So, whether its food, or an herb, or a particular type of sweet pea and discovering that it's got a scent that you like or working out what you can do with lavender after you have harvested it, all these connections are really important rather than just looking.

*Rita:* Could you tell me a little more about the design of the Community Wellbeing Garden?

*Ozichi:* There are these circular elements that I would call mini private gardens or little rooms. They have got the tall grasses, so you have got this 'fizzing' of grass, and the design came from the idea of catherine wheels [a rotating firework]. You have got the movement in the wind of the grasses and how they sprawl over onto the paths, and when they do, you find that people will automatically touch the grass. On the grass lawn area when the weather is good, we do get people having a picnic there. On the bigger circles, there are family picnic spots. So, in effect, these are all small gardens within a garden, and they are a more intimate space to be in. We have some other nooks and crannies in the garden that we call our 'solitary areas' where there is just one seat. We have had people on our wellbeing sessions who will want to go off and sit by themselves. The other thing that is noticeable is that the paths meander. Straight paths for someone who has dementia can be quite frustrating, so this garden allows you to meander, to weave, and to walk around.

Our food forage garden is based on a permaculture style, or ecological style, of gardening. It was not part of the initial design, but I asked for this because it is representative of how I work with people. So, in a way, it's a bit more freeing and it is about making use of what is in it rather than just maintaining it. If you see a strawberry plant, you must dive in and look for the strawberries; in that way, it is more of a tactile engagement with the plants. This part of the garden is designed to really wake up a lot of your senses. You do not need to ask permission, a lot of the forage garden has edible perennials and visitors learn that gardening does not have to be hard labour, it can be as simple as planting a strawberry plant…and it will last for over three years, very low maintenance. We have got redcurrants, blackcurrants, blackberries, blueberries, gooseberries, and raspberries and suddenly this is something that people see for real, and not just something that is in a punnet in a shop. We have also got a dry herb area, and we often make teas with the herbs that we harvest, in addition to the aesthetic pleasure that they bring. We are bringing people closer to nature.

*Rita:* Any final thoughts about your role as a therapeutic gardener?

*Ozichi:* I love plants because when it is about introducing people to a growing area, it is about getting to know and building up their own legacy of enjoying plants. I think what nature does is spark the plugs within us, it kicks us into a feeling of *'this is a really nice sensation and I'm enjoying it'*. It is curiosity and discovery, almost childlike fun. This is really the stuff of it for me, to allow people to be part of it, not to be just the keepers of it. The activity of gardening is very immediate. You can see straightaway what you have changed in that space and what you have achieved. And that is helpful for people who do not know if they are of any use to anyone anymore; everybody needs purpose in their life. People living with dementia need purpose in their lives. There's something about plants, we can move them around, we can shuffle them like cards, and we can play. Really, gardening is quite playful and if you have got access to plants, they may seem insignificant on their own, but you can soon start being creative and let your imagination fizz.

## Discussion

Seen from an everyday and care aesthetics lens, the four seasons of the year sit as a temporal context to our everyday interactions with the relational and sensory impact that being outdoors has in all our lives, whether we live with dementia or not. For example, once we are outside in the fresh air, we are at the mercy of the weather and the climate. Stepping into open spaces, our senses are immediately engaged and they work together to connect us to the present moment in time; for instance, we may feel the warmth of the summer sun or the coldness of the winter skies; we will get wet if it rains and feel the raindrops on our skin; we touch and remove our wet clothes; we can hear soundscapes all around us, the wind through the trees, the buzzing of the bees, the birdsong, the voices of our neighbours, the crunch of the spade as it digs into the soil, and the snip of the secateurs; we see the blue skies and the colours of nature and, in autumn, we see the daylight slowly retreating until our late afternoons are in darkness; and we dress differently to match the different seasons.

Even with the limited information and the number of pictures that could be placed on each of the seasonal posters in Images 9.6 to 9.9, it was striking how the person living with dementia's interaction with their garden positioned them away from a dependency relationship and into an active citizenship identity. In many ways, this focus adds to our understanding of an aesthetics of care insofar as it is not only the 'carer to person living with dementia' relationship that is important to consider, but also that care is a multidirectional process which includes environments as well as interhuman practices. Moreover, Images 9.6 to 9.9 also reveal that domestic garden use by people living with dementia in autumn and winter is not the same as garden use in spring and summer. Going forward, it is this intersection between seasonal time and lived time of people with dementia that is so important to consider and balance. Being outside in the domestic garden with a pair of secateurs at 10 o'clock on a summer's evening is acceptable; it is less so in the depths of winter dressed in nightwear and wanting to tend to the plants. For people living with dementia, and the sensory, embodied, and relational context of their lives, domestic gardens can also act as a barometer of their experience of lived time.

As we have intimated in the previous paragraph, and drawing on care aesthetic theory, domestic gardens are sensory, embodied, and relational spaces and the text/images on the four seasonal posters, as well as in the extracts from the conversation with Ozichi, highlight that people living with dementia continue to show care and appreciation of, and about, nature and the natural world. Care is demonstrated by people living with dementia in different ways, such as through the pruning, planting, and cultivation of plants, seeds, and the soil; in the symbolic representation and personal meaning attached to ornaments; in the care of wildlife; and in an appreciation of the beauty of created floral displays. Care is also shown in the maintenance and upkeep of garden furniture, patios, sheds, and other architecture situated in the garden. As Thompson (2023) has stated, care aesthetics must be 'of and between the bodies, objects, and environments of the world' (p. 25). Accordingly, the point we want to make here is that people living with dementia take their cumulative life experiences and expectations into their future and that future includes an embodied identity as a gardener, however full or limited that exposure may have been. Arguably, for those professionals visiting people living with dementia at home, or continuing care in other supportive environments, it is important to be aware of this identity and to cultivate it as far as it is needed or wanted. Perhaps developing a garden biography where life-long exposure to gardening practices could be documented alongside people living with dementia would be an important first step in grounding this future work.

As we have seen across the two case studies in this chapter, domestic gardens, and the act of gardening itself, can help to improve the well-being of people living with dementia by connecting the person to the natural rhythms of the seasons and, if it is not too grand a statement, to the very stuff of life itself. Perhaps these two quotations in the winter poster in Image 9.9 help to capture these points: 'the garden takes away the stress that I feel' and 'I never thought I would like gardening, but even in the winter it is quite therapeutic'. It is therefore surprising that up to the present day, so little research, practice, and policy attention has been focused on better understanding people living with dementia's interaction with the outside spaces of their domestic home and the meaning that this holds in their everyday life. As Huizenga et al. (2023) have argued, viewing the lived experience of dementia from within the frame of everyday life opens-up the importance of place, objects, and the mundanity of routine to create a sense of belonging with 'a connection to the self across past, current, and future time' (p. 10). As seen in the two case studies, being in the garden and in the outside spaces of the home is part of the experience of everyday life and an activity that has its roots deeply embedded in a person living with dementia's autobiographical and narrative identity. However, to date, it has just not been seen or nurtured as such.

For the households recruited into the study, and in extracts from Ozichi's shared conversation in case study 2, the regenerative features of a garden both showcase and instil a narrative of 'the future' into the discourse of people living with dementia. This quite simple observation has some profound implications for the caring professions. For example, outside of people living with dementia being involved in preparing legal documentation, such as a Lasting Power of Attorney to come into force once capacity has been lost at an (unknown) future time, or setting out an Advanced Directive to spell out their future needs and wishes (particularly at the end of life), most psychosocial evidence in 'caring' for a person living with dementia is focused on preserving or recalling past memories. As Section 1.4 of the National Institute for Health and Care Excellence (2018) dementia guideline illustrates, the names of some of the recommended evidence-based interventions to promote cognition, independence, and well-being include group reminiscence therapy, cognitive stimulation therapy, and cognitive rehabilitation. It would be so interesting to consider how domestic gardens and the outside spaces of the home, contextualised through the temporal dimensions of the four seasons of the year and their accompanying aesthetic practices, could start to capture and respond to a future-based caring and decision-making dynamic. Care aesthetics has such an important role to play in platforming this new approach to dementia care and in the language needed to make that happen.

## Conclusion

Spending time in the domestic garden enables people living with dementia to maintain a sense of continuity and identity by connecting to nature, people, and to the moment whilst managing everyday life. Yet, all too often, the act of gardening is seen as a series of tasks such as mowing the lawn, watering the plants, and tidying up the autumn leaves. Whilst all of these are important, by taking a care aesthetics lens to these everyday activities, it is possible to move away from seeing 'only the task' to consider the intimate, sensory, and embodied connection – and interdependent relationship – between a person living with dementia and their garden space(s) at home. A perspective that has been all too frequently overlooked in the literature and in everyday domestic garden practices.

## Acknowledgements

We would like to thank the ESRC FOSS team at The University of Manchester for their support of the exhibition; the RHS for their willingness to support the exhibition; all the visitors to the exhibition at RHS Garden Bridgewater; and to the households who took part in the study and who made the exhibition possible.

We would also like to acknowledge the support of the ESRC for funding this PhD studentship: ESRC Northwest Social Science Doctoral Training Partnership Grant Number ES/P000665/1.

## Note

Should any reader wish to see the colour representations of the postcard and the ESRC FOSS exhibition posters shared in this chapter, they can be accessed free of charge on Figshare – The University of Manchester's data repository site – at the following weblink: https://figshare.manchester.ac.uk/articles/poster/Exhibition_posters_on_Gardening_and_Dementia_for_the_ESRC_Festival_of_Social_Science_Manchester_2024/29069918; accessed 1 March 2026.

## Three Key Reading References

### *Reference 1*

Newton, R., Keady, J., Tsekleves, E. and Adams, S. (2021). 'My father is a gardener…': A systematic narrative review on access and use of the garden by people living with dementia. *Health and Place*, 68: e102516. Available: https://doi.org/10.1016/j.healthplace.2021.102516; accessed 1 March 2026.

This paper is the first published systematic narrative review on the access and use of the domestic garden by people living with dementia. The paper helped to open up the discourse on domestic gardens in dementia and provides a foundation for the development of aesthetic experiences, especially in the act of being outdoors and in establishing the importance of conducting a garden biography.

### *Reference 2*

Buse, C., Balmer, A., Keady, J., Nettleton, S. and Swift, S. (2023). 'Ways of being' in the domestic garden for people living with dementia: Doing, sensing and playing. *Ageing & Society*, First View 1–25. Available at: https://doi.org/10.1017/S0144686X22001489

This paper provides an analysis of gardening practices by people living with dementia and highlights their significant implications for 'living well' at home. The methods of study included filmed walking interviews and garden tours, diaries and sketch methods and repeat visits. Findings are presented in relation to the different 'ways of being' in the garden, namely working in and doing the garden; being in and sensing; and playing, empowerment and agency. This is the first published paper in the world to look at this area.

### *Reference 3*

Royal Horticultural Society (2023). A lifelong adventure with gardening. *RHS Strategy to 2030*. Available: https://www.rhs.org.uk/about-us/pdfs/about-the-rhs/mission-and-strategy/rhs-strategy-to-2030.pdf; accessed 1 March 2026.

Whilst not dedicated solely to dementia, this important strategy document published by the RHS highlights its enduring organisational purpose to encourage and improve the science, art, and practice of horticulture. The report is threaded with a sense of inclusivity operationalised through the goal to offer a sense of unified optimism that everyone can find joy and fulfilment in the personal and collective action of gardening. As such, the report sits as both a context and backdrop to the gardening practices of people living with dementia.

## References


Allen, F., Cain, R. and Meyer, C. (2019). How people with dementia and their carers adapt their homes. A qualitative study. *Dementia: The International Journal of Social Research and Practice,* 18 (3): 1199–1215. https://doi.org/10.1177/1471301217712294

Braun, V. and Clarke, V. (2019). Reflecting on reflexive thematic analysis. *Qualitative Research in Sport, Exercise and Health,* 11 (4): 589–597. https://doi.org/10.1080/2159676X.2019.1628806

Buse, C., Balmer, A., Keady, J., Nettleton, S. and Swift, S. (2023). 'Ways of being' in the domestic garden for people living with dementia: Doing, sensing and playing. *Ageing & Society*, First View 1–25. Available at: https://doi.org/10.1017/S0144686X22001489

Campbell, S., Clark, A., Keady, J., Kullberg, A., Manji, K., Odzakovic, E., Rummery, K. and Ward, R. (2023). 'I can see what's going on without being nosey…': What matters to people living with dementia about home as revealed through visual home tours. *International Journal of Geriatric Psychiatry*, 38 (9): e5999. Available: https://doi.org/10.1002/gps.5999; accessed 1 March 2026.

Chalmin-Pui, L.S., Griffiths, A., Roe, J. and Cameron, T.H.R. (2021). Why garden? – Attitudes and the perceived health benefits of home gardening. *Cities,* 112: Available: https://doi.org/10.1016/j.cities.2021.103118; accessed 1 March 2026.

Chung, P.Y., Ellis-Hill, C. and Coleman, P. (2017). Supporting activity engagement by family carers at home: Maintenance of agency and personhood in dementia. *International Journal of Qualitative Studies on Health and Well-being*, 12 (1): 1–14. https://doi.org/10.1080/17482631.2016.1267316

Dewing, J. (2002). From ritual to relationship: A person centred approach to consent in qualitative research with older people who have a dementia. *Dementia: The International Journal of Social Research and Practice,* 1 (2): 156–171. https://doi.org/10.1177/147130120200100204

Dewing, J. (2007). Participatory research: A method for process consent with persons who have dementia. *Dementia: The International Journal of Social Research and Practice*, 6 (1): 11–25. https://doi.org/10.1177/1471301207075625

Duggan, S., Blackman, T., Martyr, A. and Van Schaik, P. (2008). The impact of early dementia on outdoor life. *A 'shrinking world?' Dementia: The International Journal of Social Research and Practice*, 7 (2): 191–204. https://doi.org/10.1177/1471301208091158

Edwards, C.A., McDonnell, C. and Merl, H. (2013). An evaluation of a therapeutic garden's influence on the quality of life of aged care residents and dementia. *Dementia: The International Journal of Social Research and Practice,* 12 (4): 494–510. https://doi.org/10.1177/1471301211435188

Greater Manchester Population Statistics. Available: https://www.visitnorthwest.com/population/greater-manchester/; accessed 1 March 2026.

Huizenga, J., Scheffelaar, A., Bleijenberg, N., Wilken, J.P., Keady, J. and Regenmortel, T.V. (2023). What matters most: Exploring the everyday lives of people with dementia. *International Journal of Geriatric Psychiatry*, 38 (8): e5983. Available: 10.1002/gps.5983.https://doi.org/10.1002/gps.5983; accessed 1 March 2026.

Ibsen, T.L. and Eriksen, S. (2021). The experience of attending a farm-based day care service from the perspective of people with dementia: A qualitative study. *Dementia: The International Journal of Social Research and Practice*, 20 (4): 1356–1374. https://doi.org/10.1177/1471301220940107

Kaplan, S. (1995). The restorative benefits of nature: Toward an integrative framework. *Journal of Environmental Psychology*, 15 (3): 169–182. https://doi.org/10.1016/0272-4944(95)90001-2

Keady, J. (ed.) (2024). *Reconsidering Neighbourhoods and Living with Dementia: Spaces, Places and People*, Maidenhead: Open University Press/McGraw-Hill.

Kim, S., Anstey, K.J. and Mortby, M.E. (2023). Who displays dementia-related stigma and what does the general public know about dementia? Findings from a nationally representative survey. *Aging & Mental Health*, 27 (6): 1111–1119. https://doi.org/10.1080/13607863.2022.2040428

Lauwerijssen, R., Mell, I. and Barker, A. (2025). Exploring domestic garden identities: Personal histories from older people in the Netherlands. *Landscape Research*, 50 (3): 543–561. https://doi.org/10.1080/01426397.2024.2428811

Mapes, N. (2012). Living with dementia through the changing seasons. In J. Gilliard and M. Marshall (eds.) *Transforming the Quality of Life for People with Dementia Through Contact with the Natural World. Fresh Air on My Face,* London: Jessica Kingsley, pp. 30–44.

Mmako, N.J., Courtney-Pratt, H. and Marsh, P. (2020). Green spaces, dementia and a meaningful life in the community: A mixed studies review. *Health & Place*, 63: 102344. Available: https://doi.org/10.1016/j.healthplace.2020.102344; accessed 1 March 2026.

Motealleh, P., Moyle, W., Jones, C. and Dupre, K. (2019). Creating a dementia-friendly environment through the use of outdoor natural landscape design intervention in long-term care facilities: A narrative review. *Health & Place*, 58: 102148. Available: https://doi.org/10.1016/j.healthplace.2019.102148; accessed 1 March 2026.

National Institute for Health and Care Excellence (2018). *Dementia: Assessment, Management and Support for People Living with Dementia and Their Carers.* [NICE Guideline: NG97]. Available: https://www.nice.org.uk/guidance/ng97; accessed 1 March 2026.

Newton, R., Adams, S., Keady, J. and Tsekleves, E. (2023). Exploring the contribution of housing adaptations in supporting everyday life for people with dementia: A scoping review. *Ageing & Society*, 43 (8): 1833–1859. https://doi.org/10.1017/S0144686X2100136

Newton, R., Keady, J., Tsekleves, E. and Adams, S. (2021). 'My father is a gardener…': A systematic narrative review on access and use of the garden by people living with dementia. *Health and Place*, 68: e102516. Available: https://doi.org/10.1016/j.healthplace.2021.102516; accessed 1 March 2026.

Noone, S. and Jenkins, N. (2018). Digging for Dementia: Exploring the experience of community gardening from the perspectives of people with dementia. *Aging & Mental Health*, 22 (7): 881–888. https://doi.org/10.1080/13607863.2017.1393793

Noone, S., Innes, A., Kelly, F. and Mayers, A. (2017). The nourishing soil of the soul': The role of horticultural therapy in promoting well-being in community-dwelling people with dementia. *Dementia: The International Journal of Social Research and Practice*, 16 (7): 897–910. https://doi.org/10.1177/1471301215623889

Phinney, A., Kelson, E., Baumbusch, J., O'Connor, D. and Purves, D. (2016). Walking in the neighbourhood: Performing social citizenship in dementia. *Dementia: The International Journal of Social Research and Practice*, 15 (3): 381–394. https://doi.org/10.1177/1471301216638180

Royal Horticultural Society (2023). A lifelong adventure with gardening. *RHS strategy to 2030*. Available: https://www.rhs.org.uk/about-us/pdfs/about-the-rhs/mission-and-strategy/rhs-strategy-to-2030.pdf; accessed 1 March 2026.

Rushton, L., Smith, L. and Phillipson, L. (2025). Gardens, agency and citizenship of people with dementia: A critical interpretive synthesis. *Ageing and Society*, 45 (10): 2141–2163. https://doi.org/10.1017/S0144686X24000771

Thompson, J. (2023). *Care Aesthetics: For Artful Care and Careful Art*, London: Routledge.

Tsai, M., Cushing, D.F. and Brough, M. (2020). "I've always lived in a place with gardens": Residents' homemaking experiences in Australian aged-care gardens. *Health & Place*, 61: 102259. Available: https://doi.org/10.1016/j.healthplace.2019.102259; accessed 1 March 2026.

Whear, R., Thompson Coon, J., Bethel, A., Abbott, R., Stein, K. and Garside, R. (2014). What is the impact of using outdoor spaces such as gardens on the physical and mental well-being of those with dementia? A systematic review of quantitative and qualitative evidence. *The Journal of Post-Acute and Long-term Care Medicine,* 15 (10): 697–705. https://doi.org/10.1016/j.jamda.2014.05.013

# 10

# CARE AESTHETICS OR THE AESTHETICISATION OF CARE? REMINISCENCE ROOMS AND THE TENSIONS OF DEMENTIA-FRIENDLY DESIGN

*Daryl Martin, Christina Buse and Sarah Nettleton*

## Introduction

We begin our chapter with an awry glance at a parable taken from Georgi Gospodinov's International Booker Prize-winning novel 'Time Shelter', which tells the story of a 'clinic for the past' built to serve people living with dementia in the contemporary period (Gospodinov, 2022). In the novel, Dr Gaustine, the director of the clinic, is an enigmatic geriatric psychiatrist who has developed a treatment for patients with Alzheimer's disease that involves the careful curation of ornaments and relics that recreate different decades within different rooms, and then different floors, of the building. This is a project sparked by Dr Gaustine's observation of how patients with memory loss start to become more relaxed and talkative in his office after he decorates it with The Beatles memorabilia and other ornaments from the 1960s (Gospodinov, 2022, p. 16). From this point, Dr Gaustine considers the complexity, as well as the efficacy, of utilising the past in order to make the present more comfortable for his patients. When he shows the narrator around his clinic, Dr Gaustine introduces different rooms on the 1960s floor, describing the attention to detail involved in assembling artefacts that, separately and together, connote a variety of lifestyles for the benefit of residents whose biographical experiences of the time differed materially, according to whether they lived in Eastern or Western Europe or whether they were students or not at the time (Gospodinov, 2022, p. 43). Subtly, the novel articulates the powerful affective charge carried by the material culture associated with specific historical periods, as noted by the narrator in a visceral response triggered when he sees a coat in the present environment that resembles one previously worn by his mother. Strategically, the novel reflects the potential for individual artefacts of the recent past to have a therapeutic impact on people living with dementia, even if only momentarily.

DOI: 10.4324/9781003623441-14
This chapter has been made available under a (CC BY) 4.0 license.

Gospodinov's novel draws on an emerging trend in the architecture of residential settings for later life, especially when designed for people living with dementia; namely, the use of reminiscence rooms to evoke memories of the residents' pasts, in order to make them feel at home within their new communities. It should be noted that 'Time Shelter' does not aim to offer a realistic account of how people live in institutional settings, but rather takes the care home setting, and specifically reminiscence rooms within them, as the starting point for a sharp satire of how nostalgia works in the political discourses of contemporary Europe. Gospodinov suggests that the use of reminiscence rooms becomes so attractive to the families and friends of residents living with dementia that the 'past-clinics' are soon opened up to them too and thereafter to people with no connections to anyone already living there; by this point in the novel, the clinics have become metaphorical and literal shelters to those who feel disaffected through living in their contemporary times. From here, the growth of the 'past-clinic' is the spark to a series of national referenda on the past throughout the European Union (EU) whereby each country's residents vote on which year or decade they were happiest, and thus the national polities, institutions, and patterns of everyday life are reset to these dates (thus, the Scandinavian countries in the EU vote to go back to the 1970s, France, Germany, and Spain vote to go back to the 1980s, and most post-Soviet Bloc countries vote to reset to the 1990s). In the aftermath of Brexit, the novel reads as a wise fable on the political dangers of lives lived in avoidance of the present moment, of using the objects of the past as theatrical props to promote ideals of 'life as a reenactment' (Gospodinov, 2022, p. 123).

Notwithstanding its pointed political purpose, Gospodinov's novel is astute on the ways in which temporalities clash between the model of care (or, perhaps, better treatment) envisaged in the reminiscence room and the experience of time by people living with dementia. Gospodinov's (2022) narrator reflects that for people living with dementia 'the present is a foreign country, while the past is their homeland' (p. 44), before proceeding to characterise Dr Gaustine's approach as an attempt to adjust the appearance of the present throughout his clinics in order to align with the internal time of those living with Alzheimer's disease. This passage is telling, in terms of identifying the therapeutic aspirations of the novel's 'clinic of the past' specifically, and reminiscence rooms more generally; the therapeutic aim comes from staging the physical environment so accurately that it tries to meet its residents emotionally in moments of their past, as a kind of validation therapy. In this, there is at least some connection with the idea of care aesthetics described by Sarah Campbell and colleagues (2024) as a meeting 'in the moment' (p. 2) between carer and a person living with dementia. This builds on James Thompson's (2015) proposal of care aesthetics as a term that captures 'a relational process that emphasise(s) engagements between individuals or groups *over time*' (p. 437, emphasis added); in this understanding, the practice of care aesthetics involves something of a synchronicity between people in encounters of care, in which the agency of the person living with dementia is respected and enhanced and in which 'being in the moment' of care becomes part of a larger 'continuum of moments' via which care becomes concurrently created, engaged, ended, and remembered (Keady et al., 2022, p. 681). The experience of temporality is key: for people living with dementia and their carers, the relations between experiences of the past, present, and future are complex, and their lived experience of time itself is underwritten by structural constraints and power imbalances (Ward et al., 2022).

Campbell and colleagues (2024) locate care aesthetics as happening in the wider relations resulting from the assemblage of people, objects, and environments; care aesthetics may be prompted through 'the place of a body in a room and its relation to others' (p. 4). In many ways, this seems to align with the spatial strategies underlying the development of reminiscence rooms, staged as their objects are to prompt feelings of comfort and happiness in their residents, especially people living with dementia. And yet, when the topic of reminiscence rooms came up in interviews with architects as part of our research in the 'Buildings in the Making' project (Buse et al., 2018), they articulated similar feelings of disquiet about the use of these as those increasingly articulated in Gospodinov's novel. It seems to us that reminiscence rooms might offer a cautionary tale about what can happen when reminiscence activities become overwhelmed by the logics of nostalgia – a common conflation of two superficially similar but fundamentally different approaches (Dempsey et al., 2014). Reminiscence rooms, used carelessly and without due regard for the interpersonal encounters that support dementia care, illustrate how overly specifying the care environment can overwhelm the relational qualities of care aesthetics; thus, *care itself becomes aestheticised* and can become overly prescribed as a result (Nettleton et al., 2018a). In the following section, we will discuss some of the concerns about reminiscence rooms raised by architects in our study; first, though, we will offer a short reflection on the importance of architectural design in care for later life and offer further methodological detail about the research study from which the current paper is taken.

## Architecture and later life

When thinking about the role of the built environment in later life residential settings, Catharina Nord (2011) has described architecture as 'a moulding factor' in the delivery of care, with care workers using spatial strategies to strengthen a sense of agency for residents. Ken Worpole (2020) has argued that architecture and interior design 'can exert a form of soft power' in creating a sense of home, especially in institutional care settings 'where the death of life-partners and long-standing friends, along with increasing physical impairment, requires the designed environment to do more work in providing security and emotional stability' (p. 139). It is certainly the case that architectural expertise in the design of residences for later life is increasingly recognised as important to the provision of good quality care, whether in actual legislation or in the institutional norms that follow from regulations in the care sector (Nord, 2013a) or in the use of cultural traditions that are drawn upon to improve the environment for people living with dementia (Bowes et al., 2024). Within the UK, for example, principles issued by the University of Stirling's Dementia Services Design Centre are widely followed by architects and designers working in residential settings, especially with respect to how spatial layouts, lighting, and colour designs can be made sensitive to the needs of people living with dementia (Designing for Healthy Cognitive Ageing Project, 2023). Indeed, in our own research, we have argued that the work of architectural professionals is vitally important to understanding the '*feel* of ageing' in contemporary societies, given the importance of the buildings they design to the experience of age, well-being, and the overall 'atmospherics of care' for their residents, especially in later life (Buse et al., 2017, p. 1452).

One of the most notable architectural interventions within the context of later life care, and dementia design in particular, is De Hogeweyk in the Netherlands, which is a 'dementia village' located approximately 20 miles south of Amsterdam (Vinick, 2019). A collection of 23 houses, each home to six or seven residents, comprise this pedestrian friendly development, with different architectural and design features utilised to create different sites within the village to cater for residents with different lifestyles and social backgrounds; so, certain areas of the site have a more urban feel than others, and other areas have been designed with tropical plants and Buddha statues to appeal to residents with Indonesian heritage (Godwin, 2015). It contains restaurants, grocery stores, and even a non-functioning bus stop to encourage small talk, but no visible markers of institutional care. Staff do not dress in uniforms here – although they may dress as cashiers (Adams and Chivers, 2021) – and they actively encourage residents on shopping missions and other routine social encounters (Godwin, 2015). The performance of everyday activities is handled delicately for residents living with dementia, as Godwin (2015) explains:

> Where a resident absent-mindedly starts eating an apple in the supermarket, no one will accuse him or her of shoplifting. If someone selects 20 loaves of bread, the staff member will surreptitiously return 19 to the shop. No one will point out their mistake, although no one will lie to them either.
>
> *(pp. 28–29)*

For critical commentators, De Hogeweyk fabricates an architecture based on principles of reminiscence therapy, where a village-like environment is staged in an 'urge to camouflage serious illness' (Adams and Chivers, 2021). An example of the deep ambivalence De Hogeweyk prompts can be found in Phoebe Friesen's comment that there is 'just something so strange about responding to a disorder in which reality is slipping away with more unreality' (in Adams and Chivers, 2021). Adams and Chivers (2021) argue that the kind of architecture for dementia realised in De Hogeweyk marks the point 'where fictional experiences cross a line into another state, where there is no longer an awareness of enacting a fiction' (p. 6). In its powerful capacity 'to create a nostalgia for somewhere residents may have never been, but have always wanted to call home', Adams and Chivers (2021) raise concerns about the operationalisation of architecture as a form of validation therapy – just as Gospodinov does in 'Time Shelter'.

As Worpole (2020) states, De Hogeweyk combines the 'familiar domestic ornaments and small elements of architectural detailing' (p. 139) that identify as the soft power of architecture for later life. Previous research has shown the significance of personal objects in creating a sense of home for residents living with dementia in institutional settings (see, for example, Chaudhury et al., 2018, and Ferdous, 2020 for reviews of these studies). These objects may be cherished objects, or objects that offer a representation of their past lives, or more ordinary objects that often are particularly useful in maintaining engagement in everyday activities (Nord, 2013b). Developing a sensitised understanding of how material culture can help people living with dementia to play an active part in everyday life is important, given the move from previous homes to a new setting is often accompanied by the loss of objects and the downsizing of domestic environments (Lovatt, 2018). However, as Lovatt (2018) notes, it is not the having of possessions *in themselves* that make for residents' feelings of belonging within care homes, but rather the affordances of objects that allow residents to create new relationships and new routines – those that allow them to exert some control over their personal space and to 'perform' a sense of being at home (p. 374). She also notes that it is important that the needs of residents are not primarily defined in terms of their ownership of cherished objects; it may be equally important that they are free to acquire and use new objects as part of an ongoing process of developing a sense of self. We will return to the potential of objects and spaces to enable a sense of agency and identity in later life elsewhere in this chapter, via our discussion of our interviews with architects. First, we introduce some details about the wider study, our research design, and methodological approach.

## Methods

The data presented in this chapter are drawn from the 'Buildings in the Making' project, a research study funded by the United Kingdom's (UK) Economic and Social Research Council (ESRC) between 2015 and 2018. This project sought to explore how care for adults in later life is conceived and operationalised in the design and construction of residential care homes and Extra Care housing in the UK – including specialist care homes for people living with dementia. Although, as noted previously, there is a recognition of the role of architectural expertise within care and construction sectors, research focusing on the work of architects specifically remains under-explored (Bowes et al., 2024). Therefore, our project sought to address this through two core strands of data collection: interviews with 26 architectural professionals in the first stages of the project, followed by a second stage of ethnographic research observing nine live projects for later life care in which we followed the work routines of architects. This second, ethnographic strand, allowed us to collect fieldnotes, carry out documentary analysis of planning documents and project meeting minutes, and record nine discussions with architects as they talked through project plans, as well as eight further interviews with clients, developers, and building contractors collaborating with them on these projects.

The scope of the early interviews with architects covered many aspects of their professional lives, with a focus on their previous and ongoing experience designing buildings for the care sector. The interviews also explored how architects imagined the end users of their buildings, and from where they derived their understanding of the needs of those users, including older people living with dementia (for an extended discussion of the cultural scripts they worked with and reproduced, see Buse et al., 2017). Findings from these interviews informed the approach to the ethnographic research where we purposively selected projects at different stages of development. These ranged from the early stages of designs being worked up for planning purposes, right through to projects at the delivery stage, which included observational study of construction site work. To ensure maximum variation within the study, when selecting the case studies for the ethnographic strand, we sought projects with different degrees of specialist support for residents (including dementia care); projects for clients from different sectors (i.e., private, public, and third sector bodies); and projects including architectural input that varied according to different contract types. In total, 172 hours of observation were completed in multiple locations associated with the different projects (e.g., architectural offices, construction site settings, and public planning consultation events). In addition to our interview and ethnographic data, which form the basis of this chapter's analysis, we also analysed the plans of an architectural competition to design care homes of the future (findings from this strand of the project can be found in Nettleton et al., 2018a, 2018b; Martin et al., 2020a, 2020b).

Data analysis involved close reading of architectural plans, interview transcripts, and ethnographic fieldnotes supported by the use of NVivo; the generation of emergent themes; and frequent discussion within the research team at all stages of analysis (further details on the analytical approach may be found in Annandale et al., 2024). It should be noted that none of the projects observed through to completion in our research study included reminiscence rooms, but several architects interviewed in both strands of our project did mention their experience of these, and their reflections will be drawn on below. All of the following quotations and fieldnotes are anonymised, in line with the approval granted by the University of York's ELMPS ethics committee for research in the social sciences (for further information see https://www.york.ac.uk/politics/ethics/; accessed 1 March 2026).

## Findings

In this section, we will open with some general reflections by architects about the role of reminiscence rooms in residential settings for later life, before proceeding to discuss some of their concerns about their use in greater detail. Probing their concerns in more depth reveals an underlying ambivalence about how design for later life is caught up in wider sectoral norms that move their buildings away from ideals about homemaking and more towards a hospitality sector model of care homes – of which reminiscence rooms are a symptom.

### *The role of reminiscence*

The following fieldnote comes from one of the case study sites that we followed from its construction stage through to completion. It was a refurbishment of a local authority built Extra Care development scheme and at a tour around the time of the building's opening:

> We go out through the patio doors on to the balcony – there is a sign by the patio doors which reads (in reference to the mural):
>
> Encouraging Reminiscence
>
> Conversation scenes are located on each floor to aid discussion, for example the beach or the harbour.
>
> This prompts memories and the telling of life stories, to the benefit of the individual and staff.
>
> *(Fieldnote, case study 9)*

Although this care home did not include an actual room decorated with artefacts from a previous historical period, the idea of reminiscence is clearly cited here, as well as its therapeutic potential when attached to everyday objects. Reminiscence as a therapeutic strategy has been found to support people living with dementia to retain a sense of identity when used effectively in care encounters and settings (Dempsey et al., 2014).

Sometimes the conversation objects we observed in our fieldwork might be somewhat general in character, with no particular connection to the previous life residents, such as a generic image of a coastal scene which could, nonetheless, be used as a prompt to revisiting holidays from the past:

> Kay says that they went for a blue and silver scheme, lots of pictures on the wall, and the mural of a beach which can be a 'point of having conversations' e.g., 'Did you used to go to the beach?' or 'What did you used to do?'
>
> *(Fieldnote, case study 9)*

At other times, the use of objects to prompt discussion and memories of previous hobbies, likes, and interests could be highly specific, as in an Extra Care housing scheme where staff mounted photographs and objects linked to residents' histories on the walls outside their bedrooms. One example we observed was where staff pinned up football shirts next to the bedroom door of a resident who had been a keen footballer. This scheme included 'memory boxes' outside residents' rooms, which demonstrates a sensitivity to cherished or personalised objects and encourages conversations between residents and staff that are mindful of the need to consider the whole person in practices of care (Kitwood, 1993). Used with sensitivity, we see personal objects being utilised in residential settings to facilitate interpersonal encounters with the grace, craft, and skill that are markers of care aesthetics in practice (Thompson, 2015, 2023).

Some of the architects we interviewed viewed reminiscence rooms as important aspects of their designs, although they were rarely specified in their clients' brief or in building regulations, and therefore vulnerable to being squeezed out of final designs:

> From my point of view as an architect, I worked previously in school design, and you get all these building bulletins which are very prescriptive, but that then helps you provide the best possible facilities. Whereas I find the stuff we get out of them [regulations around design for later life] is very minimal. There is no, we don't have to provide half of these spaces, I don't have to give them a café or a reminiscence room or treatment space or anything, but these things are good to provide, and we want to provide the best building we can, and it would help if the inspectors would, and the commissioning people would, actually say this is necessary. But they don't.
>
> *(Interview 4 FCH14)*

This architect articulates a sense of frustration about the lack of influence they can exert on the finished design in the care sector, and what was perceived as indifference on the part of clients or inspectors to prioritise aspects of design with therapeutic potential. This sense of frustration was a wider theme with architects often unhappy about their limited capacity to consult people living with dementia about their building plans (Interview 1). Indeed, one architect we spoke to joined the board of a local care home to increase awareness and understanding of the needs of residents and staff (Interview 11), in light of her frustration about not being able to involve the primary users of buildings in their planning.

### *Reminiscence rooms, ambivalence, and deception*

The following fieldnote is from another local authority sponsored project in a different part of the country to case study 9. We followed this scheme at an early stage of development, around the time of its planning, which involved the architects working in collaboration with a wide team of other professionals – construction professionals, landscape architects, and an artist. During a walk around the site:

> The landscape architect and artist talk about having familiar objects or technologies in the garden e.g., an old phone box, lots of schemes have this. The arts

> consultant says that some of these types of schemes don't work though – e.g., in one care home they put an old car in the garden, but no-one goes out there because they are scared of being run over. Alan [the landscape architect] says that reminiscence theory is a 'bit dubious'. However, a good example of it is the pub in one of the care homes. There is a lady there who 'thought she was in a pub' – she used to sing in the pub and started singing again when she was there. Nick [the architect] adds that she 'came back to life'.
>
> *(Fieldnote, case study 3)*

In this exchange, we can see the ambivalence we typically heard from architects about reminiscence rooms and the use of familiar objects to mute the institutional aspects of care home environments. Alan expresses scepticism about the use of reminiscence theory in general (it is a 'bit dubious'), but the conversation with Nick does recollect one successful response to a care in a previous project where the location of a pub encouraged a convivial response from some residents. The conversation continues:

> The landscape architect mentions a Dutch village for people living with dementia, they have a bar, square, post office, support workers dress up as postmen etc…each resident has a flat that reflects their life.
> Nick says that is 'really sweet'.
> The artist says she has seen it, it is like 'The Truman Show'.
>
> *(Fieldnote, case study 3)*

Further conversation confirmed that this is, indeed, a reference back to De Hogeweyk, the dementia village mentioned earlier in this chapter. Again, we see the ambivalence about the strategies of validation therapy, and the architectural environment built around it, operationalised at De Hogeweyk. Nick considers the thinking behind it 'really sweet', whereas the artist, who has visited it, compares it to 'The Truman Show' film. The comparison with 'The Truman Show' is often made by visitors to the village, and it is rarely used as a compliment. 'The Truman Show' is a 1998 film about an insurance salesman who discovers that, unbeknownst to him, all aspects of his life are being filmed for a reality television show and that all his acquaintances, work colleagues, and even family members are actors. Adams and Chivers (2021) discuss De Hogeweyk with respect to 'The Truman Show' at length in their commentary on the dementia village, as a way of understanding how the architecture of the development is complicit in a wider fictional world and, to extend this point more critically, a strategic use of deception for people living with dementia there. Adams and Chivers (2021) write that whilst 'all architecture provokes some sort of fictional experience' (p. 6), De Hogeweyk crosses an important threshold because of the reduced agency it affords to people living with dementia. 'In a true fictional experience', Adams and Chivers (2021) argue, 'we know that we exist in two worlds at once: the real world in which we exist, and the fictional one we enact'; for people living with dementia in De Hogeweyk, 'the residents of the dementia village know only one world' (p. 6).

The idea of deception in residential settings for dementia care that utilise domestic and familiar objects to erase institutional markers of care, and to stage a comforting environment for residents, is highlighted in Kamphof and Hendriks's (2020) ethnography of care homes in Belgium and the Netherlands. Kamphof and Hendriks (2020) observed the use of familiar objects in their research at various care homes, such as the superimposed photographs of the front doors of residents' previous homes onto room doors in institutional homes – the 'True Doors' initiative. For these authors, such initiatives can sometimes lead to practices of deception and a kind of othering 'when they make or let people living in the care facility think, believe or expect something that puts them apart from "our" shared beliefs and expectations outside the ward' (Kamphof and Hendriks, 2020, p. 278). As these authors go on to argue, 'If making things homelike turns these people into "others"', they continue, 'core values of person-centred dementia care are threatened' (Kamphof and Hendriks, 2020, p. 278). Such a concern about reminiscence rooms perhaps lies behind Alan's concerns about the 'dubious' nature of the thinking behind them.

### *Reminiscence rooms and questions of home*

One architectural professional in our early interviews was strongly of the opinion that the use of reminiscence rooms 'goes against the grain of wanting it to be a home for people' (Interview 1). He continued to argue that these rooms involve the staging of the environment in ways that are antithetical to practices of homemaking:

> It's going to have to be neat and clean and tidy and organised and manicured, things put on the wall for effect, stuff arranged for effect, but it's not actually used. You often go into a dementia care corridor, neighbourhood, whatever they're calling it, and there'll be a reminiscence room or there'll be a coatrack with hats and scarves and all this stuff, and it's a stage set, they're props, but they don't actually use them.
>
> *(Interview 1)*

This quote reveals the role of architectural design in attempts to choreograph what we have elsewhere called an 'atmospherics of care', whether in respect to residential settings for later life (Martin et al., 2020a) or healthcare architecture more generally (Martin 2016; Martin et al., 2019). However, this interviewee had experience of seeing reminiscence rooms that he felt were underused and, indeed, unsuccessful in terms of engaging residents' interest and encouraging them in homemaking activities.

Scepticism about reminiscence therapy was repeated in our early interviews by another architect with experience of them in previous projects, where their use was linked to innovative ideas about medical treatment at the time:

> I mean 20 years ago there wasn't the internet, there wasn't, you couldn't just dial up and say design for dementia, and it would come up with something. It came from talking to people, and again, like I said, we had a few clinicians who had some ideas. I'm not sure all of them were correct, you know. There was a whole thing about reminiscence, reminiscence therapy, I'm not sure. We don't really do reminiscence rooms anymore, because where do you fix it? What era are you fixing it to? But that was a whole area that we got quite…was quite involved.
>
> *(Interview 19)*

This interviewee powerfully pinpoints the sociological complexity that belies the apparent clarity of therapeutic approaches that enrol the built environment into their treatment regimes: as this respondent muses, 'where do you fix it [the past]? What era are you fixing it to?' This is a dilemma considered in Gospodinov's (2020) 'Time Shelter' where that novel's psychiatrist, Dr Gaustine, comes up with the solution of hosting different decades in different floors of his 'past-clinic' to recreate the childhood of many different social groups via its common objects (pp. 70–71). Indeed, he goes further to split floors into different sections, to recreate the cultural reference points of Western European countries at one end of the corridor and the artefacts of Eastern European and Soviet Bloc societies at the other end. Such narrative detail is wittily observed in the novel, but it prompts serious consideration about whose pasts are being staged in reminiscence rooms, whose cultural tastes are being promoted, and what types of social norms are embedded in the pasts chosen for recreation? Moreover, is it even the case that the past holds comforting memories for all residents, as these rooms tend to suppose?

Such questions are related to architects' concerns about some of the default design cues which were embedded throughout the care home sector, because of uncertainty about who the end users of these buildings actually are:

> I think there's a tendency to design for something which is soft and inoffensive. So, actually, quite a lot of the care home environments tend to be, for one, quite feminine – not that that's necessarily a bad thing, but they just generally are, and they tend to strive to be inoffensive rather than actually…really to generate a character. So it's almost appealing to, not a lowest common denominator, because some of them are really, they're beautifully done, but with most of them you wouldn't say they're particular characterful, they're quite generic… You want people to feel comfortable in that setting, and comfort isn't just about creating something which is inoffensive and maybe physically comfortable, but somehow validates their life experience.
>
> *(Interview 16)*

This architect describes how uncertainty results in a somewhat 'inoffensive' approach to design that, in effect, is so 'generic' that it becomes blind to the 'life experience' of those using the eventual buildings. Concern about this same default-mode approach to care homes – and the cultural stereotypes that it reproduces – arose in design discussions when a local authority care home development was at an early stage of its planning:

> Carlos (art consultant) had his own ideas about what the care home should look like, saying 'I've never seen a care home that is not chintzy' and he felt they needed something 'modern' and 'slick'.
>
> At this point Adam (ENT Constructions) pointed out 'but that doesn't work with people living with dementia'.
>
> Shelley (project manager, developer) counteracted this saying, 'You can't assume they want 'chintz', why should they have 'chintz' and thick curtains?'
>
> *(Fieldnote, case study 3).*

Shelley's interjection in this discussion neatly punctures a dominant cultural script that associates people in care homes with the recent past and, in effect, fixes their identities there (Lovatt, 2021). Thinking about reminiscence rooms, the first architect we spoke to reflected upon the infiltration of other architectural trends in the design of later life care:

> You can see the cobwebs, the stuff is never used, and yet it's there so that when the walk family member around, 'Oh we have a reminiscence room and people can sit here and they can reminisce and they look at all these curios and play with the dolls and pram', all this, but that actually doesn't translate over into care practice, that's all about marketing, and if you've got a home that's looking at this model, of the hospitality model, and the hotel model, then they will have stuff, the décor and the interior designer is really big on to this sort of thing too, he'll have photographs of movie stars around the walls, things like that.
>
> *(Interview 1)*

This equation of reminiscence rooms, staged for the primary benefit of family members considering their relatives' move into care homes, resonates with a wider concern about the squeezing of architectural effort into saleable public areas, often at the expense of the bedroom areas that are, in effect, the places where many residents will spend the majority of their time (Nettleton et al., 2018a). It also echoes concern about more general and visual indicators of care, such as the dress of residents of dementia care settings, advancing a somewhat 'tick box' approach to care that overrides the principles of person-centred care (Buse and Twigg, 2018, p. 350) and, indeed, institutes a somewhat 'production line' approach to managing the appearance of care homes (Lee-Treweek, 1997). As Campbell and colleagues (2024) note in their arguments about care aesthetics within dementia settings, visual indicators cannot 'equate simplistically to the quality of care' (p. 19) within that place; moreover, they may even point to worrying power dynamics where the biographical identities of residents are elided and homogenised in the quest to make them presentable for family members and care home inspectors.

Indeed, the development of a 'hospitality model' throughout the sector (itself indicative of healthcare architecture more generally [Bromley, 2012; Martin et al., 2015]) was a significant concern for architects across our interviews, not least because of its ability to counteract other models that prioritise a phenomenological approach and the lived experience of residents feeling-at-home in their new spaces (Nettleton et al., 2018b). The first architect we spoke to compared the hospitality model with a more 'homely' approach to building and design (A=architect; I=interviewer):

> A: I've seen this when I've gone into homes in Norway and other places, the lady will be sitting out in the living room and she'll have her curlers in, feet up on the table, reading the newspaper, and it will look just like they're at home, and that's the difference between the living at home kind of a model, that care model, and the hotel thing.
> I: Do you think the home model is better, is that a better sort of thing to aim for?
> A: Yeah, definitely. Things need to be a bit messy, things need to be personalised, people need to be able to pick up stuff and move around, and if things are there they can be used, they can always be put back at the end of the shift. But the hospitality, hotel model, would have rooms that actually don't get used, they're for view, they're for effect.
>
> *(Interview 1)*

Here, again, there is an echo of concerns raised by researchers who have critiqued the narrow focus of providers on visual indicators of care 'as an endpoint to and as an objective for the provision of care' (Ward et al., 2016, p. 399). The architect we spoke to clearly distinguishes between the aspirational and (too) neat display of objects within a 'hotel model' of buildings for later life and the more 'messy', lived-in atmospheres of care homes where residents are 'able to pick up stuff and move around'. Key to this difference is the sensitivity of staff to the needs of residents to use objects in routine, performative, and playful ways (Lovatt, 2018), rather than this work being delegated to the objects in themselves, which has been a criticism of how objects for reminiscence can sometimes be rather over-determined and fixed in their use (Kamphof and Hendriks, 2020).

## Discussion

Running through our analysis of architects' interviews and ethnographic data are clashing imperatives between the regulation of care homes to ensure safe environments, especially for people living with dementia, and the need for these buildings to remain open enough in design to allow residents to make their own mark on their personal spaces. Such tensions are complicated by additional prescribed norms aiming to replicate hospitality industry models and, underpinning all these, the financial pressures to make care homes financially viable (Nettleton et al., 2018a).

Existing research has shown that allowing residents to bring household possessions from previous houses into new assisted living settings can help them adapt to their new homes and encourage an active engagement with their new communities (Nord, 2013b). The use of reminiscence rooms can be seen to be related to this growing understanding of, and respect for, the role of material culture in brokering a sense of belonging and well-being in residential settings for later life, not least for people living with dementia. However, as Lovatt (2018) has shown in her research in care homes for later life, for those living there 'possessions were not in themselves sufficient to instil a sense of being at home; that came from the work that residents did in incorporating the objects into a new sense of home through routines and new purchases' (p. 374).

Lovatt (2018) highlights the processual nature of homemaking, as mediated through the use of material culture, in an analysis that resonates with the research of Kamphof and Hendriks (2020), whose findings distinguish between practices of *home-scaping* and *home-playing* in overall homemaking strategies within care homes. Both these strategies involve the utilisation of objects and environments designed to help people living with memory loss connect with their new homes: *home-scaping* strategies, such as their superimposed photographs of residents' previous front doors onto room doors within care homes, offer examples of 'places or scenes of home [brought] within the facility that promise escape from it'; whereas *home-playing* strategies 'arise out of the imaginative engagement with objects' by residents, using props that engage 'people living with dementia and caregivers in joint discovery while keeping the process focused on the here and now' (Kamphof and Hendriks, 2020, p. 287). There is a subtle balance between practices of *home-scaping* and *home-playing*, with both drawing on artful approaches to the built environment; however, Kamphof and Hendriks (2020) sound a cautionary note about strategies that are premised on a principle of escape from the present, as they can serve the purpose of abstracting residents from the realities of life on the wards surrounding them. Regardless of best intentions, managers of some care homes in their research worried that 'care facilities may end up building mere façades or may slide into "a fake circus"' (Kamphof and Hendriks, 2020, p. 287) in which artifice within the care home environment slips into the possibility of deception, which is against principles of person-centred dementia care (Kitwood, 1993). As Worpole (2020) writes, there is a growing tendency in the design of settings for people living with dementia 'where the outside world is designed out of existence, with exit doors disguised and a make-believe interior constructed', all of which raise 'serious questions about personal freedom' (pp. 141–142). There are obvious implications for how we might think about reminiscence rooms, a spatial model designed in many respects around residents of care homes escaping their present circumstances and conditions, if only temporarily.

Kamphof and Hendriks (2020) note a concern about homemaking strategies utilising objects within care settings which might, unintentionally, raise questions of deception in the built environment; even if this is not the case for reminiscence rooms, there may be other reasons for the unease expressed by the architects in our study. At root, reminiscence rooms are based on more than just an escape from the present; they also imply a sense of feeling-at-home achieved through an active retreating into the past. And, yet, as Kamphof and Hedriks (2020) argue, it cannot be postulated that 'what constitutes "home" for people living with dementia now is the same as what it used to be when they were living in their private homes, or even what it meant yesterday' (p. 288). Arguably, we should be concerned by spatial strategies and care practices that lock people living with dementia within a nostalgic staging of the past. Again, Lovatt (2018) astutely points to the dangers of this approach, as it may reinforce the idea that 'older people are primarily past-orientated, and have no meaningful future' (p. 375). 'It is as though after a certain age', as Lovatt (2021) writes elsewhere, that 'the future is regarded as irrelevant' for residents of care homes, especially for people living with dementia (p. 2956). Such effects may not be the intention of reminiscence rooms, but these may result from the prevalent tendency to view dementia as a pathology which shifts the focus of care away from the individual and their experience (Kontos and Martin, 2013). This is a much wider discourse than those found amongst design professionals of course, but it is one that slipped in throughout our analysis of buildings plans (Nettleton et al., 2018b) and interviews (Buse et al., 2017); the challenge for architects and other professionals involved in the design of dementia-friendly environments is to 'shift the emphasis from *condition* to *experience*' in their work, in order to 'allow the person with dementia to be an active participant in everyday life rather than a passive recipient of care' (Davis et al., 2009, p. 185).

Architects as a profession are uniquely placed in their anticipation of the future for those who use their buildings. Indeed, we can go further and state that architecture as a discipline is intimately involved in the *making of time* as much as the construction of space per se (Beynon-Jones et al., 2021). As such, it is a professional discipline ideally suited to support approaches to care understood within an 'in the moment' framework in order to capture the qualities of encounter in dementia care – as in the practices of care aesthetics that occur in 'use of the lifts, holds, touches and embodied presence that are important for the quality of care that is delivered, but are too often edited out of more technical accounts' (Campbell et al., 2024, p. 2). At first glance, the development of reminiscence rooms for people living with dementia seems like a creative spatial approach, using objects from the recent past to offer comfort for people with memory loss in the present; as Dr Gaustine, the therapist in 'Time Shelter', puts it when describing his use of reminiscence rooms in disarmingly clear terms, the 'only thing we can do is create a space that is in sync with their internal time' (Gospodinov, 2022, p. 44). But, as we have shown, architects were more often sceptical than enthusiastic about using reminiscence rooms in their designs, despite their potential as a kind of validation therapy, as in the famous staged social environment of the De Hogeweyk dementia village (Adams and Chivers, 2021).

To understand the ambivalence about reminiscence rooms from the architects we spoke to, we find Kamphof and Hendriks' (2020) analysis of the use of artifice, imagination, and play in care homes useful. Whilst they found a great deal of value in *home-playing* activities involving the use of familiar objects, such as doll play, cookery classes, and craft sessions, they cautioned against *home-scaping* initiatives that involved a de-territorialisation of the care home – because these seemed to promise an escape from the present to the point of deception. For Kamphof and Hendriks (2020), 'objects and material environments become deceitful when they *exclude* people with dementia from shared, agreed reality' (p. 278). Kamphof and Hendriks (2020) sound a note of concern with initiatives in their case studies that used a 'museum-like approach' (p. 277) in the recreation of old-fashioned shop interiors with products (soaps, coffee, biscuits, etc.) in vintage tins that residents can pay for with duplicate money and which are returned by staff discreetly at night; when not handled sensitively and with the awareness of residents, such simulations may have an air of deceit, but also the effect of fixing their identities. Surrounding people living with dementia with the paraphernalia of the recent past may have an unintended consequence of locking them in an understanding of the past (Lovatt, 2018), albeit a generic version of the past which may not necessarily align with their own biographical experiences (Gospodinov, 2022).

At root, reminiscence rooms may offer interesting experiments in the *creation* of caring environments, but their objects should not be left only to their own devices, without due attention to the caring work needed to animate these spaces. Reminiscence rooms, in their recreation of the recent past through symbolic markers and the material culture of a particular point in time, may be important to establishing the context of care and may even act to trigger certain memories amongst their users. However, as Thompson (2023) argues, care 'is not a context, a theme or a set of protocols governing practice'; rather, it is a happening involving the 'creation of sensory, embodied experiences' (p. 1). Designing environments for the first moments of care is important, certainly; however, this work of planning needs to be accompanied by equal attention to how these moments of care will become engaged in the living relations between residents and carers, how these moments of care may be distracted and ended, and how these moments of care might be reanimated and relived (Keady et al., 2022).

## Conclusion

Rooms such as those described in Kamphof and Hendriks' (2020) research, and fictionalised in Gospodinov's (2022) novel, are creative orchestrations of the recent past using artefacts from a previous time. They are intended to create a therapeutic atmospheric of care in residential settings for later life, especially for people living with dementia. As such, they are involved in the effective making of a particular sense of time, as architecture is uniquely placed to do (Beynon-Jones et al., 2021). Richard Ward and colleagues (2016) have argued that we need to 'to shift the focus of care practice from a fixed, endpoint image and universally applied standard of presentation' to a more processual, culturally sensitive, and person-centred approach that can, indeed, help to 'nurture place-making in dementia care' (p. 409); again, architectural design should be key to advancing such an agenda. However, as we have seen, the sense of the past evoked in reminiscence rooms often draws from a strain of nostalgia as much as reminiscence (Dempsey et al., 2014), and their underlying understandings of time are oddly depoliticised, failing to do justice to the temporal politics of dementia, and the structural challenges faced in the lived experience of care (and practices of caring) within that context (Ward et al., 2022). There is a danger, in their attempts to help maintain past identities of residents, that they detract from ongoing processes of identity formation in the present and impede practices of homemaking for the future (Lovatt, 2021). Reminiscence rooms, it could be said, are a type of *home-scaping* initiative, to use Kamphof and Hendriks' (2020) term. Without careful handling that involves awareness of the truth of the play-worlds they construct, there is a danger that they are stage-sets that look good, but do not necessarily lead to good care. That is, they offer a 'visual indicator of care' that can be more important in terms of the impression they present to the outside world of family visitors and inspectors than what they tell about their use (Buse and Twigg, 2018, p. 350). In this way, they offer a cautionary tale that care itself can become over-determined and *aestheticised* when not sufficiently attentive to the intimate, unpredictable, and ongoing encounters central to the practice of care aesthetics (Campbell et al., 2024).

## Acknowledgements

The research reported on this chapter was supported through funding from the ESRC as part of the 'Buildings in the Making: A Sociological Exploration of Architecture in the Context of Health and Social Care' project (reference ES/M008398/1). We would like to thank the editors for their interest in our research and for their generous, supportive, and constructive suggestions for revising an earlier draft of this chapter.

## Three Key Reading References

### *Reference 1*

Buse, C., Nettleton, S., Martin, D. and Twigg, J. (2017). Imagined bodies: Architects and their constructions of later life. *Ageing & Society*, 37 (7): 1435–1457. https://doi.org/10.1017/S0144686X16000362

This journal article offers an overview of the different cultural scripts associated with ageing bodies that architects work with when designing residential settings for later life, and how they attempt to challenge cultural stereotypes about age in their work but, nonetheless, often reproduce these same stereotypes in their designs. Although not exclusively focused on dementia care, the architects interviewed reflect often on the particular needs of people living with dementia, and how these are addressed in their buildings. The paper illustrates the complexity of architectural practice, especially in the field of later life settings, as design professionals juggle the needs of residents, clients, and staff, whilst being constrained by financial pressures, material properties, and design regulations in the care sector.

### Reference 2

Gospodinov, G. (2022). *Time Shelter*, London: Weidenfeld and Nicolson.
This novel is set in a series of 'clinics of the past' designed for those living with Alzheimer's disease, in which material objects from the recent past are used strategically in rooms throughout the buildings to engage the interest of residents, provide comfort in their environments, and encourage social interaction with staff and their fellow residents. The novel's narrative arc extends far beyond this initial premise: it is, at heart, an astute satire about the political uses of nationalism and nostalgia amongst wider populations. That noted, this work does offer a left-field way of thinking about the role of architecture and design in the provision of care settings that are responsive to the needs of people living with dementia.

### Reference 3

Kamphof, I. and Hendriks, R. (2020). Beyond façade: Home making and truthfulness in dementia care. In B. Pasveer, O. Synnes and I. Moser (eds.) *Ways of Home Making in Care for Later Life*. Singapore: Palgrave, pp. 271–292.
This book chapter offers an investigation of the use of architectural elements and material objects from the recent past within contemporary care homes. The chapter draws on ethnographic fieldwork undertaken in 13 facilities for residential care in Belgium and the Netherlands, with an explicit focus on the use of objects within these facilities that incorporate aspects of make-believe and play. The authors explore questions of truthfulness whenever objects and elements of the environment are used in therapeutic approaches for people living with dementia, and deal with the important question of deception as part of their analysis. Their research prompts a consideration of where appropriate ethical lines should be drawn when material culture is used to evoke past identities for people living with dementia in residential settings today.

## References

Adams, A. and Chivers, S. (2021). Deception and design: The rise of the dementia village, 2009–2019. *e-flux Architecture*. Available: https://www.e-flux.com/architecture/treatment/410336/deception-and-design-the-rise-of-the-dementia-village; accessed: 1 March 2026.

Annandale, E., Nettleton, S., Martin, D., Buse, C. and Beynon-Jones, S. (2024). The constellations of design: Architects' practice modalities when working with embodied individuals and virtual collectives in later life facilities in the UK. *Journal of Professions and Organization*, 11 (3): 293–309. https://doi.org/10.1093/jpo/joae013

Beynon-Jones, S.M., Martin, D., Buse, C., Nettleton, S. and Annandale, E. (2021). Fixing the future? How architects make time in buildings for later life care. *The Sociological Review*, 69 (1): 139–155. https://doi.org/10.1177/0038026120952743

Bowes, A., Davison, L., Dawson, A., Pemble, C., Quirke, M. and Swift, S. (2024). Housing design evaluation research for people living with cognitive change: A systematic literature review. *Journal of Aging and Environment*, 38 (4): 347–366. https://doi.org/10.1080/26892618.2023.2223589

Bromley, E. (2012). Building patient-centeredness: Hospital design as an interpretive act. *Social Science & Medicine*, 75 (6): 1057–1066. https://doi.org/10.1016/j.socscimed.2012.04.037

Buse, C., Nettleton, S. and Martin, D. (2018). *Buildings in the Making: A Sociological Exploration of Architecture in the Context of Health and Social Care*, York: University of York. Available: https://gtr.ukri.org/projects?ref=ES%2FM008398%2F1; accessed 1 March 2026.

Buse, C., Nettleton, S., Martin, D. and Twigg, J. (2017). Imagined bodies: Architects and their constructions of later life. *Ageing & Society*, 37 (7): 1435–1457. https://doi.org/10.1017/S0144686X16000362

Buse, C. and Twigg, J. (2018). Dressing disrupted: Negotiating care through the materiality of dress in the context of dementia. *Sociology of Health & Illness*, 40 (2): 340–352. https://doi.org/10.1111/1467-9566.12575

Campbell, S., Dowlen, R., Keady, J. and Thompson, J. (2024). Care aesthetics and 'being in the moment' through improvised music-making and male grooming in dementia care. *International Journal of Education & the Arts*, 25 (si1.13). Available: https://journals.psu.edu/ijea/article/view/63522; accessed 1 March 2026.

Chaudhury, H., Cooke, H.A., Cowie, H. and Razaghi, L. (2018). The influence of the physical environment on residents with dementia in long-term care settings: A review of the empirical literature. *The Gerontologist*, 58 (5): e325–e337. https://doi.org/10.1093/geront/gnw259

Davis, S., Byers, S., Nay, R. and Koch, S. (2009). Guiding design of dementia friendly environments in residential care settings: Considering the living experiences. *Dementia: The International Journal of Social Research and Practice*, 8 (2): 185–203. https://doi.org/10.1177/1471301209103250

Dempsey, L., Murphy, K., Cooney, A., Casey, D., O'Shea, E., Devane, D., Jordan, F. and Hunter, A. (2014). Reminiscence in dementia: A concept analysis. *Dementia: The International Journal of Social Research and Practice,* 13 (2): 176–192. https://doi.org/10.1177/1471301212456277

Designing for Healthy Cognitive Ageing Project (2023). *Designing Homes for Healthy Cognitive Ageing – Hints and Tips*, Stirling: University of Stirling Dementia Services Development Centre. Available: https://www.deshca.co.uk/wp-content/uploads/2025/02/DesHCAs-Tips-and-Tricks-2024.pdf; accessed: 1 March 2026.

Ferdous, F. (2020). Positive social interaction by spatial design: A systematic review of empirical literature in memory care facilities for people experiencing dementia. *Journal of Aging and Health*, 32 (9): 949–961. https://doi.org/10.1177/0898264319870090

Godwin, B. (2015). Hogewey: A 'home from home' in the Netherlands. *Journal of Dementia Care*, 23 (3): 28–31.

Gospodinov, G. (2022). *Time Shelter*, London: Weidenfeld and Nicolson.

Kamphof, I. and Hendriks, R. (2020). Beyond façade: Home making and truthfulness in dementia care. In B. Pasveer, O. Synnes and I. Moser (eds.) *Ways of Home Making in Care for Later Life*. Singapore: Palgrave, pp. 271–292.

Keady, J.D., Campbell, S., Clark, A., Dowlen, R., Elvish, R., Jones, L., Kindell, J., Swarbrick, C. and Williams, S. (2022). Re-thinking and re-positioning 'being in the moment' within a continuum of moments: Introducing a new conceptual framework for dementia studies. *Ageing & Society*, 42 (3): 681–702. https://doi.org/10.1017/S0144686X20001014

Kitwood, T. (1993). Towards a theory of dementia care: The interpersonal process. *Ageing & Society*, 13 (1): 51–67. https://doi.org/10.1017/S0144686X00000647

Kontos, P. and Martin, W. (2013). Embodiment and dementia: Exploring critical narratives of selfhood, surveillance, and dementia care. *Dementia: The International Journal of Social Research and Practice,* 12 (3): 288–302. https://doi.org/10.1177/1471301213479787

Lee-Treweek, G. (1997). Women, resistance and care: An ethnographic study of nursing auxiliary work. *Work, Employment and Society*, 11 (1): 47–63. https://doi.org/10.1177/0950017097111003

Lovatt, M. (2018). Becoming at home in residential care for older people: A material culture perspective. *Sociology of Health & Illness*, 40 (2): 366–378. https://doi.org/10.1111/1467-9566.12568

Lovatt, M. (2021). Relationships and material culture in a residential home for older people. *Ageing & Society*, 41 (12): 2953–2970. https://doi.org/10.1017/S0144686X20000690

Martin, D. (2016). Curating space, choreographing care: The efficacy of the everyday. In C. Bates, R. Imrie and K. Kullman (eds.) *Care and Design: Bodies, Buildings, Cities. Oxford: Wiley-Blackwell, pp. 37–55.*

Martin, D., Nettleton, S. and Buse, C. (2019). Affecting care: Maggie's centres and the orchestration of architectural atmospheres. *Social Science & Medicine*, 240: 112563. https://doi.org/10.1016/j.socscimed.2019.112563

Martin, D., Nettleton, S. and Buse, C. (2020a). Drawing atmosphere: A case study of architectural design for care in later life. *Body & Society*, 26 (4): 62–96. https://doi.org/10.1177/1357034X20949934

Martin, D., Nettleton, S. and Buse, C. (2020b). Biographies, bricks and belonging: Architectural imaginaries of home making in later life. In B. Pasveer, O. Synnes and I. Moser (eds.) *Ways of Home Making in Care for Later Life*. Singapore: Palgrave, pp. 109–131.

Martin, D., Nettleton, S., Buse, C., Prior, L. and Twigg, J. (2015). Architecture and health care: A place for sociology. *Sociology of Health & Illness*, 37 (7): 1007–1022. https://doi.org/10.1111/1467-9566.12284

Nettleton, S., Buse, C. and Martin, D. (2018a). 'Essentially it's just a lot of bedrooms': Architectural design, prescribed personalisation and the construction of care homes for later life. *Sociology of Health & illness*, 40 (7): 1156–1171. https://doi.org/10.1111/1467-9566.12747

Nettleton, S., Buse, C. and Martin, D. (2018b). Envisioning bodies and architectures of care: Reflections on competition designs for older people. *Journal of Aging Studies*, 45: 54–62. https://doi.org/10.1016/j.jaging.2018.01.008

Nord, C. (2011). Architectural space as a moulding factor of care practices and resident privacy in assisted living. *Ageing & Society*, 31 (6): 934–952. https://doi.org/10.1017/S0144686X1000128

Nord, C. (2013a). Design according to the law: Juridical dimensions of architecture for assisted living in Sweden. *Journal of Housing and the Built Environment*, 28 (1): 147–155. https://doi.org/10.1007/s10901-012-9300-y

Nord, C. (2013b). A day to be lived. Elderly peoples' possessions for everyday life in assisted living. *Journal of Aging Studies*, 27 (2): 135–142. https://doi.org/10.1016/j.jaging.2012.12.002

Thompson, J. (2015). Towards an aesthetics of care. *Research in Drama Education: The journal of Applied Theatre and Performance*, 20 (4): 430–441. https://doi.org/10.1080/13569783.2015.1068109

Thompson, J. (2023). *Care Aesthetics: For Artful Care and Careful Art*, London: Routledge.

Vinick, D. (2019). Dementia-friendly design: Hogeweyk and beyond. *The British Journal of General Practice*, 69 (683): 300. Available: https://doi.org/10.3399/bjgp19X703949; accessed 1 March 2026.

Ward, R., Campbell, S. and Keady, J. (2016). 'Gonna make yer gorgeous': Everyday transformation, resistance and belonging in the care-based hair salon. *Dementia: The International Journal of Social Research and Practice*, 15 (3): 395–413. https://doi.org/10.1177/1471301216638969

Ward, R., Rummery, K., Odzakovic, E., Manji, K., Kullberg, A., Keady, J., Clark, A. and Campbell, S. (2022). Taking time: The temporal politics of dementia, care and support in the neighbourhood. *Sociology of Health & Illness*, 44 (9): 1427–1444. https://doi.org/10.1111/1467-9566.13524

Worpole, K. (2020). A home at the end of life: Changing definitions of 'Homeliness' in the hospice movement and end-of-life care in the UK. In B. Pasveer, O. Synnes and I. Moser (eds.) *Ways of Home Making in Care for Later Life*. Singapore: Palgrave, pp. 135–158.

# 11

# CARE-FULL NEIGHBOURHOODS

## Exploring the aesthetic dimension of neighbourhoods for people living with dementia

*Andrew Clark*

### Introduction

Just over 15 years ago, Richard Ward and I completed a pilot study on the neighbourhood experiences of carers who supported people living with dementia. That project (Ward et al., 2012) sparked a collaboration that continues to this day and further fuelled my ongoing interest in the meanings people attach to locations that lie just beyond their front doors. This pilot study informed a larger international, longitudinal study about the neighbourhood experiences of people living with dementia as part of a five-year programme of research led by John Keady, one of the editors of this book (see Keady, 2024). As part of that earlier pilot work, Richard and I asked care partners to take us on a walk around the neighbourhoods where they lived. Whilst that work focused on carers' experiences, those individuals living with a diagnosis who they cared for would sometimes accompany us. On an overcast, damp afternoon in early autumn, a couple led me to a somewhat unremarkable group of playing fields that backed onto their home on the outskirts of Manchester. I can no longer remember which of the couple said it, but as we trod our way through the empty football pitches, I was told that whilst this 'might look like a field to anyone else, to us it is quite beautiful'. This is a statement that has stayed with me and that has sparked this chapter. The explanation for such a declaration probably lies less in pithy statements about beauty being in the eye of the beholder and more in the ways in which we find meaning in even the most mundane and anodyne of places and landscapes. It is this noticing of the aesthetic qualities of ordinary places, the importance they play in the lives of people impacted by dementia, and the ways in which places might care for those who frequent them, that I consider here, and which has prompted me to ask whether there is a care aesthetic to the most mundane of neighbourhood experiences.

DOI: 10.4324/9781003623441-15
This chapter has been made available under a (CC BY) 4.0 license.

There is a nascent interest in understanding where environments might fit within the care-aesthetic discourse. This typically focuses on sites of conventional indoor care such as hospital wards or care homes (see, for example, Richardson and Campbell, 2024; Jones et al., 2025; although for an exception see Rita Newton and her colleagues' work in Chapter 9 of this book). Mention of aesthetics specifically in the context of dementia and neighbourhoods might pre-empt thoughts about the appearance of built environments; good and bad examples of dementia friendly architecture or design; or, perhaps, discussion about how the layouts of streets and public places might invite or exclude, enable, or disable people's engagement and interaction in the public realm. All these things are important, as much work on dementia-inclusive communities attests to, but this is not the only way to think about how 'neighbourhood aesthetics' might matter.

Taking inspiration from thinking on the aesthetics of care (Thompson, 2022, 2023) and everyday aesthetics (Saito, 2008), this chapter offers an exploratory account of how we might understand the relationality that connects people living with dementia to other people and places. I draw on re-analysed material collected during a five-year longitudinal study of the lived experience of neighbourhoods for people living with dementia (Ward et al., 2018) and reflect on what routine and habitual practices, interactions, and engagements with neighbourhoods can reveal about the meaning of neighbourhoods in the lives of people living with dementia; and how attending to the emplaced aesthetics of everyday life for people living with dementia might lead to more care-full neighbourhoods for everyone. My intention is not to reach a definitive positioning of neighbourhoods as part of the constellation of 'aesthetic' practices and environments, but to set out some preliminary thoughts about how an aesthetic lens might help us to rethink how and why neighbourhoods matter for those impacted by dementia.

## Neighbourhoods as relational practices

Recent reviews have highlighted the multifaceted nature of neighbourhoods, emphasising how they are perceived and experienced as both psychosocial and material constructs (Seetharaman et al., 2021; Sturge et al., 2021; Gan et al., 2022). Thoughtful environmental design can enhance support for people living with dementia and offer deeper insight into how they engage with their surroundings. Such studies reveal how neighbourhoods can either support or hinder daily life for those living with dementia (Sturge et al., 2021). Behavioural and psychosocial dimensions of dementia mean that individuals can encounter barriers that limit their access to neighbourhood spaces, potentially impacting their well-being and increasing feelings of vulnerability (Bartlett and Brannelly, 2019; Biglieri and Dean, 2021, 2022). Such work is vital for understanding and supporting all individuals and those impacted by dementia, but my focus here is to move beyond approaching neighbourhoods as sites that require modification, and reflect on how neighbourhoods might be understood as, and in turn be reproduced through, aesthetic attentiveness to neighbourhood-situated practices.

By neighbourhood practices, I mean the processes, interactions, and engagements that make up the constellation of people, place, and personal biography that we might then label one's neighbourhood (Ward et al., 2021; Ward et al., 2022). For neighbourhoods are relational, fluid entities, more than mere spaces through which people move to perform specific tasks. They also serve as settings for everyday social practices that help build and sustain a broader socio-dementia infrastructure and citizenship (Clark et al., 2020; Clark et al., 2024). But where, if at all, might aesthetics fit into this?

Recent developments in dementia studies have highlighted an emphasis on the aesthetics of care, which foregrounds the importance of recognising and valuing the unique identities and preferences of individuals living with dementia. This perspective prioritises relational, everyday, embodied, and present-moment experiences (Dowlen et al., 2024). Invoking the idea of aesthetics emphasises the deliberate, practised, and crafted nature of caregiving interactions and the ensuing sensory experiences. Elements such as bodily engagement, tactile interaction, vocal tone, spatial awareness, and the temporal construction of caregiving practices collectively contribute to the formation of care-aesthetic experiences. Here, care is seen as a sensory, embodied, and skilfully crafted practice, applicable across both formal and informal care contexts, rather than reducing it to merely technical or task-oriented functions (Hanlon and Carlisle, 2015; Dowlen et al., 2024). In social care, this approach draws critical attention to the nuances of interpersonal interactions, including micro-movements, touch, eye contact, tone of voice, and body posture. By paying careful attention to these sensory dimensions, in the actions of both caregivers and the responses of care recipients, it is possible to illuminate often-overlooked qualities of the care experience (Dowlen et al., 2024). Thompson (2023) takes this further to argue for an understanding of how a 'care moment' comprises interconnected, embodied practices that produce a shared sensory experience. Crucial for my thinking here, this includes the actions of everyone involved, shaped by their relationship to the surrounding environment; the spatial organisation, material interactions, and physical activity that make up settings like health and social care environments such as hospital wards and care homes, as well as locations considered beyond or outside of conventional 'care environments' such as the streets, parks, retail, and leisure places that make up the physical and social infrastructure of neighbourhood life.

## Wider study context

In what follows then, I present some indicative, rather than representative, examples to illustrate how attending to a care aesthetic might illuminate neighbourhood experiences and practices. Some material has been presented elsewhere and is reinterpreted here, and some is presented for the first time. It is drawn from a five-year study investigating the neighbourhood experiences of people living with dementia (for an overview of each of the eight work programmes that constituted the ESRC/NIHR 'Neighbourhoods and dementia study', see Keady, 2024). On Work Programme 4 of the 'Neighbourhoods and dementia study', we aimed to achieve two primary objectives: (i) to generate rich, situated understandings of neighbourhoods as experienced and lived by individuals with dementia; and (ii) to empower participants to express and represent their relationships to place in ways that were personally meaningful and contextually situated.

The study employed a participatory, longitudinal framework to investigate the intricate nature of everyday interactions and encounters that inform lived experiences within local environments. Our conceptualisation of a neighbourhood extended beyond its material and spatial characteristics to incorporate social and biographical dimensions of neighbourhood engagement. We developed a qualitative, longitudinal, and comparative research design, utilising three primary approaches that had been used in previous work (Clark, 2017):

1 Walking interviews encouraged participants living with dementia, occasionally accompanied by family carers, to guide us on 'neighbourhood walks' mostly commencing from the front door of their residence. This method facilitated an embodied and narrative exploration of place, allowing participants to articulate and demonstrate their spatial practices and affective connections to their neighbourhoods.
2 Filmed home tours were undertaken based on the premise that engagement with the neighbourhood begins with the act of exiting the home. These tours provided insights into the domestic threshold as a liminal space bridging private and public realms.
3 A participatory social network mapping technique was employed collaboratively with participants and, where possible, their carer partners. This aimed to examine the structure and significance of everyday social relationships that potentially function as sources of support, interaction, and community participation.

Walking interviews and social network mappings were conducted at two distinct time points to capture temporal changes in participants' relationships with their neighbourhoods. Home tours were generally conducted once, except in cases where participants had relocated, warranting a follow-up tour. Finally, a small subset of participants produced diaries documenting their daily movements and social interactions over specified periods. The research was conducted across two United Kingdom (UK) sites: Stirling and the Forth Valley in Scotland and Greater Manchester in England, as well as Linköping in Sweden, though I draw here on data from UK-based participants. Ethical approval was secured through the relevant governance frameworks in each locale and all names shared in the extracts that follow are pseudonyms, in line with the research protocol. In what follows, I represent and reflect on some material we have presented elsewhere (and credit our original writing accordingly) and consider other data extracts for the first time. Most (though not all) of the material presented is drawn from the Greater Manchester fieldsite.

## Illustration 1: Neighbourhoods and environmental aesthetics

Writing with my colleague Sarah Campbell and others (Campbell et al., 2023; and see Sarah's main contribution to this book in Chapter 5), I have explored how environmental factors can foster either comfort or discomfort within the home. For participant Lily, the view from the window of her modest two-room apartment offered a crucial link to the outside world. From her seat, she watched the steady movement of people entering and leaving a nearby gym. Remarking that she 'never got fed up sitting there' watching the world pass by, Lily recounted being woken by the noise of outdoor exercise and responding by shouting to the gym-goers below her window; an act that conveyed her sense of presence and belonging within the neighbourhood. Similarly, George, who lived in a high-rise building, used pocket binoculars to observe distant activity, especially on clear days. This practice allowed him to stay visually connected with the neighbourhood, reinforcing his sense of engagement with the wider community (Clark et al., 2020). Such visual connections maintained from within the home were vital to feeling included and rooted in place. Beyond the potential for observing, participants also emphasised the sensory value of their windows in connecting with nature. One described witnessing the changing seasons from inside his apartment, calling the winter landscape a 'fairy wonderland'. Another appreciated the light coming through her window which offered views of distant hills and seasonal transitions, and another remarked that her mood mirrored light levels in her home, telling us that 'when her flat [apartment] was bright, she felt bright'. And a further participant told us how she would doze in the afternoon with the curtains open so she could see her neighbour's tree from her bed, which she described as 'fabulous to watch', which points to the ongoing importance of maintaining connections to nature within the context of ageing at home (Musselwhite, 2018).

So, how a neighbourhood looks, sounds, smells, or 'feels' matters. But this does not mean that seemingly unpleasant or uncomfortable qualities need to be eradicated, or that everyone will experience the same environmental aesthetic in the same way. A walk with Albert along a busy main road enabled a connection with a career driving heavy goods vehicles:

| | |
|---|---|
| *Researcher:* | Oh, it's a bit quieter now that traffic [has reduced]. |
| *Albert:* | It is yeah. |
| *Researcher:* | How do you feel about the traffic round here? |
| *Albert:* | It never bothers me…Never bothers me because I was on heavy goods myself you see so I've always, I've always had the noise of the traffic.<br>[later] |

*Researcher:* Has it changed much around this area?
*Albert:* No not, not really no. It's got noisier.
*Researcher:* Yeah, more people have got cars I suppose.
*Albert:* Yeah, more traffic. But I mean that doesn't bother me, like I say, I used to drive heavy goods [vehicles] so I've had that in my ears all the time.

Of course, it is not that busy roads or high volumes of traffic are problem-free. Indeed, our work, and that of others, shows that they do create barriers for people living with dementia who are continually having to weigh risk against the benefits of free movement (Odzakovik et al., 2021). Too many stimuli in the surroundings can also lead to negative behavioural changes such as confusion, disorientation, agitation, and anxiety whereas a calm and serene environment can alleviate distress and minimise behavioural changes. But what is also of interest here is how Albert's experience of place is particular to him, and created through his history, and this needs to be recognised when considering how changes intended to improve life for some individuals can have unintended consequences for others. We should not make presumptions about the sorts of atmospheric aesthetics that might better suit people living with dementia without their engagement. An individual who spent a lifetime amongst traffic-noise, or the hustle and bustle of a major city, might not appreciate quiet serenity in the way someone who has lived their life in rural areas for example.

These accounts present an arguably obvious, but nonetheless important link, to how we might understand the care of neighbourhood aesthetics that has been identified in wider neighbourhood research. The perceived aesthetics of a neighbourhood – encompassing the tactile, emotional, and sensory experiences individuals encounter – are a critical determinant of place experience and have health promoting effects for everyone (Root et al., 2017). But focusing solely on such qualities is to overlook other forms of care aesthetics.

## Illustration 2: Neighbourhood and relational aesthetics

My second example concerns the ways in which neighbourhoods can offer an explicitly social aesthetic, and here I draw especially on the sense of everyday aesthetics. Thompson (2023) suggests that situating care aesthetics in 'everyday life' requires understanding the often small-scale 'interpersonal and intercommunity relations' (p. 54) that constitute the bedrock of why neighbourhoods might matter to people living with dementia. Here, for example, is Douglas telling us about a barber shop he frequents and neatly encapsulating the wider sense of connection, and belonging, that this brings:

> The barber shop is a place, a local place that people go and people sit down and people come in and chat and friends come and things like that, you know.

Returning to Albert, who produced his social network map with input from his wife and primary care partner Vera, Albert spoke of being embedded in local relations and of knowing people who live in the area with whom he can chat. The couple returned to this later in the much more emotive context of the gravesite of their daughter:

*Researcher:* So, you know a few people who live round here?

*Albert:* I know quite a few that live round here and if I see we're coming up to one of them we'll stop and have a little chat and see how things are going.

[later]

*Albert:* The paper shop which I used to go to [is] at the top of the road…

*Vera:* Oh, that was great, it's closed now, they knew him very well there.

*Albert:* They knew me, and I knew them, I could stop and have a chat with them, you know.

*Vera:* And then when he'd done that, he'd walk down to [daughter]'s grave, see if the flowers were alright.

*Albert:* Yeah, I'd walk down from the corner because it's behind there, the shop, there's the graveyard where [daughter] is, my daughter is buried and I used to go up there…

*Researcher:* Yeah. So, do you miss going up there?

*Vera:* Not now, he goes to the garage.

*Albert:* Well, I do call in occasionally, but not…I used to go every day when the paper shop was there, but it's gone, that's gone now.

*Vera:* And I don't want him to stop going, I want him to, you know, make sure that he can still go out, even though he's got his identity [card], make sure he's got his identity [card] in his pocket, just in case he gets lost. You never know.

This is an example we have discussed elsewhere as indicative of the value of such small-scale social connections to social health (Ward et al., 2018; Clark et al., 2024), and above we also see the intersection of present and past connections. But what we also glimpse is the importance these neighbourhood-based relationships are for supporting communication, affording multisensory stimulation, and enabling shared experiences through opportunities to interact – in place – with other people. Alongside, we also see the juxtaposition of immeasurably significant relationships and life-shaping events such as a child's death, alongside the irreverent banality of the greeting of a shop worker, which are both made meaningful through a habitual walk. I do not intend to trivialise the tending of a loved-one's memorial to the level of being greeted in a shop. But that both happen within a few minutes' walk neatly demonstrates the relational facets of neighbourhood-based care.

Because shop staff demonstrate an attentiveness towards Albert, he is in turn able to go on to care for his daughter's grave. The loss of those staff, brought on by the closure of the shop, in turn risks the loss of a further, more profound, care practice. For what on the surface might be a convenient serendipitous engagement borne out of a routine and habitual practice enables a care landscape of love and attachment that reaches far beyond the mundane.

### Illustration 3: Neighbourhood care as an embodied, sensorial aesthetic

Connections with local actors can provide a form of latent support or assistance that remains inactive until triggered by particular conditions. In their early research on community care, Philip Abrams and his colleagues introduced the term 'neighbourhood care' to emphasise the importance of informal support networks provided by individuals residing in close geographical proximity (Bulmer, 1986). This is especially relevant for those living with dementia where they may serve as a safety net, becoming accessible when individuals encounter circumstances requiring aid (Wiersma and Denton, 2016). Whilst neighbourhood ties play an important part in shaping individuals' social support networks, what also emerges as significant is the maintenance of these relationships through routine, locally situated practices. These practices foster opportunities for support by cultivating a sense of familiarity and mutual recognition, shaped by recurring presence in shared spaces at particular times. This familiarity constitutes an aesthetic experience, not only visually, through the recognition of familiar faces, but also performative, expressed through small but meaningful gestures such as nods, smiles, and brief greetings. Dennis took us for a walk beside a nearby canal that is cared for by the environmental charity 'Waterways' (see https://waterways.org.uk/; accessed 1 March 2026), following a route that he often takes, and which has long-time connections to key stages in his life:

*Dennis:* It's quite well looked after because the Waterways people do a lot of work… but there's lots of people who come down and do a bit of cleaning up and changing and all the rest of it just because they want to keep it really nice.

*Researcher:* Have you always been [keen on] nature?

*Dennis:* Oh yes very much so, from being a child even when you went to go and get tadpoles you know doing all that sort of stuff I was always keen and especially animals or anything like that was great and getting conkers and you know the things that you would expect and then as we got older of course I found out about girls so started, you know, but as I say it's lovely when you walk along the canal and everything.

For Dennis, the canal is more than a local beauty spot; it is a location that affords fleeting connections to others:

> Well I always think if you say good morning to someone, someone will say [back] to you 'good morning' or 'lovely day, what are you doing today?' Just to say 'good morning lovely day', you know, I love doing that down there on the canal because that's the main place where it happens to *me.*

It is often only in moments of disruption that the deeper significance of these interactions becomes fully apparent and when their value beyond the symbolic is revealed:

| | |
|---|---|
| *Researcher:* | Nowadays, would you go out for a walk locally? |
| *Viv:* | Locally on my own, yes. I'm not feared [afraid]. Because I know the area quite well, and the people know me, and I know them. |
| *Researcher:* | So, you don't get lost when you come out? |
| *Viv:* | I have been lost a few times, but that was my own fault because I've took the wrong turning, gone the wrong way, and then straight away [inaudible] 'are you all right love?' And I don't know where I am, and she was absolutely lovely. She said, 'come on in and have a cup of tea and calm down'. |

The offer of a cup of tea is more than an act of kindness. To use Viv's phrase, it is a way of engaging that was, and remains 'absolutely lovely', a gesture that Viv can remember and draws on to maintain her independence, reassured that others are looking out for her. Viv's treading the same path and frequenting the same shops build up a sense of recognition and belonging that moves from being present, to having a presence, and where she is not just noted, but noticed.

Such examples arguably risk perpetuating the idea that care is something done to others, with recipients depicted in a passive role (Tronto 1993; Milligan, 2003). Yet, care is rarely one-directional. Even the acknowledgement of strangers that Dennis told us about depends on him making that initial connection. Care is performed between dyads and across networks (Milligan and Wiles, 2010). Lily explained how she looks out for a neighbour who in turn looks out for a wider group of older residents in the supported living scheme where they lived:

| | |
|---|---|
| *Lily:* | He's one of my neighbours and he's a very devout Catholic and he fetches us all a little bottle of holy water with the picture of our Lady of Lourdes on the bottle and everybody looks out for him and he's…he looks out for everybody else. |
| *Researcher:* | Do you look out for him, Lily? |
| *Lily:* | Yes, if I thought anybody was going to take the mickey out of him, I wouldn't let them. |

Of course, Lily's 'looking out' for her neighbour is more than a visual act of care. It makes up the situated practices of her everyday routines; of noticing and noting the ordinary so as to identify when something might be amiss amongst her neighbours. What Lily also describes breaks away from conventional care-dyads; she is part of a network of care located across multiple actors. Dennis's, Viv's, and Lily's examples hint at the importance of understanding neighbourhoods as embodied experiences, produced through sensorial encounters that constitute more than behaviours and actions. Neighbourhood care aesthetics is not just about how a neighbourhood looks, or even feels, but it is also about how small gestures – the offer of a cup of tea, or looking out for someone – embody the aesthetic practices of care not between a person and an object but between people in place.

## Illustration 4: Care aesthetics and neighbourhood temporalities

My fourth illustration involves temporality as a form of care aesthetic. To write of time, and especially time-past, in the context of dementia is complex, and I do not wish to reduce that complexity here. However, we know that environments, and objects within them, can trigger remembering, both good and bad. As we saw with Dennis, this can in turn prompt neighbourhood care practices. Memories of places, and the people and activities that make them as well as remnants of changed places that might remain in the guise of a pathway or building, offer glimpses of those pasts. Such memories might, but crucially are not always, grounded in changed environments. Sal, for instance, led us down what used to be a woodland track, whilst a walk with Jean took in a shopping centre that retained strong childhood memories:

*Sal:* And at the end of the street there was the forest track, it was called, which was basically the bit that ran between the gardens of the houses and the railway embankment. And there were trees and we used to play in there. But you didn't go far.

*Jean:* This part is new, but see down there? When we go by there, you'll see that's the shopping centre, you know the shopping area? That's where…I can remember actually…I don't know. Because me and my twin, my mum had a twin pram, a Silver Cross twin pram. I always remember that twin pram and I remember it being very…where can we go? I would go back straight out this way. My mum used to walk us down there. I always remember as well, she used to put reins on us, horrid things, and then she used to walk us to the shops. That was where my mum went shopping.

It is not just being in the environment that triggered such memories, but also the process of moving through them. Such memories emerge in part from the bodily and sensual clues that carry them and are released when walking through places where they were produced. Such memorialising brings a temporal structure to life;

not just in terms of the present having a past, but also of the present having a future. For example, Mark took us to a farm that has a long-standing significance for him as a site he used to work, and where his adult son now works and visits with his own children:

| | |
|---|---|
| *Researcher:* | So, you still come to this farm, the one that we're going to? |
| *Mark:* | I come up…it's all animals up here, it's all cattle. And if my… [son] is the one that comes up. In fact, if he can't make it for any reason at all, he'll ask me to go up… His boys are still at school, but in a few years' time they'll not be boys any longer, they'll be men. And my feeling is that I want him to spend as much time as he can with them. That's the way I look at it. But apart from anything else, I don't find it, I find it just quite a pleasant trip out. I don't find it's anything… |

Mark doesn't quite finish his sentence here, and I cannot finish it for him, but his search for the right words reflects a core element of the aesthetics I have been discussing. They are unremarkable, almost to the point of being unspoken or unarticulated, yet, at the same time, they have a remarkable capacity to matter; to enable people to know that they belong to people and to place. And that is why they are so potent.

Care aesthetics and memory intertwine in dementia care where physical environments, personal items, and interactions can significantly impact a person's well-being and sense of self. Saito's (2008) everyday aesthetics also encompass the look and feel of spaces and objects, which can trigger memories and create a sense of familiarity and comfort for individuals living with dementia. Conversely, a lack of attention to aesthetics can lead to disorientation and a feeling of being disconnected from one's surroundings. Places do not need to resemble how they once were to enable memorialisation; for Sal and Jean, it is enough to *know* these places were once like this. This knowing brings a kind of comfort, even if it is one, as Mark alludes, that is difficult to articulate. Neighbourhoods are more than sites cluttered with objects that trigger memories. They are situations of ongoing social and material interaction; where memories are sometimes lucid, sometimes irrevocably lost. They bring a sense of safety and belonging associated with being known in and knowing about place; and they offer an assemblage of connections with other people, environmental features, and personal histories.

## Illustration 5: Imagining neighbourhood care aesthetics

People-object-environment interactions, recollection, and embodied experiences all intersect to create an emergent neighbourhood care aesthetic. In this final illustration, I consider the imagination. The first illustration demonstrates the potential of the aesthetics of the natural environment to enable a sense of belonging to place;

and a story from Viv crystalised how participants did not just enjoy looking at, or being amongst, nature, but contributed to its meaning (Ward et al., 2018). On a walk through her neighbourhood, Viv took us to a tree that held special meaning for her and her grandchildren:

*Viv:* There's a tree that its name is the Knock-Knock Tree because somebody has painted a white door and has put a tiny little door knocker on it. So, you knock on the door to see if the fairies are in. And, of course, they never are. They've always gone out to see to fairy business.

*Researcher:* So…every time [your grandchildren] come that's something they want to do?

*Viv:* Yeah.

*Researcher:* So, are they ever hopeful that the fairies will be there?

*Viv:* Yeah. The Knock-Knock Tree…And the seven-year-old granddaughter loves going on adventures and so as soon as we're in the valley she'll say, 'where are we today, grannie?', and I have to think. So, I've turned it round and say, 'well where do you think we are?', and we have all sorts of adventures. We're in such and such a different land and what have we got to look out for and are they goodies or baddies, and I put on different accents and voices.

The value of this tree for Viv lies not just in its environmental aesthetic, but also in the way it is caught in an assemblage of interactions between the tree itself and Viv, Viv's grandchildren, and their past experiences, and their collective narratives, with the tree a crucial actant in suspending belief or becoming enchanted 'in the moment'.

Keady et al. (2022) have argued that:

> 'Being in the moment' is a relational, embodied and multi-sensory human experience. It is both situational and autobiographical and can exist in a fleeting moment or for longer periods of time. All moments are considered to have personal significance, meaning and worth.
>
> *(p. 687)*

It is during care-full moments that aesthetics come to the fore, illuminating the individuals, actions, objects, institutions, and environments that collectively create them (Thompson, 2022). To understand the significance for Viv of a seemingly ordinary tree, we need to pay attention to this wider constellation within which it, and Viv, sit. It is only then that we can start to appreciate the mutuality of care between them both. As someone living with dementia, Viv remains an active agent contributing to and shaping the environments in which she resides, rather than a passive recipient of care and support. Tronto (1993) asserts that care should be understood as a comprehensive activity encompassing all actions that maintain, sustain, and repair our world, enabling us to live within it as well as possible (p. 103). For Viv, and indeed for others we spoke to, this world comprising memories and bodies as well as physical and social environments intricately interwoven within a complex, life-sustaining web within which neighbourhoods are also entangled.

## Discussion: care aesthetics, dementia, and the environment: from design, to feeling, to being

When approaching care aesthetics, Thompson (2023) draws upon two principal fields: everyday aesthetics and relational aesthetics. Everyday aesthetics, as articulated by Saito (2008, 2022), underscore the importance of heightened sensory and emotional experiences in daily life as central to the construction of meaning. Relational aesthetics foregrounds the aesthetic dimensions of human interactions, portraying them as flexible, evolving, and subject to refinement. Care aesthetics emerges from this as a multisensory and complex experiential domain. Rather than evaluating care solely on its visual aspects, this perspective acknowledges that care engages the full range of human senses, including touch, sound, and movement. As Jones et al. (2025) observe, such moments of care are constructed through the actions of all those present and are shaped by their relationship to the broader environment. This includes the interplay of material elements, spatial organisation, and physical activities that collectively generate an atmosphere within health, social care, or community-based settings.

The five illustrative cases presented in this chapter show in different ways how adopting a care aesthetic lens to view how individuals living with dementia interact with and experience their neighbourhoods can help us make sense of neighbourhoods as embodied, relational, experiential, and socio-temporal situations and practices. Appreciating how individuals living with dementia become emplaced in their neighbourhoods, and how they too come to know and emplace themselves in their surroundings, is mediated through shared aesthetic and personal engagement with the places and people. These reciprocal relationships contribute to 'care-full' neighbourhoods, characterised by empathetic awareness not only of the individuals receiving care but also of the spaces they inhabit. Care-full neighbourhoods, then, are distinguished by a relational sensibility, marked by a familiarity with and attentiveness to people and place, that underpins the provision and reception of care.

Neighbourhood aesthetics requires an attentiveness to the style and sensory experiences in our daily lives outside of more conventional design contexts or semblances of what constitutes 'beauty'. To draw on the illustrations presented above, neighbourhood aesthetics consist of the small things, experienced 'in the moment', that make life feel pleasant, meaningful, or emotionally rich: the sense of connection achieved by the view from a window; the feelings that accompany a stranger's greeting or a smile of recognition in the street; the offer of a cup of tea when disorientated; the associations attached to the sound of traffic; or even the collaborative suspension of reality whilst telling stories about a tree. In these and I suspect countless other cases, finding beauty in the ordinariness of something that 'might look like a field to anybody else' relies on appreciating the phenomena, activities, routines, and interactions that constitute our daily lives (Fleetwood-Smith et al., 2022). In this way, making 'meaningful moments of connection' (Fox et al., 2025, p. 9) within and to neighbourhoods can enable people living with dementia to not just feel, but actively be, present in place.

## Conclusion: care-full not carefree neighbourhoods

The concept of care is inherently complex. Conradson (2003) suggested one way might be to examine experiences of care through the 'subjectivities that emerge, or which are made possible, within a particular [...] space' (p. 509). Such space enables the development of more positive forms of selfhood and supports the consolidation of such identities. Understanding this necessitates paying close attention to the social relationships that constitute caring practices, as well as to the material dimensions and agentic capacities of space, including neighbourhoods, in which these practices occur.

Social care policy has a prevailing focus on delivering individualised interventions to people living with dementia in their own domestic environments in ostensibly 'mainstream' ways, such as through the provision of formal support for personal hygiene or domestic duties. This positions care as taking place within asymmetrical dyadic relationships, typically between a caregiver and a care recipient, and risks occluding the complex, distributed, and collective dimensions of caregiving and care-receiving. It also fails to recognise the practical and conceptual value of more collective modalities of care that can emerge organically within a neighbourhood, and in which the enactment of care becomes an embedded and constitutive aspect of everyday social-environmental relations. Such contexts underscore broadening theoretical understandings of care to encompass collective, relational, and situational forms. They also resist reducing care to the binaries of giver and receiver, to recognise the reciprocal nature of human interdependence at the heart of care aesthetic concepts. So, if there is one thing care aesthetics might bring to our attempts to better understand the neighbourhood experiences of those living with dementia, it is to help us frame care as an 'ethic of encounter, or as a set of practices' (Conradson, 2003, p. 451) in all sorts of places beyond those of more familiar dementia care.

Research and practice about the environment and dementia has a long history, and so too does that about environments and aesthetics, where a feeling, atmosphere, or sense of attachment can contribute to meaning and belonging. This has been a cautious foray into exploring how a particular kind of aesthetic (care), cast in a particular kind of environment (neighbourhoods), framed through the temporal lens of the everyday, might help us make sense of how people living with dementia experience or encounter the places where they live. My endeavour has been partial at best, but what I hope to have achieved is some sense of how we might better understand neighbourhood experiences (and indeed any kind of spatial experience) for those living with dementia beyond a narrative of inclusive street design and infrastructure improvements. In the merging of the social, material, sensorial, biographical, and routine, all whilst trying to keep individuals centre stage, attending to the aesthetics of everyday experience might just help endeavours to move beyond reducing people living with dementia to risky or vulnerable subjects each time they engage with their neighbourhood.

## Acknowledgements

The data presented here was collected in a study funded jointly by the Economic and Social Research Council (ESRC) and the National Institute for Health and Care Research (NIHR). ESRC is part of the UK Research and Innovation (UKRI). The views expressed in this article are those of the author and not necessarily those of the ESRC, UKRI, NHS, NIHR or the Department of Health and Social Care. Material from Work Programme 4 of the ESRC/NIHR Neighbourhoods and Dementia mixed methods study. Study Reference Number: ES/L001772/1. I thank all participants who generously gave their time to the research as well the many individuals and organisations working in the dementia sector who supported the work in other ways. Much of the data presented here was carefully collected by Sarah Campbell: thanks to Sarah and also to Richard Ward, who led the Work Programme 4 team, for helping me to think through how and why neighbourhoods might matter.

## Three Key Reading References

### *Reference 1*

Fox, S., Thompson, J. and Keady, J. (2025). Meaningful moments of connection: How people affected by dementia and their carers living at home understand, interpret and experience everyday aesthetics. *International Journal of Geriatric Psychiatry*, 40 (8): e70136. Available: https://doi.org/10.1002/gps.70136; accessed 1 March 2026.

This paper explores how people living with dementia at home and their carers experience and interpret everyday aesthetics; ordinary sensory, relational, and material experiences that carry personal meaning. The study identified six key types of connection: with others, with material objects, with self-image, with pride and societal value, with enjoyable activities, and with the lived environment. These oftentimes subtle moments help sustain identity, wellbeing, and personhood despite cognitive changes. The authors show how recognising and supporting these meaningful experiences in home-based dementia care can enhance person-centred support, guide carers in maintaining identity and connection, and inform policies and environments that respect the sensory and relational lives of people with dementia.

### Reference 2

Thompson, J. (2023). *Care Aesthetics: For Artful Care and Careful Art*, London: Routledge. This book examines the intersection of care and aesthetics, proposing that caring practices, be they healthcare, homecare, or community settings, can be understood as inherently artistic, requiring attention, creativity, and sensitivity. The book demonstrates how artistic practices, such as participatory arts or creative facilitation, can function as forms of care that support wellbeing, connection, and dignity. Drawing on examples from healthcare, dementia care, and arts-based interventions, the text shows how attentiveness, relational engagement, and aesthetic awareness enrich both care and art, advocating for a framework in which care and creativity mutually inform and enhance one another.

### Reference 3

Ward, R., Clark, A. and Phillipson, L. (eds.) (2021). *Dementia and Place: Practices, Experiences and Connections*, Bristol: Policy Press.

This edited book is not about aesthetics, but it is about how people living with dementia experience, navigate, and relate to the places around them. Shifting the focus from institutional care to home- and community-based living, chapters examine themes like belonging, attachment, mobility, and social connectivity, highlighting the relational and environmental dimensions of daily life. The book emphasises understanding dementia through the lens of lived experience and place, offering insights for researchers, practitioners, and policymakers to create more supportive, inclusive environments. A number of the chapters present findings from Work Programme 4 of the ESRC/NIHR-funded 'Neighbourhoods and Dementia mixed methods study' that also underpins this chapter.

## References

Bartlett, R. and Brannelly, T. (2019). On being outdoors: How people with dementia experience and deal with vulnerabilities. *Social Science & Medicine*, 235: 112336. Available: https://doi.org/10.1016/j.socscimed.2019.05.041; accessed 1 March 2026.

Biglieri, S. and Dean, J. (2021). Everyday built environments of care: Examining the socio-spatial relationalities of suburban neighbourhoods for people living with dementia. *Wellbeing, Space & Society*, 2: 100058. Available: https://doi.org/10.1016/j.wss.2021.100058; accessed 1 March 2026.

Biglieri, S. and Dean, J. (2022). Fostering mobility for people living with dementia in suburban neighborhoods through land use, urban design and wayfinding. *Journal of Planning Education and Research*, 44 (3): 1704–1718. https://doi.org/10.1177/0739456X221113796

Bulmer, M. (ed.) (1986). *Neighbours: The Work of Philip Abrams*, Cambridge: Cambridge University Press.

Campbell, S., Clark, A., Keady, J., Kullberg, A., Manji, K., Odzakovic, E., Rummery, K. and Ward, R. (2023). 'I can see what's going on without being nosey…': What matters to people living with dementia about home as revealed through visual home tours. *International Journal of Geriatric Psychiatry*, 38 (9): e5999. Available: https://doi.org/10.1002/gps.5999; accessed 1 March 2026.

Clark, A. (2017). Seeing real life? Working with the visual to understand landscapes of community. *International Review of Qualitative Research*, 10 (2): 190–210. https://doi.org/10.1525/irqr.2017.10.2.190

Clark, A., Campbell, S., Keady, J., Kuhlberg, A., Manji, K., Rummery, K. and Ward, R. (2020). Neighbourhoods as relational places for people living with dementia. *Social Science & Medicine*, 252: 112927. Available: https://doi.org/10.1016/j.socscimed.2020.112927; accessed 1 March 2026.

Clark, A., Ward, R., Campbell, S., Keady, J., Kullberg, A., Manji, K., Odzakovik, E. and Rummery, K. (2024). Experiences and contributions of people living with dementia to the social life of everyday places. In J. Keady (ed.) *Reconsidering Neighbourhoods and Living with Dementia: Spaces, Places and People*. Maidenhead: Open University Press/McGraw-Hill, pp. 28–49.

Conradson, D. (2003). Geographies of care: Spaces, practices, experiences. *Social & Cultural Geography*, 4 (4): 451–454. https://doi.org/10.1080/1464936032000137894

Dowlen, R., McPherson, D.H.J., Swarbrick, C., Hoskin, L., Thompson, J. and Keady, J. (2024). Creating and reliving the moment: Using musical improvisation and care aesthetics as a lens of connection and self-expression for younger people living with dementia. *International Journal of Environmental Research and Public Health*, 21 (8): 972. Available: https://doi.org/10.3390/ijerph21080972; accessed 1 March 2026.

Fleetwood-Smith, R., Tischler, V. and Robson, D. (2022). Aesthetics and dementia: Exploring the role of everyday aesthetics in dementia care settings. *Design for Health*, 6 (1): 91–113. https://doi.org/10.1080/24735132.2022.2074207

Fox, S., Thompson, J. and Keady, J. (2025). Meaningful moments of connection: How people affected by dementia and their carers living at home understand, interpret and experience everyday aesthetics. *International Journal of Geriatric Psychiatry*, 40 (8): e70136. Available: https://doi.org/10.1002/gps.70136; accessed 1 March 2026.

Gan, D., Chaudhury, H., Mann, J. and Wister, A. (2022). Dementia-friendly neighborhood and the built environment: A scoping review. *The Gerontologist*, 62 (6): e340–e356. https://doi.org/10.1093/geront/gnab019

Hanlon, P. and Carlisle, S. (2015). The fifth wave of public health and the contributions of culture and the arts. In S. Clift and P. Camic (eds.) *Oxford Textbook of Creative Arts, Health, and Wellbeing: International Perspectives on Practice, Policy and Research*. Oxford: Oxford University Press, pp. 19–25.

Jones, L., Cullum, N., Watson, R., Thompson, J. and Keady, J. (2025). 'Only my family can help': The lived experience and care aesthetics of being resident on an NHS psychiatric/mental health inpatient dementia assessment ward – a single case study. *Ageing & Society*, 45 (6): 1143–1164. https://doi:10.1017/S0144686X24000096

Keady, J. (ed.) (2024). *Reconsidering Neighbourhoods and Living with Dementia: Spaces, Places and People*, Maidenhead: Open University Press/McGraw-Hill.

Keady, J.D., Campbell, S., Clark, A., Dowlen, R., Elvish, R., Jones, L., Kindell, J., Swarbrick, C. and Williams, S. (2022). Re-thinking and re-positioning 'being in the moment' within a continuum of moments: Introducing a new conceptual framework for dementia studies. *Ageing & Society*, 42 (3): 681–702. https://doi.org/10.1017/S0144686X20001014

Milligan, C. (2003). Location or dis-location? Towards a conceptualization of people and place in the care-giving experience. *Social & Cultural Geography*, 4 (4): 455–470. https://doi.org/10.1080/1464936032000137902

Milligan, C. and Wiles, J. (2010). Landscapes of care. *Progress in Human Geography*, 34 (6): 736–754. https://doi.org/10.1177/0309132510364556

Musselwhite, C. (2018). The importance of a room with a view for older people with limited mobility. *Quality in Ageing and Older Adults*, 19 (4): 273–285. https://doi.org/10.1108/QAOA-01-2018-0003

Odzakovik, E., Kullberg, A., Hellström, I., Clark, A., Campbell, S., Manji, K., Rummery, K., Keady, J. and Ward, R. (2021). Everyday places and connections. In R. Ward, A. Clark and L. Phillipson (eds.) *Dementia and Place: Practices, Experiences and Connections*. Bristol: Policy Press, pp. 67–89.

Richardson, N. and Campbell, S. (2024). Sensory attunements of caregivers and care receivers: The value of an embodied and emplaced approach in everyday care encounters. *The Senses and Society*, 19 (3): 324–336. https://doi.org/10.1080/17458927.2024.2402965

Root, E.D., Silbernagel, K. and Litt, J.S. (2017). Unpacking healthy landscapes: Empirical assessment of neighborhood aesthetic ratings in an urban setting. *Landscape and Urban Planning*, 168: 38–47. https://doi.org/10.1016/j.landurbplan.2017.09.028

Saito, Y. (2008). *Everyday Aesthetics*, Oxford: Oxford University Press.

Saito, Y. (2022). *Aesthetics of Care*, London: Bloomsbury.

Seetharaman, K., Chaudhury, H. and Mahmood, A. (2021). A conceptual framework of the person–environment interaction in the neighbourhood among persons living with dementia: A focus on out-of-home mobility. In R. Ward, A. Clark and L. Phillipson (eds.) *Dementia and Place: Practices, Experiences and Connections*. Bristol: Policy Press, pp. 113–134.

Sturge, J., Nordin, S., Sussana Patil, D., Jones, A., Légaré, F., Elf, M. and Meijering, L. (2021). Features of the social and built environment that contribute to the well-being of people with dementia who live at home: A scoping review. *Health & Place*, 67: 102483. Available: https://doi.org/10.1016/j.healthplace.2020.102483; accessed 1 March 2026.

Thompson, J. (2022). Care aesthetics, coronavirus and everyday life. *Performance Research*, 27 (6–7): 54–61. https://doi.org/10.1080/13528165.2022.2197525

Thompson, J. (2023). *Care Aesthetics: For Artful Care and Careful Art*, London: Routledge.

Tronto, J. (1993). *Moral Boundaries: A Political Argument for an Ethic of Care*, New York: Routledge.

Ward, R., Clark, A. and Hargreaves, M. (2012). What does 'neighbourhood' mean for carers of people with dementia?' *Journal of Dementia Care*, 20 (2): 33–36.

Ward, R., Clark, A., Campbell, S., Graham, B., Kullberg, A., Manji, K., Rummery, K. and Keady, J. (2018). The lived neighbourhood: Understanding how people with dementia engage with their local environment. *International Psychogeriatrics*, 30 (6): 867–880. https://doi.org/10.1017/S1041610217000631

Ward, R., Rummery, K., Odzakovic, E., Manji, K., Kullberg, A., Keady, J., Clark, A. and Campbell, S. (2021). Enabling the neighbourhood: A case for rethinking dementia-friendly communities. In R. Ward, A. Clark and L. Phillipson (eds.) *Dementia and Place: Practices, Experiences and Connections*. Bristol: Policy Press, pp. 94–112.

Ward, R., Rummery, K., Odzakovic, E., Manji, K., Kullberg, A., Keady, J., Clark, A. and Campbell, S. (2022). Beyond the shrinking world: Dementia, localisation and neighbourhood. *Ageing & Society,* 42 (12): 2892–2913. https://doi.org/10.1017/S0144686X21000350

Wiersma, E. and Denton, A. (2016). From social network to safety net: Dementia-friendly communities in rural northern Ontario. *Dementia: The International Journal of Social Research and Practice*, 15 (1): 51–68. https://doi.org/10.1177/1471301213516118

**PART 4**

# New beginnings in care aesthetics

# 12

# CONCLUDING THOUGHTS AND NEXT STEPS

*John Keady, Jackie Kindell and James Thompson*

As we mentioned in the Introduction to this book, and Kate and Réka in Chapter 6, the first detailed application and development of care aesthetics was predominantly in the field of older people through the work of the Arts and Humanities Research Council-funded 'Care Aesthetics: Research Exploration' (CARE) project conducted at The University of Manchester and its associated sites in England between 2022 and 2025. Informed by James' highly influential text and writings on the topic (see, for example, Thompson, 2015, 2022, 2023), the CARE project was led by James with John and Jackie involved as co-investigators who were specifically attached to the National Health Service (NHS) healthcare support worker (HCSW) case study in the overall research design (for some of our team HCSW case study outputs to date see Kindell et al., 2025a,b and Chapter 6 of this book). However, this was not the first time that John and Jackie had worked together with our previous publications spanning a range of topic areas in dementia studies including the use and validity of life story resources (Kindell et al., 2014); the experience of living at home and/or in a care home with semantic dementia (Kindell et al., 2019 and see Chapter 4 of this book); the efficacy of everyday communication approaches in living with dementia (Kindell et al., 2017); and the need to re-conceptualise dementia care through a 'moments-based' lens (Keady et al., 2022).

That said, for the three of us as editors of this volume, it was our time together on the CARE project that led directly to the production of this book and its theoretical and applied possibilities in dementia studies (for an example of our care aesthetics and applied HCSW dissemination work in the NHS, see https://www.youtube.com/watch?v=pB7iRxnmn5c; accessed 1 March 2026). Indeed, for the last five years, it is fair to say that our time together, either individually, pairing up, or as a collective, has been a continuous journey of interdisciplinary learning and discovery that has extended from navigating and negotiating the complexities

DOI: 10.4324/9781003623441-17
This chapter has been made available under a (CC BY) 4.0 license.

of Health Research Authority ethics permissions for the HCSW case study work, through to the delivery of the Tom Kitwood Memorial Address at the UK Dementia Congress at The Bridgewater Hall in Manchester in November 2025 on the topic of care aesthetics, dementia, and person-centred practices (for a news story about this presentation, see https://dementia-united.org.uk/news/2025/11/21/uk-dementia-congress-2025-the-bridgewater-hall-manchester/; accessed 1 March 2026).

As we have seen across all the chapters in this book, care aesthetics and the lived experience of dementia have made natural partners in the processes of creative curiosity and reporting. For us, the spaces in between these two processes are important as, when we planned this book and its contents in late 2024, we had no road map to follow to provide a clear destination to an end point, only a few directional markers and signposts. These markers and signposts consisted of a handful of important papers that had directly addressed aesthetic practices in dementia studies (see, for example, Hughes, 2014; Buse and Twigg, 2018; Fleetwood-Smith et al., 2022); our research experience together on the CARE project and the lived experience and interdisciplinary links we assembled over that time; our own reflective and intuitive sensibilities on the topic area; and, not to put too finer point on it, James' guidance and conceptual thinking. Moreover, for John and Jackie in particular, in approaching several authors to take part in this book and address its overarching ambition, we drew on our networks in dementia care that had been honed and developed over many years of working, practising, teaching, supervising, and researching in the field. Put simply, we wanted to involve authors who instinctively and intuitively 'got it' without a detailed explanation of what 'it' (care aesthetics) was.

Indeed, as John and Jackie stand back today and reflect upon the completed book and its contents, it has become even clearer to us that we had been doing 'our version' of care aesthetics in dementia studies for at least the last three decades, only we never framed it or described it as such during that time. Fortunately, we have begun to address this deficit in recent years when some of our previous creative and collaborative social research work in dementia studies has been either recontextualised through a care aesthetic lens with the support of James (see, for example, Campbell et al., 2024; Dowlen et al., 2024; Jones et al., 2025) or directly commenced with care aesthetics/aesthetic practices in mind and in the title of the funded study (see, for example, Fox et al., 2025; Fox et al., 2026; Kindell et al., 2025a). But this is just the beginning.

In an attempt to further enhance this more positive positioning, we will now outline five descriptive themes that we feel summarise the narrative arc to this book; namely, that care aesthetics in dementia studies: (i) Provides a language for doing person-centred practices; (ii) Values moments and their ripple effects; (iii) Moves beyond cognition; (iv) Curates relational measurement and theory development; and (v) Applies research innovation and creativity. We do not wish to give the impression that we have followed a strict scientific method in reaching these five descriptive themes. Rather, their naming was achieved by following three broad steps: first, by acknowledging our long-standing backgrounds in undertaking and producing qualitative research; second, by repeatedly reading, and re-reading, each of the received book chapters during 2025 and writing down and mapping our thoughts about each of the chapter's contents; and third, discussing and agreeing the common threads and cross-chapter descriptive theme titles at our monthly editors' meetings that were set up to track progress on this book and to meet our submission deadline.

We will now outline each of these five descriptive themes in turn and we have provided a few bullet points under each to flesh out their meaning a little more. We will cross-reference chapters in this book as and when this is appropriate.

## Care aesthetics in dementia studies

(i) Provides a language for doing person-centred practices

- As seen across the chapters of this book, for people living with dementia and their social networks, person-centred practices have been described as happening: at home (Chapters 2, 4, and 9); in the NHS (Chapters 5 and 6); in care homes (Chapters 3, 4, 5, 7, and 10); and outside in the community and neighbourhoods where people with dementia live (Chapters 9 and 11). Care aesthetics therefore is not a static and fixed concept to place, rather it is one that is dynamic in its conceptualisation, flexible and fluid in its application, and centred on everyday life.
- With its focus on sensory, embodied, and relational practices, care aesthetics provides a focus on the micro-processes of care and starts to make visible the 'everyday' and the 'routine' nature of caring practices – the washing, shaving, cutting of hair, and trimming of fingernails, for example – into a craft with its own distinct range of skills and embodied actions. Whilst there are many illustrative examples of these practices to choose from in this book, Sarah Campbell and Rebecka Fleetwood-Smith in Chapter 5 provide a detailed and insightful framework for the 'doing' of person-centred practices when they focussed on dress, grooming, and other forms of appearance-related personal care for people living with dementia. As Sarah and Rebecka go on to state in their chapter, care extends beyond simple physical contact to 'encompass the use of the body, exercise of touch, tone of voice, awareness of space, and the construction of practice across time'. By starting to identify and distil these key elements in/of care aesthetics, *the how* of person-centred care can begin to be revealed, something that has been missing in the literature and practice context for some time (Keady et al., 2022). This focus on *the how* will shortly be taken up by Sue Ennis in the Afterword to this book in her role as a carer for her husband who lived and died with semantic dementia.

(ii) Values moments and their ripple effects

- All authors in this book have revealed an appreciation and value of the 'moment' in their writing, such as 'moments of warmth' (Introduction); 'a care moment' (Introduction and Chapters 5 and 11); 'everyday moments', 'capturing moments', 'moments of togetherness', and a 'series of moments' (Chapter 2); 'quiet moments', 'small moments', 'musical moments', and 'spontaneous moments' (Chapter 3); 'rhythmic moments' (Chapter 4); 'moments of material resistance' (Chapter 5); 'crafted moments', the 'lived moment', and 'magpie moments' (Chapter 6); 'creative moments', 'supported moments', and 'challenging moments' (Chapter 7); 'garbage moments', 'meaningful moments', and 'micro moments' (Chapter 8); 'in the moment' (Chapter 9 and throughout this book); 'present moment' (Chapter 10); 'moments of disruption' and 'care-full moments' (Chapter 11). This is not a complete list of 'moments' captured in this book or the process of cross-chapter comparison. Indeed, the use of 'moments' was also used in the title of two chapters in this book (i.e., 'changing moments' in Chapter 6 and 'creative moments' in Chapter 7) and when people living with dementia themselves coined the phrase 'meaningful moments of connection' as a proxy for everyday aesthetics (Chapter 8). Somehow, the 'moment' and its multiple meanings and application embody time and messages of being in the aesthetical experience of living with dementia. However, we suggest that this symbiotic and relational assertion requires further examination in communicating, documenting, and evaluating person-centred practices in dementia studies within an everyday life and care aesthetics register.
- Moments also have the potential to 'ripple out' from their original source meaning to create new moments of opportunity and connection within and across time. This process was eloquently described in Chapter 2 when Christina Buse outlined the act of sketching with her mum, an act that created a linked 'series of moments' from that interactional engagement. To us, this phrasing of a 'series of moments' opens a door to a new way of conceptualising and mapping everyday practices and aesthetic experiences in dementia studies and its on-going processes of evaluation and meaning-making.

(iii) Moves beyond cognition

- In Part 1 of this book, Julian C. Hughes wrote, 'practices can be considered from the perspective of their sensory qualities' and Christina Buse shared, 'My mum has not said my name for some time now, but recognition is enacted at an embodied level' before going on to say, 'She sometimes looks at me or my dad and says "ahh" and I stroke her hand and smile in return and say "ahhh" and her face still sometimes "lights up" when she sees us'. Christina then writes, 'Aesthetics like this are subtle and harder to translate into a care plan but are embodied in biographical relationships'. For us, these extracts from the two opening chapters of this book highlight that sensory, embodied, and relational practices work together in unison and that these three elements will constantly rise, or fall, in importance and value given the contextual circumstance in which they occur – but they *always* exist together and are *always* co-present. Arguably, it is this foundational sense of 'co-presence' that moves the sensory, embodied, and relational experience of living with dementia beyond its cognitive landscape and draws other pictures, values, colours, and qualities onto its canvas of possibilities.

- If Part 1 of this book could be positioned as the foundation stone for what is seen and interpreted as care aesthetics in dementia studies, then, in the chapters that follow in Parts 2 and 3 of this book, all authors have focused on the importance of the multi-sensory and the bidirectional relationality of caregiving experiences. Indeed, within our understanding and presentation of care aesthetics, aspects of materiality, the natural environment, and everyday creativity have such important stories to tell in moving beyond the cognitive in the lived experience of dementia.

(iv) Curates relational measurement and theory development

- Perhaps one of the main contributions of this book is in uncovering the applied development of care aesthetics to the field of dementia studies. This applied development is shown in numerous ways during this book, such as in Henry McPherson and his colleagues' description in Chapter 3 of the fun and enjoyment experienced by people living with dementia in co-creating and co-producing a vinyl record sleeve as a legacy object from their time on a music-based study; Sarah Campbell and Rebecka Fleetwood-Smith's descriptions in Chapter 5 of the importance of atmospheres and, separately, crafting in the everyday lives for people living with dementia in different care settings; and Rita Newton and her colleagues' description in Chapter 9 of the soundscapes in the natural world when people living with dementia are outside and gardening at home, or just sitting quietly on a garden bench in the back garden, or other outside space of the domestic home, enjoying the sunshine and the sounds and sensations of a summer's day. Uncovering and mapping this applied version of care aesthetics reveals new possibilities for relational measurement and approaches to theory development that is underpinned by biographical connections and, to slightly adapt Julian C. Hughes' terminology in Chapter 1, the *situated experience* of the person living with dementia.
- Given the preceding bullet point, and drawing on phrases used across this book by authors describing care aesthetics, 'measuring' biographical and connecting areas of lived experience would involve 'tuning in' to such elements as atmosphere, body, touch, tone of voice, spatial awareness, body movements, facial expression, hugs, holding hands, rubbing cheeks, gaze, eye contact, and the temporal construction of practice (see, also, Kindell

et al., 2025a). Going forward, new approaches are needed to raise the visibility of such elements to authentically represent their unique and interpersonal value and craft of care.

(v) Applies research innovation and creativity

- In this book, authors have used a variety of social research methods to underpin their empirical contribution on care aesthetics and dementia studies, for instance, sketching (Chapter 2); diarying (Chapter 2); video (Chapters 3, 4, 5, and 11); audio recordings (Chapters 3 and 4); fieldnotes (Chapters 3, 5, 7, and 10); producing knitted samples (Chapter 3); jewellery making (Chapter 3); tactile postcards (Chapter 3); textiles (Chapter 3); object handling (Chapter 3); object creation (Chapter 3); biographical interviewing (Chapter 4); participant observation (Chapters 5 and 9); collaborative learning groups (Chapter 6); semi-structured interviews (Chapters 6, 9 and 10); snapshot interviews (Chapters 6 and 9); reflective notes (Chapters 6 and 7); observations (Chapter 6); workshops (Chapter 7); photography (Chapter 9); reflexive journal (Chapter 9); poster development (Chapter 9); documentary analysis (Chapter 10); walking interviews (Chapter 11); and home tour interviews (Chapter 11). To complement these methods, the range of adopted methodologies and approaches includes autoethnography (Chapter 2); visual autoethnography (Chapter 2); participatory methods (Chapter 3); conversational analysis (Chapter 4); sensory ethnography (Chapter 5); ethnographic vignettes (Chapter 6); ethnography (Chapters 6, 9, and 10); applying an integrative framework (Chapter 8); reflexive thematic analysis (Chapter 9); comparative research design (Chapter 11); and participatory social network mapping (Chapter 11).
- The above range of methods and methodologies shared in this book indicates that authors have explored care aesthetics in dementia studies mainly through a qualitative, participatory, and imaginative/creative lens and many times through longitudinal engagement in underpinning their research designs. Perhaps such endeavours provide an insight into both *the how* and *the values* necessary to further develop care aesthetics and person-centred practices in the lived experience of dementia. To begin to turn a new page in care aesthetics and dementia studies means heightening the value of participatory research design and valuing the biographical, the relational, and the importance of shared and lived time.

## Final thoughts

In the Introduction to this book, we wrote: 'Being present with someone [living with dementia] is not the *soft extra*, or doing nothing, but we would argue the starting point for person-centred care'. We would like to think that this book has further developed the emphasis we originally placed on the italicised words *soft extra*. Care aesthetics begins to capture the intangible, the invisible, and the essence of what it is to both live with dementia and to care for someone with the condition, whatever and wherever the setting, circumstances, and context. And that includes people living with dementia caring for and about other people living with dementia.

To try and move with the times and the rapid advancements in technology in the first quarter of the 21st century, and as the final act in preparing this book for return to the publisher in March 2026, we asked The University of Manchester's approved artificial intelligence (AI) tool to provide us with a definition of care aesthetics in the context of dementia care/studies. Below is the result:

> Care aesthetics is an interdisciplinary approach that combines care ethics and aesthetic theory to reframe dementia care as a sensory, embodied, and relational practice rather than a purely biomedical or task-driven process.

Perhaps a task to come in the times ahead is to develop and refine that AI-generated definition and involve people living with dementia in its formulation. But for now, and together with the contents of this book, it has set a challenge and provided an emergent framework of understanding.

Finally, the text ends with an Afterword by Sue Ennis. We have not asked for the Afterword to be written as a traditional reflection on this book's contents, but more as a reflection on *the how* in care aesthetics and *the why* it is necessary for the sensory, embodied, and relational to be captured in research and everyday lived encounters, i.e., those occurring in the past; 'in the moment'; and into the future. We would like to thank Sue for her openness and honesty in responding to our request and for providing an insight into how creative social research methods could begin to be used to capture the sensory, embodied, and relational acts that underpin care aesthetics and its person-centred practices.

Thank you for reading this book and, as editors, and on behalf of all contributors, we hope that its contents have ignited your curiosity and acted as a spark to inspire further work, direction, and exploration in care aesthetics and the lived experience of dementia. It is a truly fascinating and necessary journey and one where you only need to let go and trust your own footsteps. The destination will follow.

## References

Buse, C. and Twigg, J. (2018). Dressing disrupted: Negotiating care through the materiality of dress in the context of dementia. *Sociology of Health & Illness*, 40 (2): 340–352. https://doi.org/10.1111/1467-9566.12575

Campbell, S., Dowlen, R., Keady, J. and Thompson, J. (2024). Care aesthetics and 'being in the moment' through improvised music-making and male grooming in dementia care. *International Journal of Education & the Arts*, 25 (si1.13). Available: https://journals.psu.edu/ijea/article/view/63522; accessed 1 March 2026.

Dowlen, R., McPherson, D.H.J., Swarbrick, C., Hoskin, L., Thompson, J. and Keady, J. (2024). Creating and reliving the moment: Using musical improvisation and care aesthetics as a lens of connection and self-expression for younger people living with dementia. *International Journal of Environmental Research and Public Health*, 21 (8): 972. Available: https://doi.org/10.3390/ijerph21080972; accessed 1 March 2026.

Fleetwood-Smith, R., Tischler, V. and Robson, D. (2022). Aesthetics and dementia: Exploring the role of everyday aesthetics in dementia care settings. *Design for Health*, 6 (1): 91–113. https://doi.org/10.1080/24735132.2022.2074207

Fox, S., Davies, J., Dowlen, R., Keady, J., Thompson, J. and Watson, R. (2026). Feeling safe, feeling connected: Aesthetic and polyvagal approaches to dementia care. *Frontiers in Dementia* (Perspective article), 12 January 2026: 1–7. Available: https://doi.org/10.3389/frdem.2025.1735205; accessed 1 March 2026.

Fox, S., Thompson, J. and Keady, J. (2025). Meaningful moments of connection: How people affected by dementia and their carers living at home understand, interpret and experience everyday aesthetics. *International Journal of Geriatric Psychiatry*, 40 (8): e70136. Available: https://doi.org/10.1002/gps.70136; accessed 1 March 2026.

Hughes, J.C. (2014). The aesthetic approach to people with dementia. *International Psychogeriatrics*, 26 (9): 1407–1413. https://doi.org/10.1017/S1041610214001100

Jones, L., Cullum, N., Watson, R., Thompson, J. and Keady, J. (2025). 'Only my family can help': The lived experience and care aesthetics of being resident on an NHS psychiatric/mental health inpatient dementia assessment ward – a single case study. *Ageing & Society*, 45 (6): 1143–1164. https://doi:10.1017/S0144686X24000096

Keady, J.D., Campbell, S., Clark, A., Dowlen, R., Elvish, R., Jones, L., Kindell, J., Swarbrick, C. and Williams, S. (2022). Re-thinking and re-positioning 'being in the moment' within a continuum of moments: Introducing a new conceptual framework for dementia studies. *Ageing & Society*, 42 (3): 681–702. https://doi.org/10.1017/S0144686X20001014

Kindell, J., Burrow, S., Wilkinson, R. and Keady, J. (2014). Life story resources in dementia care: A review. *Quality in Ageing and Older Adults,* 15 (3): 151–161. https://doi.org/10.1108/QAOA-02-2014-0003.

Kindell, J., Keady, J., Sage, K. and Wilkinson, R. (2017). Everyday conversation in dementia: A review of the literature to inform research and practice. *International Journal of Language & Communication Disorders*, 52 (4): 392–406. https://doi.org/10.1111/1460-6984.12298

Kindell, J., Maguire-Rosier, K., Polonyi, R., Thompson, J., Cleasby, R., Watson, R. and Keady, J.D. (2025a). Healthcare support workers working with people with dementia on mental health wards: A practice model informed by care aesthetics. *Qualitative Health Research*, 1–14. Online First (December). Available: https://doi.org/10.1177/10497323251393890; accessed 1 March 2026.

Kindell, J.A., Harman, K., Maguire-Rosier, K., Polonyi, R., Thompson, J. and Keady, J.D. (2025b). Exploring the everyday care practices of healthcare support workers when working with people with dementia admitted to National Health Service hospital wards in the United Kingdom: A qualitative systematic review of the literature. *Aging & Mental Health*, 29 (5): 915–927. https://doi.org/10.1080/13607863.2024.2447319

Kindell, J., Wilkinson, R. and Keady, J. (2019). From conversation to connection: A cross-case analysis of life story work with five couples where one partner has semantic dementia. *Ageing & Society,* 39 (10): 2322–2345. https://doi.org/10.1017/S0144686X18000533

Thompson, J. (2015). Towards an aesthetics of care. *Research in Drama Education: The Journal of Applied Theatre and Performance*, 20 (4): 430–441. https://doi.org/10.1080/13569783.2015.1068109

Thompson, J. (2022). Care aesthetics, coronavirus and everyday life. *Performance Research*, 27 (6–7): 54–61. https://doi.org/10.1080/13528165.2022.2197525

Thompson, J. (2023). *Care Aesthetics: For Artful Care and Careful Art*, London: Routledge.

# AFTERWORD

## Caring for my husband Frank who lived and died with advanced semantic dementia

*Sue Ennis*

### About Frank

Frank was a socialist to the core of his being. He was an academic. American political history was his passion … and to think he missed the second term of office of President Trump! He was kind and generous. He was funny and sexy. He was the most beautiful man I had ever met. Dealing with his semantic dementia sometimes made me forget who he really was. But I remember him with so much love, and I miss him. He was the best of us, and he loved me.

### Cutting Frank's hair

I have some practical ability. Being married to an old hippy I needed to. However, cutting hair is not in my skills set. Getting Frank to a barber was just not possible. As with many people with advanced semantic dementia he had complex needs. So, instead of trying to get him out of the house and into the car and me driving to the barbers, I watched a YouTube video on hair cutting. They make it look so easy. It was not. Frank was not keen on me cutting his hair. He seemed not to like the sound of the scissors or the feel of the cut hair nestled on his neck. Keeping him still proved nigh on impossible, so in the end I cut Frank's hair with us both sat on the floor in our lounge. We both sat facing the same way – as if we were rowers in the Oxford and Cambridge boat race – with the back of Frank's head pressed against the front of my body. That way I could cut Frank's hair a little and still reach around and hold him. From time to time, I would stop snipping away so that I could cradle his head in my arms.

### Skin on skin

You miss so much. You miss their skin on your skin. The touch of another much-loved body, holding you, touching you … and you to them. Touching for the sheer joy of it simply disappears. But, in the shower, Frank's soft skin being washed by me, could bring it all back. Sometimes, for a brief time, I had him back. But the sadness for me could be overwhelming. Touch changed.

## Voice and silence

We were never short of conversation. Never. Dementia changed that. Frank would answer questions but rarely initiated any conversation. How I phrased a question became crucial. The tone and timbre of my voice were important too. Panic and tiredness would cause my voice to rise. If my voice became high-pitched, as it increasingly did, I would receive a very limited response, if any. If I could keep my voice calm and gentle, he responded more.

There was a lot of silence in the later part of our lives together. Some silences felt so oppressive. I just wanted to scream. What Frank felt I am simply unable to hazard a guess at. How frightened he must have been not having his voice. Words were his thing and then he had so very, very few. His voice changed, as mine had.

## My red raw hands

Most days I had to change the bedding as Frank's TENA pants were not always up to the job. Changed life circumstances turned our home into a 24-hour laundry because for two years all I did was wash clothes, bedding, and protective mattress covers – and Frank's body, usually with cleaning wipes as they could be more easily rubbed and squeezed into the folds of his skin and then disposed with. Frank and I slept together in the same bed until the day he died, and I can vividly recall regularly waking to the smell and touch of urine-soaked sheets and how I would have to carefully roll and fold the mattress protector and the bed linen to strip the bed. Usually with Frank still in it. I became highly skilled at this act. The sheets always felt wet in my hands and wet when they came out of the washing machine. Thank God I had a reliable washer and dryer and a rotary line in our back garden to peg out the sheets and bedclothes when the weather in the Northeast allowed. The constant churning, tumbling, and whirring of our washing machine became the soundtrack to our home and to our everyday life. My hands soon became red raw from the constant cycle of *cleaning, folding, washing, drying; cleaning, folding, washing, drying; cleaning, folding, washing, drying* in performing acts of love, tenderness, and care for my husband. My hands stayed red raw for a long time.

## Open windows

If you passed by our home when Frank was alive, you would have seen our street-facing bedroom window constantly open to allow fresh air into the room to provide a natural filter to the smells, sounds, and fluids that were eliminated every day and every night from Frank's body; and Frank's body is all our bodies. Our private world turned public. Three years ago, straight after Frank died, I burnt our mattress protector.

# INDEX

Note: **Bold** page numbers refer to tables and *italic* page numbers refer to figures.


Adams, A. 238, 239, 243
aesthetics: art and care 43; authority and autonomy 91; of care *see* care aesthetics; communicative aesthetic practice 132–133; definition 183, 185–186, 197; of dementia care practice *see* dementia; everyday *see* everyday aesthetics; experience of 7, 32, 101, 110, 112, 114, 149, 163, 183–189, 191–192, 194–196, 263, 280; exploration of 112–114, 184; health and social care 1; history of 6; neighbourhood *see* neighbourhoods; neuroaesthetics 15, 183, 186–191, 194–196, *196*; personal and academic experiences 183–184; with Polyvagal Theory 189–191, 196, *196*; qualities 104, 110; relational aesthetics 7, 261–263, 268; sensibilities 14, 33, 72, 80, 122, 167; sensitivities 22, 72; visibility problem 131
Agich, G.J. 27; *Dependence and Autonomy in Old Age: An Ethical Framework for Long-Term Care* 27
Allan, K. 123
Alzheimer's disease 26, 35, 100–101, 180, 196, 235–236
Aristotle 22
Armstrong, P. 120
artificial intelligence (AI) 283
art(s): access to 162–163; and aesthetics 22; and care 14, 43, 60, 167; in care home 155; 'care-ful art' 61; clowning 144; and creativity 69, 161, 163, 171, 174; dance 23, 62; design 23; of everyday life 6, 43, 183; forms 1, 23; in health 8, 11; jewellery 23; literature 23; in lives of people with dementia 163; music 23, 62; photography 23; programme-based or intervention-based activities 164; public art 23; sculpture 23; storytelling 144; theatre 23; visual 23, 30, 52, 61, 187
authenticity 31–32
autobiographical memory 188, 197
autoethnography 44–46
autonomic nervous system (ANS) 183, 190–191, 194, 197

Baart, A. 12, 194
Bartlett, R. 161
Baumgarten, A.G. 6, 22, 183, 185, 190, 197
Beard, R.L. 23
Beethoven, L. 24, 34
being in the moment 46, 104, 267
Bellass, S. 164
bodywork 26, 43–44, 55–57, 61–62, 119–121, 127, 129, 133–134
Bowyer, J. 82
Bradwell, C. 166
Braun, V. 210
Bunting, M. 122

Burnham, A. 182
Buse, C. 2, 14, 49, 70, 120, 123, 125, 131, 208, 209, 280

Campbell, S. 3, 14, 78, 90, 101, 120, 122, 125, 127, 128, 131, 133, 134, 138, 144, 169, 171, 172, 236, 237, 246, 260, 270, 279, 281
*Care Aesthetics: For Artful Care and Careful Art* (Thompson) 1, 8, 30, 33, 185
'Care Aesthetics: Research Exploration' (CARE) project 2, 7–8, 11, 144–145, 148, 155, 277–278
care aesthetics (CA): ambition of 6; ambivalence and deception 242–244; appearance practices and 127–129; architecture and later life 237–239; art and everyday life 43; and care ethics 33; challenges 43, 60, 62; and creative practices 14; debates in 43; definition 3–5, 197; dementia research 1–3, 277–283; doctoral studies 125–127; doing of 124, 126–127, 137–138; dress, grooming, and appearance-related personal care 118–138; everyday aesthetics 6–7, 166–167, 185–186, 189, 193, 228; examples of analysis 9–11; expanding 124–125; expansive care 129–130; 'good' care practices 137; and living with dementia 14, 26, 100–114; methods 239–240; mundane *vs.* exceptional 54; neighbourhood experiences 256–270; neurophysiological layer 194–195; new beginnings in 15; object-handling sessions (case study) 72–80; outdoor spaces, and everyday design 15; and Polyvagal Theory 191; private spaces and public soundscapes 133–135; psychotherapeutic layer 192–194; questions of home 244–247; *Records of My Life* project (case study) 81–82; and relational citizenship 173, 237; reminiscence rooms 242–247; resistance as communication 132–133; role of creativity 161; role of reminiscence 240–241; sensory and affective elements 3, 8; spatialising practices of self-care 130–131; and structural constraints 120–121; tensions, complexities, and resistive practices 131–132; theoretical framework 121–122; through materials 129; *see also* aesthetics
care home: arts activities 144, 155; caring aesthetic 29–30; cultural stereotypes 245–246; dance intervention in 23; families 94; financial pressures 247–248; high or low quality 4; home-scaping and home-playing in 248, 250; hospitality sector model 241; importance of music in 85; participatory manner 32; for people living with dementia 25, 72, 124, 126, 144–145, 160, 161, 167–169, 192, 239, 277; residents 94, 130, 133, 185, 239, 247–249; staff 72–74, 76–77, 92, 94, 129–130, 172; woman in 11
'care-ful art' 61
care-full neighbourhoods: care-aesthetic discourse 257; carers' experiences 256; and environmental aesthetics 260–261; everyday aesthetics and relational aesthetics 268; experiences and practices 258–260; imagining care aesthetics 266–268; and relational aesthetics 261–263; as relational practices 257–258; research and practice 269–270; sensorial aesthetic 263–265; style and sensory experiences 268–269; temporalities 265–266
carers (and family carers): bodily practice 11, 13, 44, 61; and cared 7, 44; embodied practices 10; emotional labour 44; formal carers 163; living with dementia 5, 16, 22, 44, 62, 70, 150–151, 153, 181–182, 192, 208, 228, 236–237; neighbourhood experiences 256, 259; and residents 250; self-aware carer 151
Chalmin-Pui, L.S. 206
Chapman, L. 46, 52
Chatterjee, A. 187
Chesla, C.A. 25
Chivers, S. 238, 239, 243
Cinza, D. 187
Clark, A. 2, 15
Clarke, V. 210
*Client-Centred Therapy* (Rogers) 190
Conradson, D. 269
co-regulation 191, 193–197
COVID-19 pandemic 47, 49, 78, 162, 208
creative methods 14, 44, 61, 71, 72, 126
creative moments 76, 160; access to arts *see* arts; enabled creative moments 168, 169; everyday creativity *see* creativity; idealised imagining 161; importance of noticing (and feeling) 174; material moments 171–173;

PPIE project 169–171; research and practice 160–161; 'speculative route in' 161; 'speculative route out' 174–175; spontaneous creative moments 168, 169
creativity: and arts 69, 174; care aesthetics 166, 167; collective creativity 89, 91; everyday aesthetics 166, 167; everyday creativity 43–44, 52–55, 60, 62, 164–166, 168, 281; 'full-bodied' approach 122; and identity 43; object-handling sessions 76; of people living with dementia 86, 160–161, 163, 173, 174; relational citizenship and 165–166; research on 44, 278, 282; social inclusion 25
*Critique of the Power of Judgment* (Kant) 32
Cürlis, D. 70

Daly, T. 121
Damico, J.S. 106
Dana, D. 189–191, 193; *Polyvagal Practices* 193
default mode network (DMN) 188–189, 194
Dekkers, W. 28, 29
dementia: access and use of domestic (home) gardens *see* gardens; with advanced dementia 28–29; in care home *see* care home; care practice *see* care aesthetics; CARE project 11; carer, sensory practices of *see* carers (and family carers); caring aesthetic beings 29–31; case studies 145–154; creative moments and 160–175; 'dementia-friendly' design 15; embodied beings 24–26; everyday creativity 43–44, 60; friendship and love 34–36; frontotemporal dementia 47–49; The Genetic Choir (Amsterdam) 10–11; interrelated and interdependent beings 26–27; living with *see* People Living with Dementia (PWD); no aesthetics without ethics 32–34; person-centred dementia care *see* person-centred care; research 2; role of reminiscence rooms 15; in self-care practices 118–119; semantic *see* semantic dementia; sentient beings 22–24; situated persons 27–28; solicitude and authenticity 31–32; studies *see* dementia studies; vascular dementia 100
*Dementia Reconsidered: The Person Comes First* (Kitwood) 12
dementia studies: beyond cognition 280–281; care and aesthetics *see* aesthetics; care aesthetics; creative methods 44; developments in 258; neighbourhoods and 259; person-centred care 119, 279; relational approaches 119–120; relational measurement and theory development 281–282; research and practice 14, 44; research innovation and creativity 282; into social environments 15; values moments and ripple effects 280
*Dependence and Autonomy in Old Age: An Ethical Framework for Long-Term Care* (Agich) 27
*Dependent Rational Animals* (MacIntyre) 25, 27
Descartes, R. 25
Dimmock, C. 206
Don, M. 206
Donovan, J. 7
Dowlen, R. 14, 144, 169–171

Economic and Social Research Council (ESRC) 214–215, 217, 219, 223–225; Collaborative Studentship Competition (CASE) 207–208; FOSS event 209, 212
Ennis, S. 15, 279, 283
European Union (EU) 236
everyday aesthetics: and art 52; for care aesthetics *see* care aesthetics; definition 184–186, 197; people living with dementia to 6, 15, 50, 167, 187, 192, 266, 280; research 2, 181, 189; sensory and emotional experiences 268; and visibility problem 123–124; *see also* aesthetics
*The Experience of Alzheimer's Disease, Life Through a Tangled Veil* (Sabat) 27
*Experience of Awe: An Expansive Approach to Everyday Aesthetics* (Leddy) 185

feminist care ethics 2, 4, 145
Festival of Social Science (FOSS) 209
Fleetwood-Smith, R. 3, 14, 73, 126, 133, 171–173, 192, 193, 279, 281
Flowerdew, B. 206
Fox, S. 5, 15, 62, 144, 167
friendship 21, 34–36

gardens: autumn poster 222–223, *223*; care home settings 92, 208; community gardening 207; Community Wellbeing Garden 225–226, *226*; during

COVID-19 pandemic 49; domestic (home) garden 205–210, 228–230; ESRC FOSS Manchester exhibition 214–215, *216*, *218*; ESRC FOSS visitor numbers and evaluation outcome 224–225; exhibition posters, designing and showing 215–219; forget-me-nots 47, *48*, 49; and gardening 2, 15, 23, 206–207, 227; and green spaces 205–206; household demographics and property type 210, **211**; identity of 'being a gardener' 207; leaf printing *52*, 53; partnership with RHS Garden Bridgewater 212–214, *213*, *216*, *217*, 217–219, *218*, 225–228, *226*; relationship of care 13; sketching *48*, 49–52, *50*, *52*; spring poster 220–221, *221*; summer poster 221–222, *222*; support and feelings of well-being 15; visits to household 210, **212**; winter poster 223–224, *224*
Geller, S.M. 191
Gendlin, E. 190
The Genetic Choir (Amsterdam) 7, 10–12
gestural significance 25, 27–28
Gilby, T. 35; *Poetic Experience: An Introduction to Thomist Aesthetic* 35
Gilligan, C. 4
glimmers 189–191, 193–195, 197
Godwin, B. 238
Gospodinov, G. 235–237, 239, 245, 250
Gray, K. 163
Gregor, M.J. 22
Gulino, E. 189
Guzmán-García, A. 23

Hagerty, B.G.S. 43
Hamilton, H.E. 112
Hamington, M. 5, 84, 112, 122
Hammond, A. 69
Hatton, N. 167
Hayman, E. 121
Health Research Authority (HRA) 146, 210, 278
healthcare support worker (HCSW) 11, 13, 122, 146, 149, 151–154, 192, 277, 278
Heidegger, M. 30, 31, 33
Hendriks, N. 70
Hendriks, R. 244, 248, 250, 251
Highmore, B. 6
home-scaping and home-playing in care home 248, 250
Hughes, J.C. 2, 14, 280, 281
Huizenga, J. 229
Hulko, W. 168

interdependent beings 21, 26–27, 116, 124–125, 137–138, 166, 172, 230
interrelatedness 21, 26–27, 191

Jacquez, F. 82
Johannsen, T. 10–12
Johnstone, K. 149
Jones, L. 191, 192, 268

Kamphof, I. 244, 248, 250, 251
Kant, I. 32; *Critique of the Power of Judgment* 32
Kara H. 69, 78
Keady, J. 44, 78, 104, 144, 151, 168, 181, 256, 267
Kelly, L. 13
Killick, J. 123
Kindell, J. 14, 101, 122, 192, 193
King, M. 30, 31
Kitwood, T. 12, 13, 119, 182, 185, 278; *Dementia Reconsidered: The Person Comes First* 12
Kontos, P. 25, 120, 161, 165, 166

Lauwerijssen, R., 206
Lecoq, J. 123, 136
Leddy, T. 183, 185, 189, 197; *Experience of Awe: An Expansive Approach to Everyday Aesthetics* 185
Lee-Treweek, G. 121, 123, 130, 134, 135
Ligaya, K. 187
Long, S. 151
Lovatt, M. 239, 248, 249
love 21, 24; in caring relationships 12; and creativity 175; and friendship 21, 34–36

MacIntyre, A. 25–27; *Dependent Rational Animals* 25, 27
Maguire-Rosier, K. 2, 8, 14
Mapes, N. 207
*Marzahn, Mon Amour* (Oskamp) 9–10
Matthews, E. 25
McCabe, H. 34
McCall, V. 163
McPherson, D. H. J. 14, 144, 281
Menon, V. 188, 194
Merleau-Ponty, M. 25, 28, 29
mesocorticolimbic reward system 187–188, 190, 198
Mihai, M. 7

mirroring 56–57, 60–61, 107
Mol, A. 5, 125
moments 9, 11–12; aesthetic moments 14–15, 30, 186, 191–195, *196*; of care 13, 30, 44, 60, 118, 122, 124, 130, 133, 148, 154–155, 194, 250; care-full moments 267–269; case studies 145–154; co-creating and capturing 46–55, 60; connected/disconnected 55–59, 186, 193, 269; continuum of moments 237; creative *see* creative moments; everyday moments 43; fleeting moments 60; garbage moments 185; of interaction 87, 106; meaningful moments 195, 196; and memories of being together 45; object-handling sessions 78–80; recording 61–62; reflection and sharing 85; rhythmic moments 106; sketching 61; sparkling moments 60; values moments 278, 280
Murray, J. 151
Musalek, M. 22

Nadal, M. 187
National Health Service (NHS) 1, 125, 145, 146, 182, 277; Case Study 145–146, 150–151, 153; healthcare support worker (HCSW) 277; mental health wards for older people 14, 145, 152; National Research Ethics Service 105; Research Ethics Committee 72, 125, 126, 169
National Institute for Health and Care Research (NIHR) 81, 181, 230
neighbourhoods: aesthetics 15, 268; care-full *see* care-full neighbourhoods; comfort and belonging 184; and environmental aesthetics 260–261; experiences 270; imagining care aesthetics 266–268; mixed-use urban areas 210; neighbourhood walks 259; of people living with dementia 2, 15, 207, 279; and relational aesthetics 261–263; as relational practices 257–258; relationships 15, 259; residential suburbs 210; scholarship on 2; sensorial aesthetic 263–265; temporalities 265–266
neuroaesthetics 15, 183, 186–191, 194–196, *196*; aesthetic experiences 186–187; beauty and brain 187–189; everyday encounters 189
neuroception 190, 198
Newton, R. 15, 23, 208, 281
Noddings, N. 4
Nord, C. 237

object-handling sessions (case study): cycle of study 72–73; designing 73–74; dramatic 75–76; engagement with ‘things’ 77–78; moments from 78–80; narrative 74–75; physical, aesthetic, and ethical considerations 76–77; playfulness 73–74; research study 72–73; sharing words and experiences of participants 78
*On the Aesthetic Education of Man in a Series of Letters* (Schiller) 32
Open Doors Research Group 82
Oskamp, K. 9, 10; *Marzahn, Mon Amour* 9–10
Özen, Y. 44

participatory research 82, 196, 282
patient and public involvement and engagement (PPIE) 71–72, 81, 82, 84, 92–95, 169, 171, 172, 181, 188
People Living with Dementia (PLWD): attuning and attending 90–91; creative PPIE 71–72; creative research methods 69–70; curating spaces for sharing 92–94; embodied beings 24–26; improvisational and relational facilitation 91–92; sentient beings 22–24
Perry, G. 74, 75
person-centred care 1, 3, 12–13, 16, 118, 119, 126–129, 246, 279, 282; aesthetics 183–184; care aesthetics 185; everyday aesthetics 184; interests and identity 180; lived experience of dementia 183–185; research and policy 182, 185–186
Phillipson, L. 69
Phinney, A. 25
physiotherapy 7–9
Pickering, L. 78
Pink, S. 126
Plato 22
*Poetic Experience: An Introduction to Thomist Aesthetic* (Gilby) 35
Pointon, B. 22
Polonyi, R. 2, 8, 14
*Polyvagal Practices* (Dana) 193
Polyvagal Theory 189–191, 196, *196*
Porges, S.W. 190–194
Pottinger, L. 93
Puig de la Bellacasa, M. 122, 130
Pym, C. 74, 75

*Records of My Life* project (case study): emotional and sensory connections 83–85; musical bookmarks 85–87; participatory research methods 82; vinyl and paper stock samples 87–88; vinyl records as artefacts 81–82
relational aesthetics 7, 261–263, 268
Richards, R. 164
Robertson, J.M. 163
Rogers, C.R. 190; *Client-Centred Therapy* 190
Rosendal, K.A. 133–136
Royal Horticultural Society (RHS) 209; FOSS exhibition 209; Garden Bridgewater 209, 212–219, *213*, *216–218*, 224–228, *226*
Rushton, L. 209

Sabat, S. 26; *The Experience of Alzheimer's Disease, Life Through a Tangled Veil* 27
Saito, Y. 6, 7, 122, 124, 127, 129, 131, 136, 167, 183–186, 188, 189, 197, 266, 268
Scarles, C. 45
Scheibenbogen, O. 22
Schiller, F. 32; *On the Aesthetic Education of Man in a Series of Letters* 32
School for Social Care Research (SSCR) 81
Schreiber, C. 70
semantic dementia 14; care tasks 101; case study 102–109; communication abilities 100–101; conversation analytical perspectives 112; craft of connections in long-term care 109–110; data collection methods 101–102; of primary progressive aphasia 100; video, data-driven method 113, 114; ways of 'making connections' 110, *111*; *see also* dementia
semantic memory 100, 188, 198
Shakespeare, T. 162
Shusterman, R. 6
Simmons-mackie, N.N. 106
situated persons 21, 27, 36
sketchbook 43–46, 51, 56, 58, 61
sketching *47*, *48*, *50*, *52*; being with or caring with 47–49, 60, 62; bodywork 44, 55–58; as care-ful practice 44; co-creating and capturing moments 46–47; connected/disconnected moments 55–58; craft-like or artful elements 43; creativity and identity 52–55; embodied and sensory adjustments 58–60; into series of moments 50–51; sketching together 46–47; turning points 45, 46, 58–59
Skov, M. 187
social care 1–2, 4, 12, 16, 60, 71, 77, 118, 147, 155, 167, 172, 174, 181–182, 210, 258, 268, 270
socially engaged arts 2
solicitude 21, 31–36

Taylor, C. 24, 25
Taylor, J.S. 49
Thompson, J. 7, 22, 26, 46, 61, 71, 91, 92, 101, 110, 112, 113, 122–124, 132, 136, 137, 151, 167, 172, 181, 186, 197, 229, 236, 250, 258, 261, 268; *Care Aesthetics: For Artful Care and Careful Art* 1, 8, 30, 33, 185
Timmerman, G. 12, 194
Titchmarsh, A. 206
Treadaway, C. 74
Tronto, J. 268
Twigg, J. 2, 25, 51, 120, 121, 123, 125, 131

United Kingdom (UK) 60, 81, 108, 145, 160, 239, 259

Valverde, J.M. 32
Vartanian, O. 187
Vaughn, L.M. 82
Vessel, E.A. 188
visibility problem 123–124, 127, 130–132, 135
visual arts 23, 30, 52, 61, 187
Vittorio, G. 187

Ward, R. 120, 124, 125, 129, 131, 132, 250, 256
West, J. 167
Wilkinson, A. 70
Wittgenstein, L. 28
Worpole, K. 237, 239, 248

Yoshizaki-Gibbons, H. 123, 128, 130

Zeilig, H. 88
Zoom 47, 162

For Product Safety Concerns and Information please contact our
EU representative GPSR@taylorandfrancis.com Taylor & Francis
Verlag GmbH, Kaufingerstraße 24, 80331 München, Germany